Clinical Topics in Disorders of Intellectual Development

To Kara, Charlotte and Marguerite

Clinical Topics in Disorders of Intellectual Development

Edited by Marc Woodbury-Smith

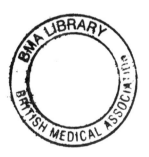

RCPsych Publications

RCPsych Publications is an imprint of the Royal College of Psychiatrists,
21 Prescot Street, London E1 8BB, UK
http://www.rcpsych.ac.uk

British Library Cataloguing-in-Publication Data.
A catalogue record for this book is available from the British Library.
ISBN 978-1-909726-39-0

Distributed in North America by Publishers Storage and Shipping Company.

The views presented in this book do not necessarily reflect those of the Royal College of
Psychiatrists, and the publishers are not responsible for any error of omission or fact.

The Royal College of Psychiatrists is a charity registered in England and Wales (228636)
and in Scotland (SC038369).

Printed by Bell & Bain Limited, Glasgow, UK.

Contents

Contributors

Neil Arnott General Practitioner, Tweeddale Medical Practice, Fort William, NHS Highland, UK

Alina Bakala Consultant Psychiatrist, Central and North West London NHS Foundation Trust (NHS), UK

Teresa (Terry) Bennett Assistant Professor, Offord Centre for Child Studies, McMaster University, Hamilton, Ontario, Canada

Tom Berney Developmental Psychiatrist, Newcastle University, UK

Penny Blake Consultant Psychiatrist in the field of Intellectual Disability Psychiatry and Honorary Lecturer for Cardiff University, School of Medicine, Cardiff, UK

Elspeth Bradley Associate Professor, Department of Psychiatry, Faculty of Medicine, University of Toronto; Psychiatrist-in-Chief, Surrey Place Centre, Toronto, Ontario, Canada

Sherva Elizabeth Cooray formerly Honorary Senior Lecturer, Faculty of Medicine, Department of Mental Health, Imperial College London, UK

Shoumitro Deb Honorary Clinical Professor of Neuropsychiatry, Imperial College London; Department of Medicine, Division of Brain Sciences, Centre for Mental Health, Hammersmith Hospital Campus, London, UK

Irene Drmic Postdoctoral Fellow, Holland Bloorview Kids Rehabilitation Hospital and the Hospital for Sick Children, Toronto, Ontario, Canada

Rachel Elvins Consultant Child and Adolescent Psychiatrist, Central Manchester University Hospitals NHS Foundation Trust, Manchester, UK

Stelios Georgiades Assistant Professor, Offord Centre for Child Studies, McMaster University, Hamilton, Ontario, Canada

Jonathan Green Professor of Child and Adolescent Psychiatry, University of Manchester; Honorary Consultant Psychiatrist, Central Manchester Foundation Trust, Manchester, UK

Simon Martin Halstead Independent Consultant Psychiatrist, UK

Anthony Holland Holder of the Health Foundation Chair in Learning Disabilities, Cambridge Intellectual and Developmental Disabilities Research Group, Department of Psychiatry, University of Cambridge, UK

Sheila Hollins Emeritus Professor of the Psychiatry of Disability, St George's, University of London, UK

Mike Kerr Professor of Learning Disabilities and Honorary Consultant in Neuropsychiatry at the Welsh Centre for Learning Disabilities, Department of Psychological Medicine, University of Wales College of Medicine, Cardiff

Marika Korossy Librarian (Retired), Surrey Place Centre, Toronto, Ontario, Canada

Gregory O'Brien (deceased) formerly Professor of Developmental Psychiatry, Northumbria University and the University of Queensland; Consultant Psychiatrist and Associate Medical Director Northumbria, Tyne and Wear NHS Trust; and Senior Psychiatrist with the Queensland Mental Health Assessment and Outreach Team of Disability Services

Jo-Ann Reitzel Clinical Director, Psychologist and Assistant Professor, McMaster Children's Hospital and McMaster University, Hamilton, Ontario, Canada

Howard Ring University Lecturer, Department of Psychiatry, University of Cambridge, UK

Anagha Sardesai, Higher Specialty Trainee (ST6) in Psychiatry of Intellectual Disability, Hertfordshire Partnership University NHS Foundation Trust, UK

Neill J. Simpson Consultant Psychiatrist, Kirkintilloch Health and Care Centre, NHS Greater Glasgow and Clyde, UK

Jane Summers Clinical Supervisor, Psychologist and Assistant Professor, McMaster Children's Hospital and McMaster University, Hamilton, Ontario, Canada

Peter Szatmari Professor of Psychiatry, Chief of the Child and Youth Mental Health Collaborative, Hospital for Sick Children, Centre for Addiction and Mental Health, University of Toronto, Patsy and Jamie Anderson Chair in Child and Youth Mental Health, Toronto, Canada

Jeremy Turk Professor of Developmental Psychiatry, Institute of Psychiatry, King's College, University of London; Consultant Child and Adolescent Psychiatrist, Southwark Child and Adolescent Mental Health Neurodevelopmental Service, South London and Maudsley NHS Foundation Trust

Fred R. Volkmar Irving B. Harris Professor, Yale University Child Study Center, New Haven, Connecticut, USA

Paul White Dual Diagnosis (Intellectual Disability) Service, Park Centre for Mental Health, Wacol, Queensland, Australia

Anusha Wijeratne Consultant Psychiatrist, Central and North West London NHS Foundation Trust (NHS), UK

Marc Woodbury-Smith Associate Professor and CIHR Clinician-Scientist, Departments of Psychiatry & Behavioural Neurosciences and Pediatrics, McMaster University, Hamilton, Ontario, Canada

Asif Zia Consultant Psychiatrist and Clinical Director, Psychiatry of Intellectual Disability, Hertfordshire Partnership University Hospital Trust, UK

Foreword

Fred R. Volkmar

Awareness of children with significant problems in intellectual development can be traced to antiquity but awareness of associated problems in mental health is a much more recent phenomenon. The increase in awareness in recent years can be related to several factors: greater inclusion of individuals with disabilities in the population, the need to support individuals of all ages in their communities, and increasing sophistication on the part of both researchers and clinicians. Sadly, and somewhat paradoxically, a diagnosis of intellectual disability in the more distant past often led to a presumption that such individuals were somehow protected from other problems – the phenomenon known as 'diagnostic overshadowing'. However, research with this population began to suggest that rather the converse was true, with persons exhibiting milder intellectual disability having 4- to 5-fold increases in rates of associated psychiatric problems (Reiss & Szyszko, 1983). Awareness also began to increase regarding the difficulty of applying the usual models of psychiatric nosology, particularly in individuals with more severe intellectual disability (Fletcher *et al*, 2007).Other work began to note significant associations between certain syndromic forms of intellectual disability and specific mental disorders (Dykens & Hodapp, 2001). This volume provides an important overview and update of the current status of the field, and areas where more work is needed.

The opening chapters of this book provide a very helpful overview of basic issues and approaches to classifying intellectual disability and characterising behavioural phenotypes. The next section summarises comorbidity, with specific chapters on commonly associated conditions in general, and anxiety disorders in particular. Relevant disorders are highlighted including behavioural difficulties, problems associated with seizure disorders, and pharmacological management.

Part three of the volume focuses on autism and related conditions. This is an area where there has been a vast increase in research, although, unfortunately, problems in adolescents and adults have been much less frequently addressed. Chapter 8 provides a helpful overview, with other chapters focused more specifically on Asperger syndrome and on pharmacological management. Chapter 11 on behavioral and psychological approaches to management is an excellent addition to the literature on this topic.

The next section of the volume is concerned with service provision. Chapters address more general health care needs as well as the important gap in linking primary and secondary care. The issue of ageing in this population is relatively infrequently addressed, and Chapter 14 providers an extremely timely summary. The final chapters address issues of services and mental health needs for children as well as forensic issues.

This book represents the current state-of-the-art in addressing issues of concern to all of us who work with individuals with intellectual disability. It will be of great value to both clinicians and researches and will be a resource for years to come.

Dykens EM, Hodapp RM (2001) Research in mental retardation: toward an etiologic approach. *Journal of Child Psychology and Psychiatry and Allied Disciplines,* **42**: 49–71.

Fletcher RJ, Loschen E, Stavrakaki C, *et al* (eds) (2007) *Diagnostic Manual – Intellectual Disability (DM-ID): A Textbook of Diagnosis of Mental Disorders in Persons with Intellectual Disability*. NADD Press.

Reiss S, Szyszko J (1983) Diagnostic overshadowing and professional experience with mentally retarded persons. *American Journal of Mental Deficiency,* **87**: 396–402.

Preface

The practice of medicine has seen significant changes in recent years, the result of scientific advances in diagnosis and treatment, as well as more general changes in the pattern of disease in our ever-expanding population. Psychiatry itself has undergone more fundamental changes, due in part to recent modifications in classification (DSM-5, and forthcoming in ICD-11) and greater clinical subspecialisation. Moreover, for a variety of reasons comprising both well-elucidated factors and those that are poorly understood, the prevalence of mental disorders continues to rise, which has major implications for the healthcare budget of the nation.

My own specialty, the psychiatry of intellectual disabilities, has itself seen innumerable changes. It has risen in status from psychiatry's Cinderella subspecialty to one that embraces new technologies and scientific advances, in addition to benefitting from new legislation. This is acutely visible in relation to the care of individuals with autism spectrum disorder (ASD), which represents a significant component of the clinical workload of healthcare professionals in the psychiatry of intellectual disabilities. Advances in ASD's conceptualisation, diagnosis, comorbidity and treatment are increasingly incorporated into clinical practice, which includes the publication of evidenced-based guidelines. Generally speaking, the psychiatry of intellectual disabilities sits neatly on the interface of child and adolescent psychiatry, neurology and genetics, and, as a matter of course, it will be affected by developments in these specialisms.

Consequently, while we find ourselves at an exciting juncture in the care of the population of those with disorders of intellectual development (DID), a large body of literature exists that could impact on the clinical care we provide. By 'we' I do not refer principally to psychiatrists, but instead to all health and social care professionals working with this population. I believe that both clinicians and allied healthcare workers can benefit from research evidence being distilled down to the most important, clinically relevant points. Both can also profit from the availability of up-to-date references, as they provide the opportunity for broader and deeper reading, and it is with this in mind that the current volume was prepared.

Several of the chapters herein are revised and updated versions of previously published articles from *Advances in Psychiatric Treatment*. Many chapters, however, have been commissioned specifically for this book. The emphasis throughout is on clinical care, and the most common presenting complaints and their diagnosis and management. Particular chapters, such as those by Tony Holland (Chapter 1) and Jeremy Turk (Chapter 2), facilitate a wider, conceptual understanding, whereas Simon Halstead's personal perspective looks beyond the forensic care of this population to articulate a growing awareness of the potential problems, ethical and otherwise, of definitional changes, and service provision for the DID population (Chapter 16). Even if his polemics are at odds with the reader's own viewpoint, there is no doubt that he raises important points that cannot be ignored, as they are fundamental to the future of caring for the DID population.

A chapter specifically focusing on Asperger syndrome is also included (Chapter 9). Despite its removal from the DSM-5, there is little doubt that this term remains clinically relevant, and will continue to be for the foreseeable future. This chapter also provides a more in-depth discussion of the characteristics of adults with higher functioning ASD, along with their mental health comorbidities. Further, in view of the importance of ASD, additional chapters provide a detailed overview of ASD (Chapter 8), and a presentation of pharmacological (Chapter 10) and psychological (Chapter 11) management.

With a particular focus on clinical care, the two broad areas of (i) comorbidity and complications of DID (Part 2 and chapters therein) and, (ii) service provision (Part 4 and chapters therein) are discussed in detail. Again, detailed exposition is given to those key areas that have most clinical valence. As such, the epidemiology, aetiology and management of psychiatric disorders are discussed (Chapter 3), along with a more detailed consideration of anxiety disorders (Chapter 4) and behaviour problems (Chapter 5). Responsibility for the diagnosis and management of epilepsy often falls to the psychiatrist; however, even if this is not the case, the neuropsychiatric complications of epilepsy are an important aspect of clinical care (Chapter 6). Finally, the use of psychotropic medications in this population for problem behaviours is considered, drawing on the recommendations from recently published national and international guidelines (Chapter 7).

Service provision focuses on several key areas, which comprise general health needs (Chapter 12), and models of primary and specialist care (Chapter 13). In addition, other chapters focus more specifically on the service needs of the ageing population with DID (Chapter 14), of children (Chapter 15), and of the interface with the criminal justice system and specialist forensic services (Chapter 16).

Of course, a single volume such as this cannot cover everything; consequently, certain areas such as legislation, education and vocational needs are not specifically included. Nor was I able to incorporate the perspectives of nursing, social work, or occupational, speech and physical therapies. This in no way reflects any judgement of perceived importance, but is merely the result of space limitation.

The reader will note that the term Disorders of Intellectual Development (DID) is used throughout. This is the term that, after much debate, was decided on by WHO for the forthcoming 11th revision of the International Classification of Diseases (ICD-11, due for publication in 2017). Clearly, terminology has not only changed over time, but also between the two principal classification systems, with the DSM-5 including the term 'intellectual developmental disorder' defined in almost identical terms (see Chapter 1 for further discussion). It is important to bear in mind these different terminologies and their relationship as discussed by Holland (Chapter 1).

During my own tenure as a clinician working with this population, I have been fortunate to have worked directly with key leaders such as Tony Holland, Peter Szatmari, Fred Volkmar and Greg O'Brien. I first met Greg in the early 2000s through our respective roles in the Society for the Study of Behavioural Phenotypes (SSBP), and I later worked more closely with him, albeit for a short time, as a colleague in Northumberland. He went on to become my College mentor until I left the UK in 2007, but I did keep in touch with him. Greg made enormous contributions to the field of developmental psychiatry as evidenced by his widely cited publications, and was well regarded and respected, both as a clinician and friend and colleague, by all those who worked with him before his death in 2014. I am deeply honoured to have known him, and for him to have contributed to this book.

Marc Woodbury-Smith MRCPsych, FRCP(C)
McMaster University, Hamilton, Ontario, Canada

Part 1
Disorders of intellectual development: concept and epidemiology

Disorders of intellectual development: historical, conceptual, epidemiological and nosological overview

Anthony Holland

There are different ways of thinking about the needs of people with disorders of intellectual development (DID); each has its place and none is perfect. The aim of this chapter therefore is to provide an overview of the various perspectives that those working in this field may use to orient themselves to the issues. In clinical practice, when seeing someone who has been referred, the starting point is to ask the question: What am I being asked to do? For the paediatrician and/or geneticist it may well focus on identifying whether a single major cause for a child's developmental delay can be identified. For a psychiatrist, clinical psychologist or community nurse it may be about identifying the reasons for, and treatment of, a particular constellation of problem behaviours. The task, through history taking, observation, examination and investigation, is to arrive at an understanding – a formulation – that then informs intervention through the integration of information about the individual within an accepted theoretical and conceptual framework that has been developed through research.

While DSM-5 uses the term 'intellectual developmental disorders' (American Psychiatric Association, 2013), the term generally used in this book is the one due to be used in ICD-11: 'disorders of intellectual development'. It is the latest in a long line of labels that have included a range of unacceptable and derogatory terms, from idiot, imbecile, feeble-minded and moral imbecile to mentally retarded, mentally handicapped and mentally subnormal, and, more recently, learning disabled and intellectually disabled. Many of these terms were incorporated into laws, such as the Mental Deficiency Act 1913 in England. At that time, a method of classification was considered to be necessary to make possible the segregation of people whom science had deemed to be harmful to the population as a whole and a major source of criminality (Goddard, 1912). However, despite this inauspicious past, there have been substantial positive changes in the way society as a whole perceives and wishes to engage with people with DID, and with this there have also been changes in almost every aspect of the lives of these individuals, with a focus on community inclusion and support. This chapter sets these changes in a historical context and seeks to integrate what have been very divergent and conflicting approaches. It also considers the 'models' that are helpful in thinking about the needs of people with DID and the various classification systems used.

Background

Understanding the causes and prevalence of any specific illness or disability requires that it can be accurately defined and identified. This is the bedrock of epidemiology and the investigation of aetiology and the underlying pathophysiology of ill health. Although such an approach works particularly well for investigating specific illnesses and has been central to the development of treatments, it fits less comfortably in the case of potentially lifelong disabilities such as DID. The term DID is not fundamentally a diagnosis, as its use implies very little understanding about cause, pathophysiology or likely prognosis. Furthermore, as described above, classification in DID has been associated with negative stereotyping and labelling has been used to justify actions such as segregation from society. The application of any system of classification is inevitably contradictory; on the one hand, it enables needs to be defined and for groups of people so 'labelled' to act together to argue for recognition (as seen through advocacy organisations) yet, on the other hand, the outcomes can be negative, such as dismissive attitudes. Over the years, this approach of defining and classifying has resulted in tensions between what are referred to as the 'biomedical' and the 'social' models of disability. In the papers advocating different perspectives, the language and concepts used and the conclusions drawn at times appear irreconcilable. However, although debate has been polarised, the value of each perspective and the need for a more nuanced understanding of the value of each have been increasingly recognised (Shakespeare, 2006). While each of us, with our very different professional backgrounds, places a different emphasis on the interplay between different conceptual views, there is a necessary coming together of these perspectives.

In addition to the biomedical and social models of disability, there is also a systemic model that guides understanding by seeking specifically to set disability in the context of what is often considerable complexity. The purpose of these conceptual and theoretical perspectives is that they provide a means for structuring our thinking about the needs of people with DID and, in turn, how we might respond to those needs. I very briefly consider each of these models below, before moving on to definitions and systems of classification that, at their best, provide the means for an informed and valid understanding of the person concerned and of the issues that have brought that person to the attention of services.

Theoretical models that may inform understanding

The biomedical model, central to all branches of medicine, is fundamentally diagnostic in its approach, addressing very specific questions in a particular context. For example, early in childhood this may be attempting to answer the questions that parents may ask, such as 'Why has my child not developed like other children? What are the chances that any future children will be similarly affected?' To answer these questions the approach is largely a diagnostic one – is the child's developmental trajectory atypical and does the child have a known neurodevelopmental disorder? In high-resource countries the focus is now generally on genetic disorders (and on the complex ethical issues that come with this), but in many parts of the world this biomedical approach has identified potentially preventable causes of disability, such as maternal iodine deficiency. In the latter case significant disability can be prevented through nutritional supplementation. Such an approach also seeks to understand and characterise the 'developmental trajectories' that people with specific neurodevelopmental syndromes are likely to follow across their life span, setting this understanding in the context of typical and atypical developmental profiles, such as those characteristic of autism spectrum conditions. As discussed later, this biomedical approach also provides a framework for identifying specific comorbid conditions, such as sensory impairments or physical or psychiatric illness, the treatments of which may bring benefits and reduce secondary disabilities.

The social model of disability is generally seen as the model that should drive our understanding of how social support should be structured and the philosophy that underpins policy and practice. The basic tenet of this model is that specific impairments (e.g. sensory, motor or intellectual) do not in themselves have to result in disability or disadvantage. Consequently, the social model requires individuals and society as a whole to address attitudinal and practical barriers to the full inclusion and participation of people with DID. By doing so, such disadvantage can be minimised and even eliminated. By viewing 'impairment' solely as a failure in 'an organ system' (as the biomedical model is seen to do), which in the case of people with DID may not be amenable to medical treatment, the concern is that the state may decide to abrogate any responsibility to help that person have a better life.

A further conceptual perspective that may be of value in orienting ourselves towards understanding and meeting the needs of people with DID is that described as the systemic model. It places emphasis on the idea that human behaviour should be considered and is best understood in the context of people's lives being part of a complex system. People with DID may be dependent on others for their very survival or, at the least, for enabling them to have a good life. From a health perspective, for people with DID, assessments and interventions are frequently delivered at the interface with social care. Family members or those paid to provide support are necessarily the intermediaries between those working in healthcare, such as the general practitioner (GP), and the individuals themselves. In addition, perspectives such as that of applied behavioural analysis, which help elucidate the factors that predispose to, precipitate or maintain challenging behaviour, are very much concerned with the 'complex system' that is social care, in terms of how particular behaviours are shaped and maintained (I will return to this later in the chapter). Thus, the needs of people with DID and how best to understand and meet such needs cannot be readily separated from the wider network that surrounds each individual.

Historical context

An increasingly rapid rise in new medical and scientific knowledge took place during the 19th and 20th centuries. For example, Pasteur put forward the germ theory of disease and developed the first vaccines in the late 19th century and, in the early 20th century, Garrod proposed the concept of 'chemical individuality', recognising that individuals are importantly different in their make-up. He described alkaptonuria, an inborn autosomal recessive error of metabolism, and in doing so brought together the emerging science of genetics, as pioneered by Mendel in the 19th century, with that of chemistry (Prasad & Galbraith, 2005). Subsequently, this work on 'inborn errors of metabolism' led to the description by Følling in 1934 of phenylketonuria, an example of a rare biological cause of DID, the consequences of which are largely preventable, provided that there is early diagnosis and appropriate dietary treatment.

The accelerating nature of scientific advances is very well illustrated in the field of genetics. The structure of DNA was elucidated by Watson and Crick in 1953, and in 1956 the normal human complement of 23 pairs of chromosomes was established (Tjio & Levan, 1956). Three years later Lejeune and colleagues identified trisomy 21 as the cause of Down syndrome (Lejeune et al, 1959). Technologies were subsequently developed for identifying genetic variants (polymorphisms) at particular loci in the genome, which in turn led to genetic linkage studies, which were prominent in general psychiatric research by the end of the 20th century. In the year 2000, the first draft of the sequencing of the human genome was announced (International Human Genome Sequencing Consortium, 2001). DNA sequencing is now becoming increasingly possible. Over this period, the chromosomal and molecular genetic basis for many neurodevelopmental syndromes associated with DID were described. Most recently, the emphasis in genetics has moved to the expanding field of epigenetics and to an understanding of the mechanisms that regulate gene expression and the potential mechanisms whereby environmental and biological factors interact (Jirtle & Skinner, 2007).

The early 20th century saw the development of tests of intelligence. These IQ tests were initially developed as a means of distinguishing those whom we now see as having an intellectual disability from those with mental illness, as well as for screening particular populations, such as people enlisting in the armed forces. The importance of these tests was that they provided a standardised way of comparing particular abilities and individuals' levels of performance. However, as is well known, their use was not without controversy, as IQ tests were adopted by the eugenics movement and were also used to argue the case for the belief in the inferiority of certain races (Hermstein & Murray, 1994). Wechsler tests eventually became the most established. They were standardised to a median of 100 with a standard deviation of 15 points (Wechsler, 1997). The score for any individual could then be ranked against the standardised sample for that age. Subsequent twin and family studies suggest that IQ is under considerable genetic influence and, like height, many genes may each have a small effect, a fact that is relevant when considering the aetiology of mild intellectual disability (Davis *et al*, 2010; but as a challenge to this interpretation see also an earlier paper by Devlin *et al*, 1997). Although IQ has some ability to predict an individual's level of functioning, education and opportunity are clearly of paramount importance, and perhaps the most significant advance in the 20th century for people with DID was the requirement placed on education authorities in many countries to provide education for them. Thus, as so often occurs in this area of study, developments such as the IQ test were contentious, but psychometrics in its increasingly sophisticated forms remains an important tool.

In the later 20th century there was a backlash against the over-classification and over-medicalisation of DID, particularly given the application of dubious scientific ideas to the detriment of those to whom they were applied. The horror of the consequences of misunderstanding and misapplication of scientific theory was most vividly demonstrated by the treatment of people with mental disorders, of whatever form, in Nazi Germany and afterwards by programmes of forced sterilisation.

However, despite an extremely problematic start, the 20th century was to end in very significant improvements in the lives of people with DID and in the conceptual frameworks that informed thinking, through the development of a social model of disability and an increased emphasis on human rights. Among the most striking was the changing philosophy initiated by the normalisation movement, away from segregation and towards integration and social inclusion, initially put forward by Nirje and developed by Wolfensberger (Wolfensberger, 1972). There has also been the recognition that people with DID represent a highly complex and heterogeneous group with a varied range of needs, together with an appreciation that special education, skills and communication training, and appropriate social support, can lead to levels of independence and a quality of life that were never aspired to or attained in the large institutional settings that had predominated in the care of such individuals. In the UK the scandal of abuse uncovered at Ely Hospital in Cardiff, Wales, led to the government White Paper *Better Services for the Mentally Handicapped*

(Department of Health and Social Security, 1971) and the start of the closure of long-stay institutions, once established as 'colonies' and later reborn as hospitals with the start of the National Health Service (NHS) in 1948. To the credit of successive UK governments, this enlightened and progressive approach continued with the publication of *Valuing People* in 2001 (Department of Health, 2001). In the 21st century, this fundamentally rights-based approach was established internationally in 2006 through the United Nations Convention on the Rights of Persons with Disabilities, which has now been ratified by the majority of countries across the world.

The present day

The background to developments in the understanding of intellectual disability has therefore been problematic, with systems being devised for the purpose of classification (considered below) using labels that certainly would now cause offence. Where such systems became part of the law, they were then used to legally segregate and isolate those to whom they applied. At the same time, there was an uncomfortable juxtaposition between those propounding the social model of disability, on the one hand, and, on the other, the biomedical approach and advances that were identifying specific single major causes of DID, one outcome of which was the possibility of prenatal testing. In high-resource countries, major environmental causes such as congenital rubella were identified and have essentially been eliminated through vaccination programmes, and elsewhere in the world public health measures are tackling nutritionally determined causes. Moreover, to be able to target educational support or to address some of the concerns that a family may raise when it is clear that something is wrong with their child does require a means of describing and characterising those people being referred to, and thus definitions are necessary. In addition, the variability and potential complexity of need among children and adults with DID has been highlighted by epidemiological studies that have demonstrated high rates of secondary disability due to the presence of sensory and physical impairments, behavioural and psychiatric disorders, and/or a developmental profile indicative of autism (e.g. Rutter *et al*, 1976; Cooper *et al*, 2007). The identification of such secondary impairments and disabilities and their treatment or amelioration through a range of interventions have helped to replace a feeling of therapeutic nihilism that had perhaps previously been all too pervasive. It became apparent not only that good education and social support services were required, but also that multidisciplinary and community-based specialist health support should be available to people with DID, particularly those with challenging behaviour and/or mental health problems.

The social model of disability underpins models of support for both children and adults. The biomedical model enables the identification of specific causes of developmental delay in children. For adults with DID, it becomes important for different reasons, as the attention moves away from identifying the cause of the person's disability towards understanding, for example, the reasons for apparent ill health or the emergence of problem behaviours. Here again, different conceptual models of understanding have arisen, from the developmental to the biomedical and the psychological. One of the most influential of these has been an approach informed by learning theory that is commonly referred to as applied behavioural analysis. Applied behavioural analysis was initially developed by Lovaas as a form of intensive behavioural modification to facilitate skills development and reduce maladaptive behaviours (for a review see Matson *et al*, 1996). The importance of this approach is the contrast with the traditional biomedical model, moving attention away from the individual towards an understanding of the interaction between the individual and the environment, and how particular behaviours are shaped and maintained through reinforcement. The methods of observation developed and the subsequent coding of behaviour in order to identify antecedents and consequences now underpin much of our present-day approach to support, particularly of children and adults with autism spectrum disorders. In turn, this has led to perspectives such as those of positive behaviour support (Allen *et al*, 2005).

What the various approaches illustrate is the complexity of this field and the need for conceptually clear thinking. The challenge is to integrate different perspectives and to be able to judge what frameworks are best applied in any particular set of circumstances. Within this complex field, with its potentially competing systems of understanding, is there a role for the process of classification using systems such as DSM-5 and ICD-11? Or are there other ways of thinking about classification that might provide a better and more productive perspective?

Classification: a cautionary tale

As argued at the beginning of this chapter, the process of defining and classifying what is meant when someone is said to have a disorder of intellectual development has been a source of debate. From a positive perspective, the central principle of any system of classification is to bring order to disparate knowledge in a manner that may then enable further advances or the instigation of interventions that research has shown to be effective. In the field of DID there is no ideal or universal system – the system of classification used depends on the reasons for its use. These reasons range from the predominately administrative to the guiding of interventions and the use or not of specific treatments; definitions may also be enshrined in law, bringing with it specific powers.

During a research project that involved tracing family members (Holland & Gosden, 1990), a form was found in a file completed many years earlier, which enabled the detention of a person in a long-stay institution under the Mental Deficiency Act 1913. The evidence used to justify segregation included the phrase 'was simple in appearance'. This phrase demonstrated both the attitudes of the time and the dangers of ill-informed and prejudicial thinking, made worse by the power that such classification has when incorporated into law. What the completed form illustrated was that being 'simple in appearance' and also being 'unable to work out change' – using the complex monetary system the UK had at the time ('doesn't know how many pennies there are in half a crown') – were essentially sufficient for the state to incarcerate this person in an institution for many years. Her four children were taken from her and placed in different families across the UK.

The dilemma, therefore, is how to target resources to those with special needs, but also to identify those with such needs in a manner that is valid and reliable and respects individual rights in a non-discriminatory way. Any system of classification inevitably has to focus on a few specific characteristics to the potential exclusion of others, and no system can impart a truly comprehensive picture. Methods of classification have therefore inevitably changed over time in an attempt to clarify the key issues and to minimise the stigma that might be associated with any given label. Some are clearly informed by one or other of the models mentioned at the beginning of this chapter, such as the biomedical model.

Conceptually, there are difficulties, as classification systems are by their very nature categorical, yet intellectual ability is clearly dimensional and continuous. Any cut-off is defined, at least partially, on the basis of IQ, and a point below which someone might be considered to have an intellectual impairment is statistically determined (two standard deviations below the mean). In contrast, particular neurodevelopmental syndromes that may be associated with DID are categorical – you have it or you do not – but even there, such obvious categorical distinctions have begun to break down as the genetic bases for syndromes are more clearly elucidated. For example, in fragile-X syndrome there is variation in the number of repeat sequences in the FMR1 mutation, in both carrier and affected individuals and across particular groups. The accepted significance of the exact number of repeat sequences, although being informed by their predictive value, in the end requires a decision as to some cut-off (below 50, above 200, etc.) (Nolin *et al*, 2003). As the significance of chromosomal copy number variants (CNVs) of various sizes is elucidated, a similar problem is likely to arise. Thus, as with conditions such as high blood pressure or diabetes mellitus, exactly what is considered normal or typical and what is considered abnormal or atypical is a judgement based on observation and research, but without necessarily a distinct separation between one and the other. I will now examine different systems of classification and then consider the relationship between assessment and classification.

The DSM and ICD systems

As set out in the Introduction to DSM-5, the first *Diagnostic and Statistical Manual* was published in 1844, to be used for the classification of the mental disorders of patients in institutional settings (American Psychiatric Association, 2013). This led to the various iterations of the DSM, most recently DSM-5, published in 2013. The ICD-11 classification is due to be published in 2017.

Both DSM-5 and ICD-11[1] place intellectual disabilities/disorders of intellectual development (DID) within the broad framework of what are termed 'mental disorders', and in that regard both are 'biomedical' in their approach. However, in DSM-5 the structure of the classification proposed has been shaped around developmental and life-span considerations and within a cultural context that recognises the dimensional nature of psychiatric disorder and how factors in the environment in which the person lives influence whether a particular symptom has functional significance or not, thereby moving beyond simply a diagnosis. Its predecessor, DSM-IV (American Psychiatric Association, 1994), provided a framework of multi-axial diagnosis, with Axis II for personality disorders and what was then termed 'mental retardation'. This is no longer the case in DSM-5. Box 1.1 summarises the DSM-5 criteria for IDD, which in essence remain as in DSM-IV, although differently worded. IDD is included in a section headed 'Neurodevelopmental disorders', which also includes communication disorders, autism spectrum disorder (without distinguishing between Asperger syndrome and autism), attention-deficit hyperactivity disorder (ADHD), specific learning disorders, motor disorders and 'other neurodevelopmental disorders'. The focus is not primarily on aetiology but rather on quantifying the extent of disability, by defining the level of intellectual impairment and listing the range of adaptive functions that might be impaired. The definition makes it explicit that the onset is in the developmental period and that IDD is the final common pathway of a number of potential aetiologies. Significant subaverage intellectual function is defined as an IQ of 70 or below (using standard IQ tests). IQ is also used to help determine the level of intellectual disability (mild, moderate, severe or profound). Adaptive functioning has to be measured against what would be expected for a person of that age, and the social and cultural experience of the person has to be taken into account. The Wechsler Intelligence Scales (to establish IQ) and the Vineland Adaptive Behavior Scales or the American Association on Intellectual and Developmental Disabilities revised Adaptive Behavior Scale (for characterising functioning) are established instruments for the measurements of these abilities and for which there are normative data for comparison.

---

1. It is likely that ICD-11, currently under preparation, will use the term 'disorders of intellectual development', within the category of 'Mental and behavioural disorders', but the broad framework will remain the same (http://apps.who.int/classifications/icd11/browse/l-m/en).

> **Box 1.1** Summary of the DSM diagnostic criteria for intellectual disabilities
>
> • Onset during the developmental period
> • Deficits in conceptual, social and practical domains
> • Deficits in intellectual functions on both clinical assessment and intelligence testing (the choice of testing instrument should take into account the individual's socioeconomic background, native language and other associated handicaps)
> • Deficits in adaptive functioning – how effectively individuals cope with common life demands and how well they meet the standards of personal independence expected of someone in the particular age group, sociocultural background and community setting
>
> The degree of severity of mental retardation may be specified on the basis of intellectual impairment, taking into account other aspects of functioning.
>
> • Mild mental retardation: IQ level 50–55 to approximately 70
> • Moderate mental retardation: IQ level 35–40 to 50–55
> • Severe mental retardation: IQ level 20–25 to 35–40
> • Profound mental retardation: IQ level below 20 or 25

The inclusion of definitions of IDD in a manual designed to inform 'diagnosis', however, has its problems. Even where any categorisation is subdivided according to severity, it tells us very little about the cause, nor does it significantly help with intervention. Its value is to bring consistency and a degree of rigour to the classification process. Thus, it can reasonably be assumed that when properly used there will be a degree of reliability to the conclusion that someone has an IDD. It will not simply be based on appearance or educational abilities (as described earlier), but rather take into account evidence for a delayed and atypical pattern of development and the continuing presence of intellectual and functional impairments. Depending on circumstances, the next question might well be whether there is a single major cause for the developmental delay (genetic or environmental) or whether that is unlikely and a combination of factors have contributed to a person's atypical developmental history. However, in many ways, the limitations of such an approach are readily exposed, and for this reason other conceptual models have been proposed.

International Classification of Impairments, Disabilities and Handicaps

In 1980 the World Health Organization proposed a system of classification that attempted to overcome the limitations of other systems and, most importantly, aimed to guide intervention (World Health Organization, 1980). Box 1.2 summarises the terms. In this system DID can be conceptualised at different levels. In the case of *impairment*, the organ system involved is the central nervous system. It is impairment of this system for genetic, chromosomal or environmental reasons that has primarily affected the acquisition of developmentally determined skills and the ability to learn.

Box 1.2 Definitions of impairment, disability and handicap

The *International Classification of Impairments, Disabilities and Handicaps* (World Health Organization, 1980) uses the following definitions:

Impairment

- Is any loss or abnormality of psychological, physiological or anatomical structure or function
- Represents deviation from some norm in the individual's biomedical status
- Is characterised by losses or abnormalities that may be temporary or permanent
- Includes the existence or occurrence of an anomaly, defect or loss in a limb, organ, tissue or other structure of the body, or a defect in a functional system or mechanism of the body, including the systems of mental functioning
- Is not contingent upon aetiology

Disability

- Is any restriction or lack (resulting from impairment) of ability to perform an activity in the manner or within the range considered normal for a human being
- Is concerned with compound or integrated activities expected of the person or of the body as a whole, such as represented by tasks, skills and behaviours
- Is the excesses or deficiencies of customarily expected activities and behaviour, which may be temporary or permanent, reversible or irreversible, and progressive or regressive
- Is the process through which a functional limitation expresses itself as a reality in everyday life

Handicap

- Is a disadvantage for a given individual, resulting from an impairment or disability that limits or prevents the fulfilment of a role that is normal for that individual
- Places some value upon this departure from a structural, functional or performance norm by the individual or his or her peers in the context of their culture
- Is relative to other people and represents discordance between the individual's performance or status and the expectations of his or her social/cultural group
- Is a social phenomenon, representing the social and environmental consequences for the individual stemming from his or her impairment and disability

Certainly, a key task is to identify the reasons for any abnormality of brain development and therefore intellectual impairment, and this is best done as early in the person's life as possible. It may have treatment implications, may guide prognosis and, most important, may help the parents of those affected to make sense of the disability. It may also have important implications for genetic counselling.

The associated *disability* is the effect of the impairment on a person's ability to learn and to acquire new skills that come with development. These in turn enable the acquisition of increasingly advanced skills necessary for an independent life. The exact nature and extent of the disability may include not only intellectual disabilities but also physical and sensory disabilities. The extent to which a given impairment results in a loss of function (disability) may well be influenced by the extent and nature of interventions such as special education or the correction of hearing loss by means of a hearing aid.

The final level, that of *handicap*, is a result of an interaction between the disability and the extent to which support is available or environmental adjustments are made. It is a measure of disadvantage that can be ameliorated through, for example, the provision of support or environmental modifications (e.g. wheelchair ramps) that diminish the impact of physical disabilities. Such interventions maximise independence and thereby reduce disadvantage by ensuring that the impact of any given disability on an individual's independence and quality of life is minimised. Shakespeare (2006) has argued that such a structure helps to bring together the biomedical and the social models of disability.

International Classification of Functioning, Disability and Health (ICF)

The WHO introduced this new system of classification (World Health Organization, 2001) to replace the above-mentioned International Classification of Impairments, Disabilities and Handicaps. The focus switched from a system that had been seen as just characterising the negative to a system that also emphasised the positive – what people are able to do, rather than just what they cannot do. The ICF was developed to enable the characterisation of 'health domains' across the whole population and therefore has universal application, which includes people with DID. The ICF organises information in two parts. Part 1 ('Functioning and disability') is the means whereby body functions and structures and activities and participation can be characterised. Part 2 relates to 'Contextual factors', whether in the environment or pertaining to the individual. Fig. 1.1 illustrates the relationship between the different components of this system. The WHO emphasises that it enables a multiperspective approach and, for this reason, that it provides 'the building blocks for users who wish to create models and study different aspects of

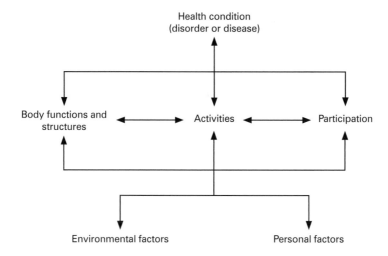

Fig. 1.1 Schematic representation of the structure of the ICF (World Health Organization, 2001: p. 18). This provides a framework for comprehensive data collection about an individual or a group of people so that needs can be characterised and comparisons made.

this process' (World Health Organization, 2001: p. 18). Thus, different disciplines can use it creatively to link to their specific scientific orientation.

Part 1 is divided into organ systems. With respect to people with DID the sections on mental functions and structures of the nervous system may be of particular relevance, but problems in these areas may be compounded by secondary disabilities, such as sensory impairments, consequent on abnormalities in the structure and function of other organ systems. All of these categories are extensively subdivided. In Part 2 the focus is very much on the specific personal circumstances and the characteristics of the individual's environment, including the health system and support available.

This system seeks to do two things. First, it aims to provide a reliable structure for the description of the complex effects of ill health and those factors that might moderate its impact, thereby enabling accurate comparisons across countries, between cultures and throughout the life span. Second, it aims to provide a more comprehensive framework to aid intervention, which moves beyond the single word or brief phrase of classification systems such as ICD and DSM, to a more structured and meaningful description of an individual's strengths and difficulties, in order to aid intervention. In this respect, it seeks to incorporate aspects of the biomedical and social models of disability and also to take a more systemic perspective, setting the person within the context of his or her support network and culture.

The prevalence and aetiology of DID

As argued, the above classification systems are not truly diagnostic. In addition, these different ways of conceptualising DID indicate that the path to functional impairments is not simply to do with biology; there are interactions with respect to the extent and nature of the statutory provision of education, opportunities in adult life and societal attitudes, all of which have an impact on ability and quality of life. The biomedical perspective is fundamentally about understanding the reasons for problems at birth or in childhood and in this regard there have been significant advances. It has been recognised for some time that there are fundamentally two broadly distinct groups, identified through population-based studies such as the Aberdeen children's cohort study of the 1950s (Birch *et al*, 1970). First, there are children who have a definite or likely genetic abnormality or specific environmental causes with major effects on subsequent development. Second, there are those in whom there is no obvious single major cause for their early developmental delay and subsequent intellectual disabilities. Here, the small effects of many genes combined with social disadvantage may be crucial. The broad differences between these two groups are summarised in Box 1.3. This 'two-group' perspective also illustrates the difficulty in arriving at a true prevalence of DID in any given community, given the fact that more than an IQ below 70 is required when determining

---

Box 1.3 Differences between biologically determined and subcultural DID

Biological

- Moderate/severe impairment
- Significant impairment in adaptive functioning
- Equal distribution across families of different socioeconomic status
- Parents and siblings usually of normal intelligence
- Dysmorphic characteristics common
- Other impairments and disabilities common
- Neglect unusual

Subcultural

- Mild or borderline impairment
- Minor or no impairment in adaptive functioning
- More common in families of lower socioeconomic status
- Intellectual ability impaired in family members
- Dysmorphic characteristics unlikely
- Other impairments and disabilities unusual
- Neglect more common

---

that someone should be considered to have a DID. The distribution of IQ in the general population is near normal, but with a skew to the left from the presence of neurodevelopmental disorders, which are generally associated with a downward shift in IQ. Given this, a figure of 2% to 2.5% is estimated as the proportion of the population with an IQ below 70. The problem then is to know how many of this group truly should be considered to have DID. To address this question there have been studies of the 'administrative prevalence' of people with DID – that is, the percentage of any given geographical population known to DID services. Figures of between 0.4% and just under 1% are arrived at, depending on a number of factors, including: whether active screening for people with DID in the population was attempted; whether it was just those people already known to DID services; whether children and adults were included; and specific geographical factors, such as levels of deprivation. Studies indicate that there is a peak in prevalence in childhood (Fryers, 2000), and that there may be significant regional variations in any given country. Examples of studies from different countries include: Sondenaa et al (2010) in Norway; McConkey et al (2006) in the island of Ireland; the European Intellectual Disability Research Network (2003) in Spain; Larson et al (2001) in the USA; and Wen (1997) in Australia. In an important study in the USA, Fujiura & Taylor (2003) estimated that there were a further 1.27% of people with mild intellectual disabilities who had very substantial needs and were effectively falling through the net of DID services.

The striking feature about this population is its heterogeneity, in terms of the nature and severity of disability but also of the presence or not of individuals whose DID is due to one of many possible single major causes. Making up this population there are those with conditions resulting from specific environmental factors, such as fetal exposure to alcohol, very low birth weight, congenital infections and maternal iodine deficiency (which, worldwide, is of major significance – see Zimmerman, 2009), and those with chromosomal and single-gene disorders that arise either de novo or are inherited. Down syndrome, due to trisomy 21, and fragile-X syndrome, due to X-linked FMR1 mutations, are two relatively common examples of the latter. Other neurodevelopmental syndromes due to copy number variants have been identified (Kaminsky et al, 2011) and advances in genetics using microarray technologies (sometimes referred to as molecular karyotyping) readily enable the identification of copy number variants of various sizes, including chromosomal rearrangements, deletions and duplications (Miller et al, 2010). There are some well-recognised deletion syndromes (e.g. Williams syndrome and cri du chat syndrome), but some previously unrecognised chromosomal abnormalities are still to be properly phenotypically characterised. Whether such copy number variants should be considered to be pathogenic or a normal polymorphic variation has to be judged using established databases such as DECIPHER (Firth et al, 2009). With improvements in DNA sequencing technology, the identification of specific gene mutations is now more readily available. These technologies together make possible the characterisation and subsequent identification of an increasing number of neurodevelopmental syndromes of genetic origin.

Why does this matter to psychiatric practice? People with some of these syndromes have been shown to have specific developmental profiles and to be at high risk of developing certain comorbid conditions. Well known examples include the excessive eating behaviour and risk of psychopathology associated with Prader–Willi syndrome (Holland *et al*, 2003), the high rates of Alzheimer's disease affecting people with Down syndrome (Holland *et al*, 1998), anxiety disorders affecting people with Williams syndrome (Woodruff-Borden *et al*, 2010) and severe self-injurious behaviour in people with Lesch–Nyhan and Smith–Magenis syndromes (Arron *et al*, 2011). These observations, famously described by Nyhan as the 'behavioural phenotype of organic genetic disease' (Nyhan, 1971), have very significantly altered our understanding of the aetiology and pathophysiology of such behaviours and psychiatric disorders. Conceptually, comparative studies across these neurodevelopmental syndromes have challenged the orthodoxy of applied behavioural analysis; more complex models are needed, recognising the role of the syndrome-specific developmental profiles and brain mechanisms in the aetiology of syndrome-specific behaviours – see for example Karmiloff-Smith & Thomas (2003) on Williams syndrome and Reiss & Dant (2003) on fragile-X syndrome. Oliver and colleagues have, for instance, reported very different behavioural and developmental profiles across different neurodevelopmental syndromes, and they propose specific models to account for the occurrence and maintenance of specific behaviours in particular syndromes (Oliver *et al*, 2013). Holland *et al* (2003) proposed different mechanisms to account for the various components of the behavioural phenotype in Prader–Willi syndrome. High rates of psychotic illness developing in early adult life were found in the those with the syndrome, although the particularly high rates were limited to those with the chromosome 15 maternal uniparental disomy (UPD) subtype, indicating that it is not simply having Prader–Willi syndrome that increases the risk; rather, it is something unique to having a chromosome 15 maternal UPD that accounts for the increase (Boer *et al*, 2002).

The challenge is to integrate the expanding knowledge base, so as to make both conceptual and practical advances that bring real benefits to people with DID. For mental health professionals working with people with DID the focus is on the prevention and treatment of secondary disabilities that may arise in the form of maladaptive behaviours or mental ill health. Research in this area has moved from the descriptive to the epidemiological and, as indicated above, is now focusing on understanding mechanisms. Studies addressing mechanisms have been diverse and have included detailed observational clinical studies and the construction and study of genetic knockout mouse models of neurodevelopmental syndromes. The significance of this latter approach was recognised by the award of the

Nobel Prize to Mario Capecchi, Martin Evans and Oliver Smithies in 2007. The message fundamentally from these very diverse areas of research is that we must pay attention to both biology and environment when we are seeking to understand the factors that give rise to, and maintain, different constellations of problem behaviours and psychiatric disorders as they affect people with DID. Our approach to the understanding of maladaptive behaviours therefore draws from diverse perspectives including: the developmental, whereby such behaviours (e.g. repetitive behaviours) are seen as a direct consequence of a delayed or atypical developmental trajectory and may be syndrome specific (behavioural phenotype); applied behavioural analysis; and the possibility that such problems may be secondary to comorbid physical or psychiatric illness. Assessments should draw on these different perspectives and seek to arrive at an understanding in the context of the individual's life experiences and their emotional and physical environment.

The integration of perspectives

Given the complexity and heterogeneity of DID, it is clear that attempts to describe and categorise, although having their place, also have very significant limitations and, when incorporated into law, unless very carefully framed, may be misused. Tensions exist between wishing to respect an individual's autonomy and wishing to protect from harm a person seen as vulnerable. These tensions are universal. Stigma, lack of resources and punitive laws, policies and practices prevail to varying degrees in different countries and societies. Particular forms of guardianship legislation and the labelling that such laws require are still the means in some countries of enabling the lifelong segregation of individuals in large institutional settings. It is for these reasons, and because difficult judgements may have to be made, that an approach is required that can articulate and make explicit such tensions. Despite the complex ethical challenges, and through accepting the core principles that underpin approaches to community support within a social model, there have been considerable advances in our understanding of the nature and extent to which comorbid physical and mental health problems exist and how maladaptive behaviours may arise and are maintained.

References

Allen D, James W, Evans J, *et al* (2005) positive behavioural support: definition, current status and future directions. *Tizard Learning Disability Review*, **10**: 4–11.

American Psychiatric Association (1994) *Diagnostic and Statistical Manual of Mental Disorders (4th edn) (DSM-IV)*. APA.

American Psychiatric Association (2013) *Diagnostic and Statistical Manual of Mental Disorder (5th edn) (DSM-5)*. APA.

Arron K, Oliver C, Berg K, *et al* (2011) Prevalence and phenomenology of self-injurious and aggressive behaviour in genetic syndromes. *Journal of Intellectual Disability Research*, **55**: 109–20.

Birch HG, Richardson SA, Baird D, *et al* (1970) *Mental Subnormality in the Community: A Clinical and Epidemiologic Study*. Williams & Wilkins.

Boer H, Holland AJ, Whittington J, *et al* (2002) Psychotic illness in people with Prader Willi syndrome due to chromosome 15 maternal uniparental disomy. *Lancet*, **359**: 135–6.

Cooper SA, Smiley E, Morrison J, *et al* (2007) Mental ill-health in adults with intellectual disabilities: prevalence and associated factors. *British Journal of Psychiatry*, **190**: 27–35.

Davis OS, Butcher LM, Docherty SJ, *et al* (2010) A three-stage genome-wide association study of general cognitive ability: Hunting the small effects. *Behavior Genetics*, **40**: 759–67.

Department of Health (2001) *Valuing People: A New Strategy for Learning Disability in the 21st Century*. Department of Health.

Department of Health and Social Security (1971) *Better Services for the Mentally Handicapped* (Cmnd 4683). HMSO.

Devlin B, Daniels M, Roeder K (1997) The heritability of IQ. *Nature*, **388**: 468–71.

European Intellectual Disability Research Network (2003) *Intellectual Disability in Europe: Working Papers*. Tizard Centre, University of Kent at Canterbury.

Firth HV, Richards SM, Bevan AP, *et al* (2009) DECIPHER: Database of Chromosomal Imbalance and Phenotype in Humans using Ensembl Resources. *American Journal of Human Genetics*, **84**: 524–33.

Følling A (1934) Über Ausscheidung von Phenylbrenztraubensäure in den Harn als Stoffwechselanomalie in Verbindung mit Imbezillität. *Hoppe-Seyler's Zeitschrift Fuer Physiologische Chemie*, **227**: 169–76.

Fryers T (2000) Epidemiology of mental retardation. In *Oxford Textbook of Psychiatry* (eds MG Gelder, J Lopez-Ibor, NC Andreasen). Oxford University Press.

Fujiura GT, Taylor SJ (2003) Continuum of intellectual disability: demographic evidence for the 'forgotten generation'. *Mental Retardation*, **41**: 420–9.

Goddard HH (1912) *The Kallikak Family: A Study in the Heredity of Feeble Mindedness*. Macmillan.

Hermstein RJ, Murray C (1994) *The Bell Curve: Intelligence and Class Structure in American Life*. Free Press.

Holland AJ, Gosden C (1990) A balanced chromosomal translocation partially co-segregating with psychotic illness in a family. *Psychiatry Research*, **32**: 1–8.

Holland AJ, Hon J, Huppert FA, *et al* (1998) Population-based study of the prevalence and presentation of dementia in adults with Down's syndrome. *British Journal of Psychiatry*, **172**: 493–8.

Holland AJ, Whittington JE, Butler J, *et al* (2003) Behavioural phenotypes associated with specific genetic disorders: evidence from a population-based study of people with Prader–Willi syndrome. *Psychological Medicine*, **33**: 141–53.

International Human Genome Sequencing Consortium (2001) Initial sequencing and analysis of the human genome. *Nature*, **409**: 860–921.

Jirtle RL, Skinner MK (2007) Environmental epigenomics and disease susceptibility. *Nature Reviews Genetics*, **8**: 253–62.

Kaminsky EB, Kaul V, Paschall J, *et al* (2011) An evidence-based approach to establish the functional and clinical significance of copy number variants in intellectual and developmental disabilities. *Genetics in Medicine*, **13**: 777–84.

Karmiloff-Smith A, Thomas M (2003) What can developmental disorders tell us about the neurocomputational constraints that shape development? The case of Williams syndrome. *Development and Psychopathology*, **15**: 969–90.

Larson SA, Lakin CL, Anderson L, *et al* (2001) Prevalence of mental retardation and developmental disabilities: estimates from the 1994/1995 National Health Interview Survey Disabilities Supplements. *American Journal on Mental Retardation*, **106**: 231–54.

Lejeune, J, Gautier M, Turpin R (1959) Les chromosomes humains en culture de tissus [Human chromosomes in tissue culture]. *Compte Rendus Hebdomadaires des Séances de l'Académie des Sciences*, **248**: 602–3.

Matson J, Benavidiz D, Compton L, *et al* (1996) Behavioral treatment of autistic persons: a review of research from 1980 to present. *Research in Developmental Disabilities*, **17**: 433–65.

McConkey R, Mulvany F, Barron S (2006) Adult persons with intellectual disabilities in the island of Ireland. *Journal of Intellectual Disability Research*, **50**: 227–36.

Miller DT, Adam MP, Aradhya S, *et al* (2010) Consensus statement: Chromosomal microarray is a first-tier clinical diagnostic test for individuals with developmental disabilities or congenital anomalies. *American Journal of Human Genetics*, **86**: 749–64.

Nolin SL, Brown WT, Glicksman A, *et al* (2003) Expansion of the fragile X CGG repeat in females with pre-mutation or intermediate alleles. *American Journal of Human Genetics*, **72**: 454–64.

Nyhan W (1971) Behavioral phenotypes in organic genetic disease: Presidential address to the Society for Pediatric Research, May 1, 1971. *Pediatric Research*, **6**: 1–9.

Oliver C, Adams D, Allen D, *et al* (2013) Causal models of clinically significant behaviors in Angelman, Cornelia de Lange, Prader–Willi and Smith–Magenis syndromes. *International Review of Research in Developmental Disabilities*, **44**: 167–211.

Prasad C, Galbraith PA (2005) Sir Archibald Garrod and alkaptonuria – 'story of metabolic genetics'. *Clinical Genetics*, **68**: 199–203.

Reiss AL, Dant CC (2003) The behavioural neurogenetics of fragile-X syndrome: gene–brain–behaviour relationships in child developmental psychopathologies. *Development and Psychopathology*, **15**: 927–68.

Rutter M, Tizard J, Yule W, *et al* (1976) Isle of Wight Studies, 1964–1974. *Psychological Medicine*, **6**: 313–32.

Shakespeare T (2006) *Disability Rights and Wrongs*. Routledge.

Sondenaa E, Rasmussen K, Nottestad JA, *et al* (2010) Prevalence of intellectual disabilities in Norway: domestic variation. *Journal of Intellectual Disability Research*, **54**: 161–7.

Tjio JH, Levan A (1956) The chromosome number of man. *Hereditas*, **42**: 1–6.

Watson JD, Crick FHC (1953) A structure for deoxyribose nucleic acid. *Nature*, **171**: 737–8.

Wechsler D (1997) *Wechsler Adult Intelligence Scale – Third Edition (WAIS-III)*. The Psychological Corporation.

Wen X (1997) *The Definition and Prevalence of Intellectual Disabilities in Australia*. Australian Institute of Health and Welfare, Canberra.

Wolfensberger W (1972) *The Principle of Normalization in Human Services*. National Institute on Mental Retardation, Toronto.

Woodruff-Borden J, Kistler DJ, Henderson DR, *et al* (2010) Longitudinal course of anxiety in children and adolescents with Williams syndrome. *American Journal of Medical Genetics: Part C Seminars in Medical Genetics*, **154(C)**: 277–90.

World Health Organization (1980) *International Classification of Impairments, Disabilities and Handicaps*. WHO.

World Health Organization (2001) *International Classification of Functioning, Disability and Health (ICF)*. WHO.

Zimmerman M (2009) Iodine deficiency. *Endocrine Reviews*, **30**: 376–40.

CHAPTER 2

Behavioural phenotypes

Jeremy Turk

The first modern use of the term 'behavioural phenotype' was by Professor Bill Nyhan in his 1972 paper on the challenging behaviours manifested by individuals with Lesch–Nyhan syndrome (Hall *et al*, 2001), and Cornelia de Lange syndrome (Berney *et al*, 1999). Nyhan, with the aid of cine film footage, argued persuasively that the characteristic behaviours of children with these genetic anomalies were sufficiently consistent, irrespective of the children's social backgrounds, to suggest that they were primarily attributable to the underlying genetic anomaly (Nyhan, 1972). It is now surprising to reflect on just how unacceptable such a proposal was at the time. There are a number of reasons for this. First, there was a high degree of scepticism regarding the possibility of genetically predetermined behavioural and developmental profiles, attributable to concerns regarding earlier eugenics philosophies, coupled with the rise of sociopolitical movements and a focus on the psychosocial determinants of development and behaviour. Second, the definitive Isle of Wight epidemiological neuropsychiatric study of children (Rutter *et al*, 1970) concluded that there were just two factors influencing the nature and severity of psychological dysfunction and challenging behaviour: the degree of intellectual disability; and the quality of the social environment of upbringing, social relationships and social experiences. These influences are not in dispute. Indeed, Emerson and colleagues, in a series of publications, reported their findings that social factors are just as important for individuals with developmental disabilities as for the general population in determining physical as well as mental health (Emerson *et al*, 2007). Furthermore, they identified that the cumulative risk from exposure to social disadvantage is associated with increased prevalence of psychopathology, primarily autism spectrum conditions, hyperkinesis and conduct disorders (Emerson & Hatton, 2007). They concluded that socioeconomic disadvantage may account for a significant proportion of the poorer physical and mental health of children and adolescents with intellectual disabilities. However, at the time of the Isle of Wight study, the aetiology (cause) of an individual's disorder of intellectual development was not seen as determining the nature and severity of the associated developmental, temperamental, emotional and behavioural challenges. This may have been because of limited understanding of biological, and indeed psychosocial, causality in developmental disabilities. It may also have arisen because of consequent conceptual reliance on *clinical–phenomenological* symptom-based descriptions of developmental and psychiatric disorders, as opposed to *aetiological* classifications as used in much of the rest of the health sciences.

In summary, the determinants of the severity and nature of psychological and psychiatric dysfunction in individuals with disorders of intellectual development can be listed as (Dykens, 2000):

- the severity of the intellectual disability
- the quality of the social environment, social relationships, social experiences and upbringing
- the underlying cause of the disorder (although this may not be ascertainable).

The influence of comorbid autism spectrum conditions on the likelihood, nature and severity of psychopathology and challenging behaviour remains controversial (Tsakanikos *et al*, 2006). However, there is evidence for autism spectrum conditions associated with intellectual disability having clinically significant detrimental effects on independent living skills and adaptive behaviours (Matson *et al*, 2009).

The concept of behavioural phenotypes, and their emanation from specific underlying aetiologies, differs from traditional classificatory approaches to the mental health of children and adolescents, and of individuals who have disorders of intellectual development. For such people, classificatory categories ('diagnoses') are based on the presenting clinical features ('phenomena') as well as, where accessible, personal reports of internal mental states, and reports from people who know the client well. These 'clinical–phenomenological' diagnoses make little if any reference to aetiological factors, rely on the presence, nature, number and persistence of certain clinical features, and hence represent common final clinical pathways and end-points with, presumably, multiple (even many) possible underlying aetiologies, acting simultaneously, as in the biopsychosocial model of mental illness.

In contrast, an aetiological model bases diagnosis on, primarily, underlying cause. This has been the popular and accepted approach for some time in general medicine, where we have had the benefit of greater understanding of causation. For example, breathlessness may have a variety of aetiologies, including cardiovascular, respiratory, 'otherwise physical' (as in obesity-related respiratory function compromise), malignant and even psychogenic. The exact nature of the breathlessness and associated investigatory findings will clarify which cause or causes are operating and hence there is greater potential for a rational treatment plan. Conversely, inferring a cause erroneously will risk inappropriate and potentially detrimental interventions and supports, and possibly the exclusion of appropriate and beneficial ones.

We are now benefiting from increasing understanding of causation in mental health and disorders of intellectual development, but there is an associated potential for conceptual confusion, whereby aetiological and clinical–phenomenological diagnoses may be viewed as contradictory rather than complementary or, even worse, with one viewed as primary and others secondary, rather than all diagnoses being seen as comorbid (Bax & Gillberg, 2010).

In child and adolescent mental health, and more recently in the field of intellectual disabilities, this predicament has been eased by the utilisation of multi-axial classification systems, whereby different axes are used to describe different diagnostic components:

1 psychiatric diagnostic label(s)
2 specific developmental delays (specific learning difficulties)
3 general level of intellectual functioning
4 medical associations
   - causal
   - consequential
   - co-occurring
   - coincidental and complicating
5 social factors
6 degree of functional impairment.

An example of how this might work is:

1 psychiatric diagnostic label(s): *attention-deficit hyperactivity disorder (ADHD), combined type*
2 specific developmental delays (specific learning difficulties): *impairments in working memory, visuospatial skills, numeracy and fine motor control*
3 general level of intellectual functioning: *IQ = 63*
4 medical associations:
   - causal: *fragile-X syndrome*
   - consequential: *repetitive bruising and fractures*
   - co-occurring: *epilepsy*
   - coincidental and complicating: *eczema and hay fever*
5 social factors: *single parent, financial hardship, racial and cultural discrimination*
6 degree of functional impairment: *extreme.*

A major argument against promoting the concept of behavioural phenotypes, and challenging the importance of diagnosis, has been the erroneous suggestion that an understanding of aetiology brings no benefits with it, and might even be detrimental in increasing the likelihood of 'self-fulfilling prophecies' regarding possible developmental, temperamental, emotional and behavioural challenges. However, knowing the causes of an individual's challenges is vital, for a number of reasons. These include, but are not confined to: the right of the individual and family to know the cause of the challenges they face; relief from uncertainty; and facilitation of grief resolution, with an associated enhanced ability to look to the future rather than dwelling on the past; genetic counselling, which may be crucial to the families of people with inherited conditions (Turk, 2013); information on likely strengths, needs and challenges to be faced, allowing families and individuals to be forewarned and forearmed; the potential for appropriate and targeted early interventions and supports; and the ability to link with appropriate support networks (Turk, 2003).

Definition

Historically, some authors have taken a very narrow view of what constitutes a behavioural phenotype. For example, it has been argued that to qualify for having a behavioural phenotype, certain clinical features must be present in all individuals with the underlying aetiological agent and must be absent from individuals with other underlying aetiologies, and the causal relationship between aetiology and clinical features must be verifiable beyond reasonable doubt (Flint & Yule, 1994). Applying these criteria, Flint and Yule identified only three conditions worthy of the description:

- Lesch–Nyhan syndrome, with its associated severe and mutilatory self-injury (Robey *et al*, 2003)
- Prader–Willi syndrome, with its associated voracious appetite, hyperphagia and consequent gross obesity (Descheemaeker *et al*, 2002)
- Rett syndrome, with its associated midline stereotypical 'handwashing' behaviour, rocking and hyperventilation (Colvin *et al*, 2003).

For practical clinical purposes, a broader and more inclusive definition is preferable (O'Brien, 2007; Turk, 2007), which might be formulated as follows:

> A behavioural phenotype refers to those aspects of an individual's psychiatric, psychological, cognitive, emotional and behavioural functioning which can be attributed to an underlying, discrete, usually biological (including genetic) abnormality which has occurred early in development.

It is of note that behavioural phenotypes can have psychosocial aetiologies, as in the frozen watchfulness and over-clinginess of the anxious and insecurely attached infant, or of the child who has experienced abuse and neglect. However, most research has focused on biological causality, and this will be concentrated on in this chapter.

Most research has focused on genetically determined behavioural phenotypes. However, other biological agents and processes are often implicated. These include infections of the central nervous system, often antenatal (e.g. toxoplasmosis, rubella, cytomegalovirus, herpes simplex, syphilis and the human immunodeficiency virus), toxins, especially fetal alcohol (Mukherjee *et al*, 2006, 2011; Chandraseena *et al*, 2009), maternally taken medications (e.g. anticonvulsants), brain malformations and occasionally autoimmune processes, as occur in the rare but well recognised opsoclonus–myoclonus ('dancing eye') syndrome (Klein *et al*, 2007).

Genetic causes

There is strong evidence for a largely genetic basis to the developmental disabilities, including intellectual disability, autism spectrum conditions (Abrahams & Geschwind, 2008) and ADHD (Sharp *et al*, 2009). Supportive data have derived from family, twin and adoption studies as well as from more recent research into molecular biology and the human genome. A range of genetic aetiologies has been found to be associated with autism (Turk, 2007) and ADHD (Turk, 2009).

Gender has an important influence on presenting psychological profiles. For example, recent research suggests that while girls and boys have similar patterns of core and coexisting autism spectrum features, speech articulation is less impaired in girls (Limnaiou & Turk, 2012). Also, the same study found that boys with ADHD are significantly more restless and fidgety than girls with the condition, and that the boys fight and bully more, as well as being more generally aggressive otherwise. In contrast, girls with ADHD presented with more emotional features, including school refusal and school phobia, mood lability, somatisations and social disinhibition.

Individual aetiologies tend to produce their own profiles of intellectual functioning, social and communicatory impairments and attentional challenges. This *genotypic* (as opposed to *phenotypic*) approach allows for more refined identification of psychological profiles, with correspondingly increased ability to fine tune interventions and supports to specific aetiological groups.

Down syndrome

The most common identifiable cause of intellectual disability is Down syndrome, usually attributable to having an extra chromosome 21 in addition to the normal complement of 46 chromosomes in each cell. Apart from a rare translocation form, all instances consist of new mutations, the main risk factor being older maternal age. Levels of intelligence are normally distributed, with the mean IQ being in the moderate–severe intellectual disability range, equivalent to an IQ of 35–70. The presence of a characteristic personality stereotype involving a pleasant, affectionate and passive behavioural style (Gibbs & Thorpe, 1983) is still equivocal, despite the earliest descriptions by Langdon Down of individuals having considerable powers of imitation, humorousness, a lively sense of the ridiculous, obstinacy and amiability. More recent research suggests that some aspects of the Down syndrome behavioural phenotype even appear in infants and toddlers, including emerging relative strengths in some aspects of visual processing, receptive language and non-verbal social functioning, and relative weaknesses in gross motor skills and expressive language skills (Fidler, 2005). Rates of autism spectrum conditions and ADHD are somewhat lower than expected for a population with this level of intellectual disability. However, the rates are considerably higher than in the general population. At least 10% of individuals with Down syndrome have a comorbid autism spectrum condition in addition to intellectual disability (Turk & Graham, 1997; Rasmussen *et al*, 2001) and 6–8% have comorbid ADHD (Green *et al*, 1989), while 10–15% of children and young people with Down syndrome have conduct and oppositional defiant disorders (Dykens, 2007). These associated disorders often go undiagnosed and untreated because the problem behaviours are attributed to the intellectual disability or are perceived as inevitable and immutable correlates of the underlying cause. These behaviours can indeed be very difficult to manage, and when present usually persist into adulthood (McCarthy & Boyd, 2001). In late adolescence and through into early adulthood, individuals with Down syndrome have been found to be more vulnerable to clinical depression, even when the effects of stressful life events and daily hassles have been accounted for (Collacott *et al*, 1998). Later, from middle age onwards, individuals are more prone to Alzheimer presenile dementia (Holland *et al*, 2000). Other psychological challenges including obsessional slowness (Charlot *et al*, 2002) and deficits in working memory have also been reported (Numminen *et al*, 2001).

Fragile-X syndrome

Fragile-X syndrome is the most common identifiable inherited cause of intellectual disability and autism spectrum conditions (Turk, 2011). There have been no recorded instances of the condition being attributable to a new genetic mutation; the condition or the liability to it is always inherited from one or other parent. Intellectual disability is usually in the mild–moderate range, although some individuals are more severely affected. It is caused by abnormal expansion of a run of DNA CGG triplet repeats just above the tip of the X chromosome's long arm, at position Xq27.3. Hypermethylation of an adjacent gene inhibits production of the fragile-X mental retardation protein (FMRP), which has adverse effects on the development of the central nervous system. The protein is known to be important in nucleus–cytoplasm movement of intracellular materials, and in messenger RNA/endoplasmic reticulum binding. A 'full mutation' consists of in excess of 200 repeats and usually the absence of the FMRP. A shorter abnormal expansion of approximately 55–200 repeats is known as a 'premutation' and this may or may not be associated with intellectual disability. However, even in the presence of good intellectual functioning, premutation carriers can experience the characteristic verbal–performance discrepancy, with particularly special needs in relation to numeracy, visuo-spatial skills, executive functioning skills and working memory and sequential information processing deficits which become increasingly noticeable as the individual approaches adolescence (Cornish *et al*, 2009). In middle age, premutation carriers can develop the fragile-X tremor–ataxia syndrome (FRAXTAS), which manifests as insidiously progressive ataxia, intention tremor, features of atypical Parkinsonism and loss of cognitive skills (Kogan *et al*, 2008).

Some 4–6% of individuals with autism spectrum conditions have fragile-X syndrome, while as many as two-thirds of individuals with fragile-X syndrome are diagnosable as having an autism spectrum condition as well (Clifford *et al*, 2007). Males and females may be affected, as may premutation as well as full-mutation individuals (Aziz *et al*, 2003; Cornish *et al*, 2005). The prevalence of autism spectrum conditions and the ease of their identification probably increase with age. Characteristic features include delayed echolalia, repetitive speech, hand flapping, insistence on routine, self-injury in the form of biting of the base of the thumb in response to anxiety and excitement, social anxiety, avoidance of direct eye contact ('gaze aversion') and delayed imitative skills and symbolic play. Most individuals with fragile-X syndrome display the paradoxical juxtaposition of a friendly and sociable, albeit shy and socially anxious, personality in the presence of a number of autistic-like social, linguistic, communicatory, ritualistic, obsessional and sensory features (Cornish *et al*, 2007). Theory-of-mind abilities, face recognition skills, emotion perception and executive function appear reasonably consistent with general levels of developmental abilities (Turk & Cornish, 1998; Garner *et al*, 1999).

Speech and language are characteristically affected, with frequently rapid up and down swings of pitch, perseverations, repetitiveness and cluttering (rapid and dysrhythmic speech) (Cornish *et al*, 2004). There are also raised rates of ADHD (Turk, 1998). Levels of intellectual functioning remain stable over time but difficulties with sequential information processing and working memory increase. Gross motor overactivity diminishes but inattentiveness, impulsiveness and distractibility persist, as do the language tendencies and anomalies.

Recent research has highlighted the importance of the metabotropic glutamate 5 receptor (mGlu5R) pathway in central nervous system inter-neuronal transmission. An up-regulation appears to underlie abnormal over-excitatory and hyper-arousing glutaminergic activity. This has led to exploration of glutamate antagonists as possible therapeutic agents. GABA agonists are also being explored, given GABA's role as a synergistic inhibitory neurotransmitter. Minocycline and arbaclofen, both suspected of having GABAergic properties, have been researched (Wang *et al*, 2010; Berry-Kravis *et al*, 2012) along with more novel selective mGlu5R inhibitors, with some evidence of improved behavioural symptoms in fragile-X syndrome studied in a randomised, double-blind, two-treatment, two-period, crossover study (Jacquemont *et al*, 2011).

Microdeletion syndromes

In addition to the possibility of a chromosome duplication, as in Down syndrome and Klinefelter (XXY) syndrome, a chromosomal deletion, as in Turner (XO) syndrome, and a DNA expansion, as in fragile-X syndrome, genetic disorders may be caused by a microdeletion of DNA. These are usually unidentifiable on light microscope examination of chromosomes. Diagnosis depends on the use either of fluorescing probes linked with specific DNA sequences ('fluorescent *in situ* hybridisation') or of DNA techniques involving southern blots for DNA sequences, northern blots for messenger RNA and western blots for protein products. Polymerase chain reaction technology allows the amassing of substantial quantities of specific DNA and gene sequences, and this facilitates identification not only of the presence or absence of an anomaly, but also of the exact DNA expansion size, as in fragile-X premutation status.

An example of a microdeletion condition is Smith–Magenis syndrome, attributable to loss of DNA on the short arm of chromosome 17 (Gropman *et al*, 2006). The condition presents with: intellectual disability, often mild or moderate; social and linguistic anomalies, which often fall short of the severity and nature required for an autism spectrum diagnosis yet nonetheless are debilitating and handicapping; severe sleep disturbance, characterised by inverted circadian rhythm of melatonin secretion; extreme self-injury; aggressive and disruptive outbursts (Taylor & Oliver, 2008); and a tendency towards ADHD. In addition to common forms of self-injury such as head banging and eye poking, individuals reportedly engage in extreme behaviours, including nail pulling and insertion of objects into bodily orifices. The multiple and severe behavioural challenges result in often low levels of attainment and adaptive behaviour in adulthood, with levels of dependency on carers in excess of what might be expected from the general levels of intellectual functioning (Udwin *et al*, 2001).

Parental inheritance and imprinting

The relevance of parental inheritance of the genetic anomaly is exemplified by Angelman syndrome and Prader–Willi syndrome. In Angelman syndrome, there is a microdeletion on the long arm of the chromosome 15 deriving from the mother. Alternatively there may be *uniparental disomy*, where both chromosome 15s derive from the father (Clayton-Smith & Laan, 2003). This results in moderate–severe intellectual disability (Beckung *et al*, 2004), a jerky ataxic gait, paroxysmal laughter and markedly delayed social, language and communication abilities (Jolleff & Ryan, 1993).

In contrast, individuals with Prader–Willi syndrome may experience a microdeletion at exactly the same gene locus, but inherit it from their father, or alternatively inherit both of their chromosome 15s from their mother (Descheemaeker *et al*, 2002). As infants, children with Prader–Willi syndrome tend to be floppy, to be poor feeders and fail to thrive. However, this is soon replaced with voracious overeating, lack of satiety, sudden and impulsive tantrums, skin picking and gross obesity, which predispose individuals to a range of physical adversities, including respiratory compromise, cardiovascular disease, diabetes, arthritis and sleep apnoea (Cassidy *et al*, 2012). It has also been suggested that individuals with Prader–Willi syndrome lack a need for stimulus novelty, and so for instance will not seek a shift from a savoury proteinacious main course to a sweet calorific dessert.

Prader–Willi syndrome is associated with raised rates of psychotic disorders in adulthood. These disorders usually present with atypical phenomenology and are said to be more common in individuals with uniparental disomy.

The importance of genetically determined neurochemical pathways: the Rasopathies

The Rasopathies are a group of genetic conditions caused by neurochemical anomalies in the Ras/mitogen-activated protein kinase (Ras/MAPK) genetic pathway. The group includes well-recognised and researched conditions such as neurofibromatosis and Noonan syndrome. Less researched and understood conditions such as Costello syndrome, cardio-facio-cutaneous syndrome, Leopard syndrome and Legius syndrome are also included. There is already good evidence for neurofibromatosis type 1 being associated with raised rates of autism spectrum conditions (Garg *et al*, 2013), even when intelligence is within the average range. Other research (Adviento *et al*, 2014) suggests that all the Rasopathies are associated with increased rates of autism spectrum conditions. A study of individuals with Noonan syndrome (Freeman *et al*, 2008) showed intellectual functioning to be largely in the low average range but with raised rates of intellectual disability and high rates of developmental coordination disorder. Social abilities were impaired, with decreases in social flexibility, and less ability to defuse tense situations or to maintain dialogues. Thirty per cent of the sample had problems making friends, had difficulties understanding emotional traits and made poor eye contact. Features of ADHD were common, as were anxiety states, mood disorders, oppositional defiant disorder, obsessive–compulsive features and conduct disorders.

Toxic causes: fetal alcohol spectrum disorders

The profound and catastrophic impacts of neurotoxins on human brain development are exemplified by the consequences of intrauterine alcohol exposure producing fetal alcohol spectrum disorders, also known as alcohol-related neurodevelopmental disabilities (Mattson *et al*, 2011). Alcohol is the most common major toxin to which the human fetus is exposed. It results in pre- and postnatal growth retardation and diminished intellectual abilities, so that IQ usually falls in the borderline/mild intellectual disability range, equivalent to an IQ of approximately 50–85. There are raised rates of: fine motor and visuospatial difficulties; tremulousness; problems with executive function, numeracy and mental abstraction; expressive and receptive language difficulties; infantile irritability; features of childhood ADHD; social challenges, including impaired perception of social cues; and autism spectrum conditions (Mukherjee *et al*, 2011). All these neurodevelopmental challenges are complicated and magnified further by the usually highly unstable family environments.

Infective causes

Rubella encephalopathy

The incidence of congenital rubella in the UK is generally about 1 per 50 000 live births, but it can become epidemic. The risk of epidemics has been heightened by the withholding of rubella immunisation in response to the false belief that the immunisation might raise the risk of autism spectrum conditions. In reality, by rendering the individual immune to rubella (as well as mumps and measles as in the MMR vaccination), potential causes of abnormal neurodevelopment and autistic disturbances are prevented. The fetuses of women who contract the condition within two months of conception are most at risk (95%), but the risk is said to have diminished very substantially by the end of the fourth month of fetal life.

Commonly occurring sequelae of rubella encephalopathy are ophthalmic conditions (especially cataract), a wide range of neurological disorders, microcephaly, heart defects, sensorineural deafness and enlargement of the liver and spleen. Disorders of intellectual development occur in about 50% of cases; among these children, autism is particularly common (Chess & Fernandez, 1980). Autism is usually of neonatal-onset type, but may occur after a period of apparently normal development, perhaps because the live virus persists after the child's birth. The great majority of children with rubella-induced autism have been identified as suffering from rubella at birth. Co-occurrence of often severe intellectual disability, autism spectrum conditions and sensory impairments results in particularly severely affected individuals, who often require intensive, long-term support.

Cytomegalovirus

Cytomegalovirus (CMV) is the most common worldwide cause of congenital and perinatal infections (Alford *et al*, 1990). Infection is usually a mild condition in adults, but the vertically transmitted infection from mother to fetus may produce serious defects. In the UK about one in 200 babies is born showing evidence of active infection (excreting virus in urine) and about 10% of these show subsequent evidence of damage. The child may be born with low birth weight, enlargement of liver and spleen, purpura and eye defects, but most are normal at birth. In one study (Ramsey *et al*, 1991) 45% of children with symptomatic, confirmed cytomegalovirus infection had neurological impairment, most showing gross motor or psychomotor abnormalities, and some having sensorineural deafness. The remaining 55% were neurologically normal at follow-up. The presence of neurological signs in the neonatal period predicted a poor prognosis. A long-term longitudinal follow-up study of those with neurological signs in the neonatal period (Pass *et al*, 1980) identified substantially raised rates of microcephaly, intellectual disability, hearing impairment, neuromuscular disorders and visual pathology.

Other infections

Other infections, such as HIV infection, herpes simplex and syphilis, may also impair fetal development and, if they do not result in fetal death and miscarriage, may be followed by severe disorders of intellectual development and other developmental disabilities.

Opsoclonus–myoclonus ('dancing eye') syndrome: an example of an autoimmune aetiology

Opsoclonus–myoclonus syndrome (OMS), also known as dancing eye syndrome, is a rare and debilitating condition usually commencing in infancy that has an autoimmune pathophysiology and results in both acute and chronic neuropsychiatric phenomena (Gorman, 2010). The name derives from the abnormal, involuntary and often continuous conjoint eye movements horizontally, vertically and diagonally, with equal speed in all directions, in association with marked ataxia and, in the acute phase, emotional extremis. Approximately half of recorded cases seem to be secondary to a thoracolumbar autonomic neuroblastoma, with the remaining cases of unknown origin but suspected of having either an undiscovered neuroblastoma or an infective, usually viral, trigger. A family history of autoimmune disease is also identified in many instances (Krasenbrink *et al*, 2007). The course of the illness is variable, but generally follows the pattern of a non-specific prodrome with subtle personality and temperament change in association with diminished emotional and behavioural responsiveness, followed by a characteristic acute phase of opsoclonus (rapid, involuntary, multi-vectoral eye movements), myoclonus (rapid, involuntary muscle contraction), ataxia, extreme irritability, sleeplessness and rage, followed by more chronic, less well defined and less well differentiated symptom clusters that can include extreme insomnia, self-injurious behaviour and aggression, obsessive–compulsive disorder (OCD), ADHD, social and communicatory impairments, and cognitive decline. These can often result in lifelong severe disability (Ki Pang *et al*, 2010).

The condition is suspected to occur through an autoantibody B-lymphocyte-mediated cross-sensitivity 'friendly fire attack' on the brain. It is presumed that this process is provoked either by antigens that are shared by a known or unknown tumour and the brain, or by viral induction. The combination of ataxia, abnormal and involuntary eye movements and emotional lability has historically led researchers to suspect damage to the cerebellum (Hayward *et al*, 2001). However, damage to the brain-stem and prefrontal cortex connections has also been implicated.

There is evolving evidence that the prodromal phase, characterised by non-specific illness, also presents with irritability, fever, gastric upset and symptoms in the upper respiratory tract. This then develops into the initial acute phase of illness over hours to days. The acute phase is often characterised by pronounced neurological symptoms and emotional and behavioural extremis, including the pathognomonic opsoclonus, myoclonus and ataxia, accompanied by extreme psychological distress, often with rage attacks, inconsolable crying, negative and aversive responses to carer efforts at calming and consoling, and insomnia. Mitchell *et al* (2002) found that almost all of the children they studied showed irritability and inconsolable crying during the acute phase, as well as night terrors, other sleep disturbances and severe tantrums with self-injurious behaviour. Persistent irritability, dysphoric mood and poor emotional regulation were also identified. In a similar study, severe tantrums, aggression and self-injurious behaviours were seen, along with persistent night terrors and enuresis. Attention difficulties and hyperactivity were also reported by schools, although this was not quantified by the authors (Turkel *et al*, 2006). This impulsive, aggressive and emotionally labile behavioural phenotype is also reported by parents.

The acute phase usually abates over a period of weeks to months but the individual is frequently left with a more chronic constellation of neurological, cognitive and neuropsychiatric difficulties that can often be more insidious yet highly disabling and difficult to treat. Longer-term neurodevelopmental and neuropsychiatric sequelae include obsessive–compulsive features, oppositional-defiant behaviours, rage attacks, hyperactivity, depression, attentional deficits, social impairments and expressive and receptive language difficulties. Sleep induction difficulties with repeated night-time waking also persist. Mean IQ is in the low-average range, with many experiencing more severe intellectual disability. Approximately 80% of children continue to have long-term, often lifelong neurological and/or behavioural deficits following the acute illness and these are often very disabling.

Immunomodulatory agents such as steroids, cytotoxic agents and intravenous immunoglobulin have been researched and are thought to reduce illness severity and risk of relapse. However, most treatments are symptom-based, comprising multimodal and multidisciplinary approaches relevant to individuals with persisting complex and multiple developmental disabilities.

Novel interventions

Current research is starting to focus on specific mediating psychological states which determine different behavioural responses to similar triggers, and specific receptor anomalies relating to particular genetic and other conditions as a means of identifying and developing more targeted drug interventions.

Examples of the former include research showing that the challenging behaviours in fragile-X syndrome can be understood in terms of the high and rapidly escalating *anxiety* levels associated with the condition (Woodcock *et al*, 2009). In contrast, problem behaviours in Prader–Willi syndrome are more understandable in terms of underlying evolving *aggression*, while in Angelman syndrome the *drive for adult attention* is a potent motivator for the behavioural disturbances; aggression serving both to initiate and to maintain social contact (Strachan *et al*, 2009). Understanding of such mediating psychological states between stimulus and observed behaviour facilitates the refinement of psychosocial interventions.

Medically, the immunosuppressant rapamycin, and other agents that act on the mammalian target of rapamycin receptors (mTOR), appear to benefit individuals with tuberous sclerosis through its actions on postsynaptic cascade pathways, whereby cerebral tuber shrinkage can be dramatic (Franz *et al*, 2006). However, whether this also leads to amelioration of cognitive, temperamental, emotional and behavioural impairments remains uncertain.

In fragile-X syndrome, as described above, pharmacologically promising developments are based on our recently developed awareness of the importance of the glutamate–GABA synergistic neurotransmitter systems in maintaining psychological stability and balance in many ways, and in particular the relevance of the postsynaptic metabotropic glutamate receptor 5 (mGluR5) pathways for fragile-X syndrome (Michalon *et al*, 2012). GABA-ergic agents (Heulens & Kooy, 2011), and by implication glutamate antagonists, are producing promising findings in scientific laboratory, small-mammal and preliminary human studies. These agents include a range of already available and frequently prescribed products, including lithium salts (Liu *et al*, 2011), minocycline (Paribello *et al*, 2010) and arbaclofen (Berry-Kravis *et al*, 2012). Such neurochemical models and research findings are promoting discussion of the possibility of making in-roads into the features of autism spectrum conditions more generally (Hampson *et al*, 2011). The underlying neurophysiology and neurochemistry of these novel, targeted, interventions is complex. However, awareness of the developing potential to focus medication on condition-specific, neurochemical deficits and imbalances allows for hope that biomedical treatments for disorders of intellectual development may be a real possibility rather than merely a dream.

Conclusion

The principles of behavioural phenotype research and clinical practice are now accepted and are important parts of developmental medicine and psychology, offering benefits for the mental health of children, young people and adults with disorders of intellectual development. Understanding of aetiology and how it affects presenting clinical features and hence effective and targeted psychological and medical interventions and supports now extends well beyond specifically genetic aetiologies, to include toxic, infective and autoimmune phenomena, as well as psychosocial causality. Psychological and medical treatments are undergoing ever increasingly refined developments, giving further promise in the treatments and supports available for this range of conditions.

References

Abrahams BS, Geschwind DH (2008) Advances in autism genetics: on the threshold of a new neurobiology. *Nature Reviews Genetics*, **9**: 341–55.

Adviento B, Corbin IL, Widjaja F, *et al* (2014) Autism traits in the RASopathies. *Journal of Medical Genetics*, **51**: 10–20.

Alford CA, Stagno S, Pass RF, *et al* (1990) Congenital and perinatal cytomegalovirus infections. *Clinical Infectious Diseases*, **12** (suppl 7): s745–53.

Aziz M, Stathopulu E, Callias M, *et al* (2003) Clinical features of boys with fragile X premutations and intermediate alleles. *American Journal of Medical Genetics Part B: Neuropsychiatric Genetics*, **121B**: 119–27.

Bax, M, Gillberg C (2010) *Comorbidities in Developmental Disorders*. MacKeith Press.

Beckung E, Steffenburg S, Kyllerman M (2004) Motor impairments, neurological signs, and developmental level in individuals with Angelman syndrome. *Developmental Medicine and Child Neurology*, **46**: 239–43.

Berney TP, Ireland M, Burn J (1999) Behavioural phenotype of Cornelia de Lange syndrome. *Archives of Disease in Childhood*, **81**: 333–6.

Berry-Kravis EM, Hessl D, Rathmell B, *et al* (2012) Effects of STX209 (arbaclofen) on neurobehavioral function in children and adults with fragile X syndrome: a randomized, controlled, phase 2 trial. *Science Translational Medicine*, **4**: 152ra127.

Cassidy SB, Schwartz S, Miller JL, *et al* (2012) Prader–Willi syndrome. *Genetics in Medicine*, **14**: 10–26.

Chandraseena AN, Mukherjee RAS, Turk J (2009) Fetal alcohol spectrum disorders: an overview of interventions for affected individuals. *Child and Adolescent Mental Health*, **14**: 162–7.

Charlot L, Fox S, Friedlander R (2002) Obsessional slowness in Down's syndrome. *Journal of Intellectual Disability Research*, **46**: 517–24.

Chess S, Fernandez P (1980) Neurologic damage and behavior disorders in rubella children. *American Annals of the Deaf*, **125**: 998–1001.

Clayton-Smith J, Laan L (2003) Angelman syndrome: a review of the clinical and genetic aspects. *Journal of Medical Genetics*, **40**: 87–95.

Clifford S, Dissanayake, C, Bui QM, *et al* (2007) Autism spectrum phenotype in males and females with fragile X full mutation and premutation. *Journal of Autism and Developmental Disorders*, **37**: 738–47.

Collacott RA, Cooper S-A, Branford D, *et al* (1998) Behaviour phenotype for Down's syndrome. *British Journal of Psychiatry*, **172**: 85–9.

Colvin L, Fyfe S, Leonard S, *et al* (2003) Describing the phenotype of Rett syndrome using a population database. *Archives of Disease in Childhood*, **88**: 38–43.

Cornish, K, Sudhalter V, Turk J (2004) Attention and language in fragile X. *Mental Retardation and Developmental Disabilities Research Reviews*, **10**: 11–16.

Cornish K, Kogan C, Turk J, *et al* (2005) The emerging fragile X premutation phenotype: evidence from the domain of social cognition. *Brain and Cognition*, **57**: 53–60.

Cornish K, Turk J, Levitas A (2007) Fragile X syndrome and autism: common developmental pathways? *Current Pediatric Reviews*, **3**: 61–8.

Cornish KM, Kogan CS, Li L, *et al* (2009) Lifespan changes in working memory in fragile X premutation males. *Brain and Cognition*, **69**: 551–8.

Descheemaeker MJ, Vogels A, Govers V, *et al* (2002) Prader–Willi syndrome: new insights in the behavioural and psychiatric spectrum. *Journal of Intellectual Disability Research*, **46**: 41–50.

Dykens EM (2000) Annotation: psychopathology in children with intellectual disability. *Journal of Child Psychology and Psychiatry*, **41**: 407–17.

Dykens EM (2007) Psychiatric and behavioral disorders in persons with Down syndrome. *Mental Retardation and Developmental Disabilities Research Reviews*, **13**: 272–8.

Emerson E, Hatton C (2007) Mental health of children and adolescents with intellectual disabilities in Britain. *British Journal of Psychiatry*, **191**: 493–9.

Emerson E, Hatton C, MacLean WE Jr (2007) Contribution of socioeconomic position to health inequalities of British children and adolescents with intellectual disabilities. *American Journal on Mental Retardation*, **112**: 140–50.

Fidler DJ (2005) The emerging Down syndrome behavioral phenotype in early childhood: implications for practice. *Infants and Young Children*, **18**: 86–103.

Flint J, Yule W (1994) Behavioural phenotypes. In *Child and Adolescence Psychiatry: Modern Approaches* (3rd edn) (eds M Rutter, E Taylor, L Hersov), pp. 666–87. Blackwell Scientific.

Franz DN, Leonard J, Tudor C, *et al* (2006) Rapamycin causes regression of astrocytomas in tuberous sclerosis complex. *Annals of Neurology*, **59**: 490–8.

Freeman L, Turk J, Patton M (2008) An exploration into a possible behavioural phenotype of Noonan syndrome. *Society for the Study of Behavioural Phenotypes, Annual Conference, Cologne: Abstracts*. Society for the Study of Behavioural Phenotypes.

Garg S, Lehtonen A, Huson SM, *et al* (2013) Autism and other psychiatric comorbidity in neurofibromatosis type 1: evidence from a population-based study. *Developmental Medicine and Child Neurology*, **55**: 139–45.

Garner C, Callias M, Turk J (1999) The executive function and theory of mind performance of young men with fragile X syndrome. *Journal of Intellectual Disability Research*, **43**: 466–74.

Gibbs MV, Thorpe JG (1983) Personality stereotype of noninstitutionalised Down syndrome children. *American Journal of Mental Deficiency*, **87**: 601–5.

Gorman M (2010) Update on diagnosis, treatment, and prognosis in opsoclonus–myoclonus–ataxia syndrome. *Current Opinion in Pediatrics*, **22**: 245–50.

Green JM, Dennis J, Bennets LA (1989) Attention disorder in a group of young Down's syndrome children. *Journal of Mental Deficiency Research*, **33**: 105–22.

Gropman AL, Duncan WC, Smith ACM (2006) Neurologic and developmental features of the Smith–Magenis syndrome (del 17p11.2). *Pediatric Neurology*, **34**: 337–50.

Hall S, Oliver C, Murphy G (2001) Self-injurious behaviour in young children with Lesch–Nyhan syndrome. *Developmental Medicine and Child Neurology*, **43**: 745–9.

Hampson DR, Adusei DC, Pacey LKK (2011) The neurochemical basis for the treatment of autism spectrum disorders and fragile X syndrome. *Biochemical Pharmacology*, **81**: 1078–86.

Hayward K, Jeremy R, Jenkins S, *et al* (2001) Long-term neurobehavioral outcomes in children with neuroblastoma and opsoclonus–myoclonus–ataxia syndrome: relationship to MRI findings and anti-neuronal antibodies. *Journal of Pediatrics*, **139**: 552–9.

Heulens I, Kooy F (2011) Fragile X syndrome: from gene discovery to therapy. *Frontiers in Bioscience (Landmark Edition)*, **16**: 1211–32.

Holland AJ, Hon J, Huppert FA, *et al* (2000) Incidence and course of dementia in people with Down's syndrome: findings from a population-based study. *Journal of Intellectual Disability Research*, **44**: 138–46.

Jacquemont S, Curie A, des Portes C, *et al* (2011) Epigenetic modification of the FMR1 gene in fragile X syndrome is associated with differential response to the mGluR5 antagonist AFQ056. *Science Translational Medicine*, **3**: 64ra1.

Jolleff N, Ryan MM (1993) Communication development in Angelman's syndrome. *Archives of Disease in Childhood*, **69**: 148–50.

Ki Pang K, de Sousa S, Lang B, *et al* (2010) A prospective study of the presentation and management of dancing eye syndrome/opsoclonus–myoclonus syndrome in the United Kingdom. *European Journal of Paediatric Neurology*, **14**: 156–61.

Klein A, Schmitt B, Boltshauserm E (2007) Long-term outcome of ten children with opsoclonus–myoclonus syndrome. *European Journal of Paediatrics*, **166**: 359–63.

Kogan CS, Turk J, Hagerman RJ, *et al* (2008) Impact of the fragile X mental retardation 1 (FMR1) gene premutation on neuropsychiatric functioning in adult males without fragile X-associated tremor/ataxia syndrome: a controlled study. *Neuropsychiatric Genetics*, **147B**: 859–72.

Krasenbrink I, Fühlhuber V, Juhasz-Boess I, *et al* (2007) Increased prevalence of autoimmune disorders and autoantibodies in parents of children with opsoclonus–myoclonus syndrome (OMS). *Neuropediatrics*, **38**: 114–16.

Limnaiou ML, Turk J (2012) Gender differences in autism spectrum disorders and hyperkinetic disorders: a cross-sectional item sheet study. In *Abstracts: 15th Society for the Study of Behavioural Phenotypes International Research Symposium, Leuven, Belgium.* Society for the Study of Behavioural Phenotypes.

Liu ZH, Chuang DM, Smith CB (2011) Lithium ameliorates phenotypic deficits in a mouse model of fragile X syndrome. *International Journal of Neuropsychopharmacology*, **14**: 618–30.

Matson JL, Dempsey T, Fodstad JL (2009) The effect of autism spectrum disorders on adaptive independent living skills in adults with severe intellectual disability. *Research in Developmental Disabilities*, **30**: 1203–11.

Mattson SN, Crocker N, Nguyen TT (2011) Fetal alcohol spectrum disorders: neuropsychological and behavioral features. *Neuropsychology Review*, **21**: 81–101.

McCarthy J, Boyd J (2001) Psychopathology and young people with Down's syndrome: childhood predictors and adult outcome of disorder. *Journal of Intellectual Disability Research*, **45**: 99–105.

Michalon A, Sidorov M, Ballard TM, *et al* (2012) Chronic pharmacological mGlu5 inhibition corrects fragile X in adult mice. *Neuron*, **74**: 49–56.

Mitchell W, Davalos-Gonzalez Y, Brumm V, *et al* (2002) Opsoclonus-ataxia caused by childhood neuroblastoma: developmental and neurologic sequelae. *Pediatrics*, **109**: 86–98.

Mukherjee RAS, Hollins S, Turk J (2006) Fetal alcohol spectrum disorder: an overview. *Journal of the Royal Society of Medicine*, **99**: 298–302.

Mukherjee RAS, Layton M, Yacoub E, *et al* (2011) Autism and autistic traits in people exposed to heavy prenatal alcohol: data from a clinical series of 21 individuals and nested control study. *Advances in Mental Health and Intellectual Disabilities*, **5**: 42–9.

Numminen H, Service E, Ahonen T, *et al* (2001) Working memory and everyday cognition in adults with Down's syndrome. *Journal of Intellectual Disability Research*, **45**: 157–68.

Nyhan WL (1972) Behavioral phenotypes in organic genetic disease. *Pediatric Research*, **6**: 1–9.

O'Brien G (ed) (2007) *Behavioural Phenotypes in Clinical Practice (Clinics in Developmental Medicine No. 157).* MacKeith Press.

Paribello C, Tao L, Folino A, *et al* (2010) Open-label add-on treatment trial of minocycline in fragile X syndrome. *BMC Neurology*, **10**: 91.

Pass RF, Stagno S, Meyers GJ, *et al* (1980) Outcome of symptomatic congenital cytomegalovirus infection: results of long-term, longitudinal follow-up. *Pediatrics*, **66**: 758–62.

Ramsey ME, Miller E, Peckham CS (1991) Outcome of symptomatic, confirmed cytomegalovirus infection. *Archives of Disease in Childhood*, **66**: 1068–9.

Rasmussen P, Börjesson O, Wentz E, *et al* (2001) Autistic disorders in Down syndrome: background factors and clinical correlates. *Developmental Medicine and Child Neurology*, **43**: 750–4.

Robey KL, Reck JF, Giacomini KD, *et al* (2003) Modes and patterns of self-mutilation in persons with Lesch–Nyhan disease. *Developmental Medicine and Child Neurology*, **45**: 167–71.

Rutter M, Graham P, Yule W (1970) *A Neuropsychiatric Study in Childhood* (*Clinics in Developmental Medicine*, Nos 35/36). Heinemann/Spastics International Medical Publications.

Sharp SI, McQuillin A, Gurling HMD (2009) Genetics of attention-deficit hyperactivity disorder. *Neuropharmacology*, **57**: 590–600.

Strachan R, Shaw R, Burrow C, *et al* (2009) Experimental functional analyses of aggression in children with Angelman syndrome. *Research in Developmental Disabilities*, **30**: 1095–106.

Taylor L, Oliver C (2008) The behavioural phenotype of Smith–Magenis syndrome: evidence for a gene–environment interaction. *Journal of Intellectual Disability Research*, **52**: 830–41.

Tsakanikos E, Costello H, Holt G, *et al* (2006) Psychopathology in adults with autism and intellectual disability. *Journal of Autism and Developmental Disorders*, **36**: 1123–9.

Turk J (1998) Fragile X syndrome and attentional deficits. *Journal of Applied Research in Intellectual Disabilities*, **11**: 175–91.

Turk J (2003) The importance of diagnosis. In *Educating Children with Fragile X Syndrome* (ed D Dew-Hughes), pp.. 15–19. Routledge Falmer.

Turk J (2007) Behavioural phenotypes: their applicability to children and young people who have intellectual disability. *Advances in Mental Health in Learning Disabilities*, **1**: 4–13.

Turk J (2009) Behavioural phenotypes in relation to ADHD. *ADHD in Practice*, **1**(3): 8–12.

Turk J (2011) Fragile X syndrome: lifespan developmental implications for those without as well as with intellectual disability. *Current Opinion in Psychiatry*, **24**: 387–97.

Turk J (2013) Communicating with children who have intellectual disability. In *Getting the Message Across: Communicating with Diverse Populations in Clinical Genetics* (eds J Wiggins, A Middleton), pp. 140–50. Oxford University Press.

Turk J, Cornish KM (1998) Face recognition and emotion perception in boys with fragile-X syndrome. *Journal of Intellectual Disability Research*, **42**: 490–9.

Turk J, Graham P (1997) Fragile X syndrome, autism and autistic features. *Autism*, **1**: 175–97.

Turkel S, Brumm V, Mitchell W, *et al* (2006) Mood and behavioral dysfunction with opsoclonus–myoclonus ataxia. *Journal of Neuropsychiatry and Clinical Neurosciences*, **18**: 239–41.

Udwin O, Webber C, Horn I (2001) Abilities and attainment in Smith–Magenis syndrome. *Developmental Medicine and Child Neurology*, **43**: 823–8.

Wang LW, Berry-Kravis E, Hagerman RJ (2010) Fragile X: leading the way for targeted treatments in autism. *Neurotherapeutics*, **7**: 264–74.

Woodcock K, Oliver C, Humphreys G (2009) Associations between repetitive questioning, resistance to change, temper outbursts and anxiety in Prader–Willi and fragile X syndromes. *Journal of Intellectual Disability Research*, **53**: 265–78.

Part 2
Disorders of intellectual development: comorbidity and complications

CHAPTER 3

Psychiatric illness and disorders of intellectual development: a dual diagnosis

Marc Woodbury-Smith and Sheila Hollins

The psychiatrist plays a pivotal role in multidisciplinary teams that provide support and services for adults with disorders of intellectual development (DID). More than simply a historical artefact, however, this undoubtedly reflects the significance of the behavioural, medical and neuropsychiatric 'complications' of DID in terms of their prevalence and complexity, as well as the dynamics of families and support systems. These points notwithstanding, the psychiatrist is only one member of the multidisciplinary team, and the complexity inherent in 'dual diagnosis', alongside the important contributions made by relational and environmental factors, demands a range of skills, as will become apparent during the course of this chapter.

The aim of this chapter is to provide an overview of the comorbidity of DID and additional psychiatric illness. The wider concept of 'mental health problems' includes the large category of 'behaviours which are experienced as challenging', which are the subject of Chapter 5, while the pharmacological treatment of psychiatric illness in this population is discussed by Deb in Chapter 7. Therefore, the present chapter will focus on epidemiology, aetiology, assessment and diagnosis, and will give some overriding principles to consider in designing a management plan.

Epidemiology of psychiatric disorder

Although estimates of the prevalence of psychiatric disorder among individuals with DID vary widely, as a general rule it seems to be higher than in the general population. The variation in prevalence figures reflects bias in ascertainment, the diagnostic methods used and the characteristics of the populations studied, including the sample size (Smiley, 2005). Moreover, the prevalence in institutionalised samples tends to be higher. The most robust studies in epidemiological terms are summarised in Table 3.1. Even within this small number of studies, different methodologies have been employed and the prevalence figures vary widely (e.g. as low as 10% in California in the 1990 study of Borthwick-Duffy & Eyman, and as high as 31.7% in the 2008 study by Morgan and colleagues in Perth, Australia). It should be pointed out that some studies have calculated point prevalence (the studies by Rutter *et al*, Lund and Cooper *et al*), while, by their very methodology, others must be considered estimates of lifetime prevalence (the study by Morgan *et al* and both US studies).

Table 3.1 Studies of the prevalence of mental illness among people with disorders of intellectual development (DID)

Study (location)	Description of sample	Diagnostic methods	Prevalence
Rutter *et al*, 1970 (Isle of Wight, UK)	59 children aged 9–10 years with an IQ two or more standard deviations below the mean, representing 2.5% of the total population of children	Questionnaires completed by parents and teachers and direct assessment by a psychiatrist	30–42% with psychiatric disorder (seen in 6.7% of controls)
Lund, 1985 (Denmark)	302 people aged 20 years or over from one county, representing 0.43% of the county population	Direct examination of individual and interview with staff/carer by a psychiatrist	28.1% with psychiatric disorder (see discussion in the text)
Jacobson, 1982 (New York, USA)	42 479 children and adults registered on the New York State register of people receiving services for intellectual disabilities; comprised 0.22% of the state population	Examination of records for any psychiatric diagnosis given by a qualified professional	20% with psychiatric disorder (see discussion in the text)
Borthwick-Duffy & Eyman, 1990 (California, USA)	78 603 children and adults receiving services from the California Department of Developmental Services; comprised 0.23% of the state population	Examination of records for any psychiatric diagnosis given by a qualified professional	10% with psychiatric disorder
Cooper *et al*, 2007 (Glasgow, UK)	Population-based study identifying administrative sample of adults with DID that comprised 0.33% of the Greater Glasgow population	Direct examination of individual and interview with carer	15.7% cross-sectional with DSM-IV psychiatric disorder
Morgan *et al*, 2008 (Perth, Australia)	Western Australian population-based psychiatric and intellectual disability registers	Cross-linking of the two registers	31.7% had a lifetime psychiatric disorder (see discussion in the text)

In general, however, the type of prevalence figure being calculated is not explicitly described, making it difficult to run comparisons with the general population. Indeed, although the point prevalence figures, as estimated by, for example, Cooper *et al* (2007), are significantly higher than those in the general population, the lifetime prevalence does seem to be comparable to the general population figures.

Further insight can be gained by considering the rates of specific psychiatric diagnoses. The studies by Lund (1985) and Cooper *et al* (2007) are particularly insightful for this purpose, as the authors, psychiatrists, directly examined the study participants, thus facilitating true estimates of the cross-sectional point prevalence. Lund identified behavioural disorders in 10.9%, affective disorders in 1.7% and schizophrenia in 1.3%. A further 5% had psychosis of uncertain type and 2% were described as having 'neurosis'. Cooper *et al* examined psychiatric diagnosis according to a number of different diagnostic systems, including those made clinically, according to the Diagnostic Criteria – Learning Disabilities (DC-LD) (Royal College of Psychiatrists, 2001) and using DSM-IV criteria (American Psychiatric Association, 1994). As expected, DSM-IV yielded the lowest prevalence estimates, but even using these criteria, 3.4% were diagnosed with a psychotic disorder (3.8% using DC-LD), 3.6% with an affective disorder (5.7% using DC-LD) and 2.4% with an anxiety disorder (3.1% using DC-LD). The rate of 'problem behaviour' according to DC-LD was 18.7%.

Prevalence as a function of level of disability

Cooper *et al* (2007) showed that rates increase with increasing severity of intellectual impairment. Similarly, Lund (1985) demonstrated an increase in prevalence associated with lower IQ scores.

Prevalence as a function of age

Studies have, on the whole, not examined rates across the age spectrum. However, Deb *et al* (2001) did report a significant association between rates of mental health problems and increasing age in a study of 101 adults with DID aged 16–64 years. Although other studies have, for example, found that rates of depression increase with age (Shooshtari *et al*, 2011), one study has suggested the rates remain fairly stable as people age (Hove & Havik, 2010). Moreover, that study reported that problem behaviours seem to decrease with age.

Cohort effects

The study by Morgan *et al* (2008) compared the prevalence of mental health problems between two birth cohorts born between (a) 1950 and 1964 and (b) 1965 and 1979 and did not identify any birth cohort effects for the prevalence of comorbid mental health diagnoses.

The specific association with psychotic disorders

The studies described above, and a number of others, all point towards a raised prevalence of psychotic disorders among individuals with DID. The presentation may be modified by the impact of the cognitive and communication impairment, and, as we will discuss below, specific features may be characteristic in a small subgroup. Moreover, at IQs below 45, where there is often very significant communication impairment, the diagnosis may be almost impossible to make with any certainty (Reid, 1980).

In 1919, Kraepelin estimated that 7% of cases of dementia praecox (later termed schizophrenia) occurred in individuals with an intellectual impairment of a mild to moderate degree (termed 'imbecility' in Kraepelin's original text). He used the term *pfropfschizophrenie* to describe such cases (from the German *pfropf* meaning engrafted, i.e. a psychotic disorder engrafted on the premorbid intellectual disability). The features of *pfropfschizophrenie* include 'naïve childish type' delusions (Milici, 1937) and more general hebephrenic features, with the onset of illness coinciding with a significant life event (for a more in-depth discussion see Mack *et al*, 2002). Little has been written of this diagnosis since the early descriptions of Kraepelin and Milici, although one study has attempted to delineate its features using a case–control design (Doody *et al*, 1998). Although the study was small, the authors demonstrated more 'negative' symptoms, episodic memory deficits, soft neurological signs and epilepsy among people with *pfropfschizophrenie* than among people with schizophrenia alone or DID alone. Moreover, those with *pfropfschizophrenie* tended to have a stronger family history of schizophrenia and/or DID than the other two groups and to show more karyotyping abnormalities.

Trauma

It is now recognised that individuals with DID are more likely than their counterparts in the general population to experience traumatic events, including sexual and physical abuse. Moreover, developmental level has been found to have a significant impact on a person's ability to cope with such events (Mevissen & de Jongh, 2010). However, established diagnostic criteria for PTSD emphasise the self-report of symptoms (such as flashbacks and hallucinations), making it potentially problematic to diagnose in the population with DID. Furthermore, there is also the suggestion that, as a diagnosis, it may be overlooked in this population (Hollins & Sinason, 2000; Sequeira & Hollins, 2003; Turk *et al*, 2005). However, adapted criteria are available (e.g. in the DC-LD), and previous work has identified a number of potential presenting symptoms that may help the clinician in diagnosis (McCarthy, 2001). These range from sleep disturbances to disruptive behaviour, and include depression and aggression.

Suicidality

Individuals with DID may engage in self-harming behaviour and may complete suicide, but the epidemiology of suicidality in this population has not been well researched. The studies that do exist indicate that rates may be lower among men with DID than among their general population counterparts, but similar in the two groups of women (Patja *et al*, 2001). The factors associated with the propensity for actual suicide in this population are not well understood, but one study comparing those with DID who only threatened suicide and those with DID who attempted suicide indicated that the latter group were younger and more likely to have visited an accident and emergency department.

Aetiology of psychiatric disorder

The frequent overlap between problem behaviour and psychiatric illness means that there is significant overlap in aetiology. The aetiology of problem behaviour is discussed in detail in Chapter 5, and so the discussion here will focus on psychiatric disorder and consider aetiology in terms of biological, psychological and social factors (Table 3.2).

Biological factors

Behavioural phenotypes

Since the description by Nyhan in 1972 of serious, unrelenting self-injurious behaviour in the context of an X-linked genetic syndrome now known as Lesch–Nyhan syndrome (Nyhan, 1972), research has unravelled a series of behavioural and psychiatric associations with particular genetic syndromes (see Chapter 2). A number are of particular interest from a psychiatric point of view. For example, depressive disorder occurs commonly in association with Down syndrome during late adolescence and early adulthood, independent of life events (Collacott *et al*, 1998). Social anxiety is often seen in individuals with fragile-X syndrome (Cordeiro *et al*, 2011), and repetitive behaviours, notably skin picking, are observed among

Table 3.2 Summary of factors associated with psychiatric illness

Biological	Psychological	Social
Genetic syndromes ('behavioural phenotypes')	Coping	Living circumstances
	Self-esteem	Daily structure and routine
Epilepsy	Social comparison	Social support
Autism spectrum disorder		Life events
Physical illness		
Medication		

individuals with Prader–Willi syndrome (Clarke *et al*, 2002). Perhaps the most striking neuropsychiatric association is psychosis in velo-cardio-facial syndrome: it occurs in about 25% of individuals with this 22q deletion syndrome (Gothelf *et al*, 2009).

Epilepsy

Epilepsy is a common neuropsychiatric disorder characterised by episodic disturbances of consciousness, sensorimotor function, behaviour and emotion presumed to result from paroxysmal abnormalities of the electrical activity of the brain. The prevalence of epilepsy in the general population is 0.5–1.0% (Banerjee *et al*, 2009), with a lifetime prevalence of 1.5–5.0%. Among those with DID, however, this prevalence is increased several-fold. For example, among those with severe intellectual disability (IQ < 50), a prevalence of 30% has been observed, and even among those with milder intellectual disability (IQ ≥ 50), the prevalence is still inflated, at 15% or more (Lhatoo & Sander, 2001; McGrother *et al*, 2006). The risk appears higher among those with additional neurological diagnoses, such as cerebral palsy (Singhi *et al*, 2003), and among those with autism spectrum disorder (Spence & Schneider, 2009).

Mood disorders are commonly seen in association with epilepsy, with as many as 13–26% of a community sample being diagnosed (Hoppe & Elger, 2011). The exact reason for this association is not well understood. Psychotic symptoms are also not infrequently seen in association with epilepsy, occurring ictally, post-ictally and inter-ictally (Toone, 2000). The post-ictal group is the largest, with symptoms of psychosis seen among 7% of individuals with a diagnosis of temporal lobe epilepsy. The psychotic symptoms are usually florid, although self-limiting. In inter-ictal psychosis, symptoms bear no relation to the occurrence of the seizures themselves and they are phenomenologically indistinguishable from schizophrenia. (For a more detailed discussion of psychiatric correlates of epilepsy see Chapter 6.)

Autism spectrum disorder

Many people with DID also have a diagnosis of autism spectrum disorder. Affected individuals are at specific risk of a number of mental health problems, including mood and anxiety disorders (see Chapter 8).

Physical illness

Physical symptoms such as pain are known to affect mental well-being, and chronic illness of any nature is known to be associated with an increased risk of mental health problems in the general population. The association between medical illness and psychiatric disorder may be due to a specific biological risk (e.g. hypothyroidism or heart disease and depression), a side-effect of long-term use of medication or the adjustment involved in living with a chronic illness.

Among individuals with DID, there may be an increased risk of certain medical disorders, either in association with the underlying genetic abnormality (e.g. Down syndrome and hypothyroidism) or due to lifestyle issues (e.g. obesity and type 2 diabetes), which in turn may be compounded by the reduced uptake of screening and preventive measures at the population level. (See chapter 13 for a discussion of primary and secondary care and Chapter 12 for a discussion of the general health needs of people with DID.)

Medication

People with DID are often maintained on polypharmacy. Certain medications may increase the risk of psychiatric symptoms and disorders (e.g. levetiracetam and mood disorder, vigabatrin and psychosis), and certain side-effects may affect mental and physical well-being (e.g. abdominal symptoms in association with non-steroidal anti-inflammatory drugs).

Psychological factors

Coping behaviour

Coping is defined as the cognitive and behavioural efforts employed by an individual to manage everyday situations that may evoke positive or negative emotions. In this respect, coping reflects the strategies employed by individuals to regulate their emotions. For a number of reasons, individuals with DID may have a limited range of coping strategies in different situations (for a more detailed discussion see Hartley & Maclean, 2008). For example, cognitive vulnerabilities such as slow language processing, autistic traits or difficulties with executive functioning may impair their ability to recognise or reflect on their emotions, and this may be compounded by learned helplessness with regard to their circumstances. Research has demonstrated that avoidant coping styles (i.e. disengaging from the stressful experience) among individuals with DID are positively related to symptoms of depression and anxiety (Hartley & Maclean, 2008). Moreover, people with DID are more likely to use avoidant than more positive coping styles (such as making efforts to gain control over the situation).

Self-esteem

Self-esteem refers to an overall positive sense of self-worth, self-respect and acceptance (Crocker & Major, 1989). A number of factors may have a negative impact on self-esteem in this population. For example, from an early age children with DID find it difficult to keep up academically with their peers and this, coupled with marginalisation and stigmatisation, may undermine their development of a positive self-image and associated self-esteem. Bullying is still a problem for this population, despite efforts to place the issue high on the public health agenda, and there is increasing awareness of the high prevalence of disability hate crime.

Although there is very little literature exploring the relationship between self-esteem and mental illness in the DID population (e.g. Dagnan &

Sandhu, 1999; MacMahon & Jahoda, 2008), the relationship is well documented in the population at large.

Social comparison

A concept related to self-esteem is social comparison, which is deemed a specific psychological process that can affect self-esteem and other indicators of well-being. It captures people's evaluations of themselves in comparison with others in their environment, such as peers, teachers and work colleagues. In people with DID, this has been shown to be significantly associated with self-esteem.

Social factors

The social milieu in which a person lives is crucial to day-to-day well-being. The environment can have a negative impact on well-being if it is, for example, overcrowded, noisy or dirty. A person's immediate surroundings are also relevant. For example, if their home is located in an unwelcoming environment, or if there is poor public transport or limited availability of activities and services such as shops and libraries, then it is unlikely to be conducive to a sense of mental contentment. Day-to-day structure and routine through scheduled activities or employment are also important.

In the epidemiological study by Cooper *et al* (2007), a number of factors were investigated for their association with psychiatric disorder. Those that were significantly associated with increased psychiatric disorder were: living with paid carer support (in comparison with living with family, in a group or independently), number of life events in the preceding 12 months, higher number of family physician appointments in the preceding 12 months, the absence of physical disability, being fully mobile and being incontinent of urine. Although some of these apparent associations are intuitive, and reflect the experiences of the general population in terms of risk factors, others are less so. It may be that, for example, being fully mobile and/or being without a physical disability affect the level and/or quality of support received, which in turn directly affects mental well-being. Cause and effect cannot be established by this type of study; for instance, having a significant mental illness may result in the requirement for expensive support packages (i.e. having a paid carer).

Social support

The relationship between social support and mental well-being in this population is not straightforward. In one study, level of social support was correlated with quality of life but not with the experience of depressive symptoms. However, the level of social strain was significantly correlated with both somatic and depressive symptoms but not with quality of life (Lunsky & Benson, 2001). Perhaps the most detailed study of social support and environmental circumstances and risk of mental health problems was based on the analysis of survey data on children collected by the Office for National Statistics (UK). In this study of children with and without DID (Emerson & Hatton, 2007), the presence of psychiatric disorders was identified using the Development and Well-Being Assessment (DAWBA; Goodman *et al*, 2000), with additional information collected on social and family circumstances. Briefly, significant association was observed between 'emotional disorder' and a number of social factors, for children both with and without DID. These factors included (but were not limited to) being from a lone-parent family, 'income poverty' in the family, poor family functioning, possible maternal mental disorder and negative life events. Importantly, exposure to social and environmental risk factors was higher among children with DID, and controlling for their effect resulted in a 51% reduction in attributable risk for 'emotional disorder'. It seems reasonable to conclude, at least for children with DID, that social disadvantage is an important correlate of psychiatric illness. Of course, the social and environmental circumstances for many adults with DID are substantially different from those during childhood, and so further research is needed to examine this relationship for adults.

Life events

It has previously been stated that people with DID are more vulnerable to stress than the general population, owing to a number of psychological factors, including prior negative coping experiences, limited environmental supports and a low belief in their abilities (Lunsky, 2008). Studies from the UK, Canada and the USA have indicated that interpersonal stress is most commonly reported in this population. Moreover, there appears to be a discrepancy between the levels of stress observed by caregivers and the stress that is experienced by individuals themselves. This is particularly noticeable among paid caregivers rather than family members providing direct care. People with DID may experience more stressful life events, particularly in relation to factors such as loss or instability of place of residence, primary care staff and employment (Lunsky & Elserafi, 2011). Research among people with DID has shown a positive correlation between behaviour and the experience of life events such as bereavement (Hollins & Esterhuyzen, 1997) and sexual abuse (Sequeira *et al*, 2003); life events have also been linked to mental illness (Esbensen & Benson, 2006) and suicidality (Lunsky, 2004).

Assessment

As evidenced above, the assessment of people with DID demands consideration of a number of competing factors that, to a greater or lesser degree, are relevant in the aetiology and/or management of the presenting complaint. History will be obtained from both the patient and carer(s), and may be complemented by carer-completed monitoring forms (regarding sleep, oral intake and so forth) and more formal assessments and investigations. The presenting complaint is often behavioural, particularly among individuals who are non-verbal, and the task of the diagnostician is therefore in its differential diagnosis. This will be fully afforded only by a detailed history in which the behaviour is expounded in terms of its predisposing, precipitating and perpetuating factors of a biological, psychological and social nature. Box 3.1 provides a thumbnail sketch case scenario and an example schema for extracting information from a clinical dilemma. The benefit of approaching a case in this way is that no stone is left unturned, as it were, and management can then target each aetiological domain in a systematic manner.

Multidisciplinary assessment

Assessment will necessarily be multidisciplinary in nature, with the person and family or chosen representative at its centre and each clinician performing their component of the assessment while being aware of the whole. It could include any or all of the following professionals (and the list is not exhaustive): a psychologist, nurse, psychiatrist, speech and language therapist, occupational therapist and social worker. While the psychiatrist may focus on diagnosis and the aetiology in general terms, a psychologist will be able to consider psychological factors relevant in aetiology and offer insight into which neuropsychological assessments may be appropriate and the interpretation of their results. For individuals with communication difficulties, a speech therapist may be able to make specific recommendations regarding management (e.g. in situations where the person has an additional diagnosis of an autism spectrum disorder). The occupational therapist can offer expertise in the areas of motor and sensory problems, as well as informing treatment in terms of provision of daily routine and structure, environmental modifications and management of sensory-related factors that may be affecting mental well-being. Finally, the social worker will play a pivotal role in ensuring that relevant care and support services are in place. In reality, there is likely to be some overlap of roles and one member of the team would usually become the main person to liaise with the individual and family, whose opinions and expertise will be extremely valuable.

Use of diagnostic instruments

Although the gold-standard diagnostic method is expert-based clinical assessment using a combination of history, physical and mental state evaluation and relevant investigations, diagnosis can be facilitated by the use of structured diagnostic instruments. Instruments such as the Schedule for Affective Disorders and Schizophrenia (SADS; Endicott & Spitzer, 1978) and the Diagnostic Interview Schedule (DIS; Robins *et al*, 1981) provide standardised interview 'cues' for structuring the diagnostic assessment, but their usefulness in the population with DID

Box 3.1 Differential diagnosis of presenting behaviour in intellectual disability

Case summary Mr A is a 47-year-old male with Down syndrome who lives in a group home with three others and, until recently, 1:1 staffing. He presents with a 2-month history of change of behaviour with recurrent episodes of agitation and physical aggression towards his environment. He is also noted to be tearful at times, and is spending more and more time in his room. Until recently he was attending a workshop 3 days a week, but his escalating behaviour, compounded by staff shortages, has resulted in exclusion from this service.

Differential diagnosis

1 Medical (constipation, infection, pain, thyroid dysfunction, neurodegenerative)
2 Psychiatric (depression, adjustment reaction)

Aetiology of differential diagnosis

	Predisposing	*Precipitating*	*Perpetuating*
Biological	Down syndrome Disorder of intellectual development	Thyroid dysfunction Infection/constipation	Thyroid dysfunction Infection/ constipation
Psychological	Possible communication impairment Probable impairment of planning, problem-solving and emotion regulation	Lack of understanding of circumstances, inability to monitor and regulate emotional response to circumstances Relationship difficulties	Learned helplessness/loss of control over his circumstances
Social	Staff shortages	Specific life event Staff shortages	Lack of daily structure Staff shortages

Management

	Predisposing	*Precipitating*	*Perpetuating*
Biological		Medical treatment (liaise with general practitioner, e.g. thyroid replacement, antidepressant medication)	Medical monitoring (e.g. serial thyroid function)
Psychological	Facilitate communication, understanding and emotion regulation	Facilitate communication, understanding and emotion regulation Arrange psychotherapy	Advocacy, facilitate involvement
Social	Advocacy with service commissioners/ providers	Ensure no recurrence of life event such as bullying Manage staffing levels and consistency	Manage staffing levels and consistency

may be somewhat limited. The Psychiatric Assessment Schedule for Adults with Developmental Disabilities (PAS-ADD) offers an alternative. This schedule is a semi-structured interview for use with people with DID and their carers or other suitable informants, and it facilitates DSM-IV and ICD-10 diagnoses (Moss *et al*, 1997). In addition to the diagnostic scale, there are screening questionnaires that allow 'potential caseness' to be identified.

Diagnosis

It is widely recognised that DSM-IV and its replacement, DSM-5 (American Psychiatric Association, 2013), and similarly ICD-10 (World Health Organization, 1992) and its eventual replacement, ICD-11, may not adequately capture the presentation of psychiatric symptomatology among people with DID, owing to the modifying effect of the communication and cognitive difficulties on symptom manifestation. For example, people with DID, even if verbal, may have difficulty articulating their emotional, perceptual and thought-related experiences. Another potential challenge is the problem of 'diagnostic overshadowing'. This describes the tendency of carers, clinicians and others to overlook the presence of psychopathology, instead attributing behaviour or any change in presentation to the underlying developmental vulnerability. Importantly, it is incorrect to conceptualise behaviour experienced as challenging as simply a feature of intellectual impairment, except for the rare cases of specific behavioural manifestations of single-gene disorders such as Cornelia de Lange syndrome, Smith–Magenis syndrome and, of course, Lesch–Nyhan syndrome. Unfortunately, the DSM and ICD classification systems are based on symptom descriptions reported by verbally capable individuals, and therefore researchers have sought to create modified criteria to facilitate diagnosis when behaviour or any other change of function may be the result of an underlying mental illness. The Diagnostic Manual – Intellectual Disability (DM-ID; Fletcher *et al*, 2007) and DC-LD (Cooper *et al*, 2003) are two such diagnostic systems developed in the USA and UK respectively. The DC-LD, for example, was created by an expert panel and subsequently piloted by 52 field researchers drawing on 709 clinical cases. In this way reliability and validity were established, with 96.3% of diagnoses fully concordant with clinical opinion.

Assessment of functioning

The *International Classification of Functioning, Disability and Health* (ICF; World Health Organization, 2001) is a complex classification system for representing dimensions of disability and health (expounded in Chapter 1). The strength of this classification scheme lies in its focus on functioning rather than disability and its attempt to unite the social and biological modes into a unitary biopsychosocial model. It has particular attraction for use with individuals with DID, especially those with comorbid mental health problems, because of the complex interplay between the many different biological, psychological and social factors impacting on functioning in such individuals.

Management

The management of dual diagnosis is described in detail elsewhere in this volume (see Chapter 7 for a discussion of medical interventions, and Chapters 11 and 5 for a discussion of psychological interventions in the context of autism spectrum disorder and challenging behaviour respectively). This brief discussion will therefore concern itself only with some overarching themes and heuristics.

Management will most likely combine medical/psychiatric, psychological and social components, and will consequently be multidisciplinary in nature. The psychiatrist often has a central role in coordinating and overseeing the various management approaches, including their implementation and the response of the patient's symptoms over time, sometimes in association with a 'case manager'. A written treatment plan is of paramount importance, and the patient and carer must be agreeable to the recommendations made. This raises the issue of capacity and consent.

Capacity and consent

A detailed discussion of capacity in relation to making healthcare decisions is beyond the scope of this chapter, and the reader is referred to other resources that expound this important issue (e.g. Brindle *et al*, 2013). With reference to the psychological/behavioural and psychopharmacological treatment of psychiatric illness, if a person is deemed to lack capacity to make this decision, steps should be taken to help the person understand the matter in hand, through, for example, the use of assistive methods such as the Books Beyond Words series, designed to support informed decision-making on a variety of health and social care topics (www.booksbeyondwords.co.uk). If appropriate, treatment may be delayed until a person's capacity has improved. Ultimately, however, particularly among those with more severe cognitive impairment, treatment may need to go ahead. It is important that such treatment is the least restrictive and that it is in the best interests of the person concerned. A legal framework now exists in England and Wales for acting and making decisions on behalf of adults who lack decision-making capacity (the Mental Capacity Act 2005), and for non-capacitous adults there is a requirement for a 'best interests' meeting to be held. In some circumstances the local authority will appoint an independent mental capacity advocate to assist in reaching a decision about management.

Psychological management

The psychological management of core cognitive difficulties and associated challenging behaviours among individuals with autism spectrum disorder has been well researched, and there is now a reasonable evidence base supporting psychological interventions in this population. Such interventions comprise behavioural approaches with or without the addition of 'cognitive' strategies (e.g. cognitive–behavioural therapy). Behavioural therapy encapsulates a set of approaches predicated on reward contingencies. Approaches are described elsewhere in this volume (Chapters 5 and 11) and an overview is provided by Allen *et al* (2005). Introducing a cognitive component to therapy may be problematic with individuals who have DID, but there is a growing body of literature supporting its use in individuals with DID and psychiatric comorbidity – for a discussion of the literature see Hollins & Sinason (2000) and Willner (2005). The use of psychodynamic strategies has also been considered in the literature (Hollins & Sinason, 2000; Willner, 2005; Cottis, 2008) and there is sustained interest and expertise in the UK in adapting proven psychodynamic treatments for use with people with DID.

Medication

Individuals with DID are often prescribed psychotropic medication, and its use is dictated by a number of factors beyond diagnosis, including, for example, availability of psychosocial interventions, level of social support and availability of appropriately resourced specialist DID mental health teams. Although the use of medication to manage behaviour may be problematic from an ethical and evidence-based point of view, it may have a place as part of a detailed treatment plan (Oliver-Africano *et al*, 2009). When a specific psychiatric disorder has been diagnosed, the use of psychotropic medication should be based on the evidence-based principles set out for the general population, with some well-described caveats such as starting at lower doses and titrating much more slowly. Medication use is described in more detail in Chapter 7.

Conclusion

Despite the limitations of the available research literature, it does seem reasonable to conclude that people with DID are at an increased risk of a range of psychiatric disorders, although these may present differently from presentations in the general population. Some of the factors associated with this risk are unique to this population, whereas others seem to occur at increased frequency in this population. However, with an appropriate multidisciplinary team that has expertise in the diagnosis and assessment of people with DID, this aetiological knowledge can inform appropriate management strategies.

Acknowledgements

Marc Woodbury-Smith acknowledges the support of both the Canadian Institutes of Health Research (CIHR) and Scottish Rite Charitable Foundation during the preparation of this chapter.

References

Allen D, James W, Evans J, *et al* (2005) Positive behavioural support: definitions, current status and future directions. *Learning Disability Review*, **10**: 4–11.

American Psychiatric Association (1994) *Diagnostic and Statistical Manual of Mental Disorders* (4th edn) (DSM-IV). APA.

American Psychiatric Association (2013) *Diagnostic and Statistical Manual of Mental Disorders* (5th edn) (DSM-5). APA.

Banerjee PN, Filippi D, Allen Hauser W (2009) The descriptive epidemiology of epilepsy: a review. *Epilepsy Research*, **85**: 31–45.

Borthwick-Duffy SA, Eyman RK (1990) Who are the dually diagnosed? *American Journal on Mental Retardation*, **94**: 586–95.

Brindle N, Branton T, Stansfield A, *et al* (2013) *A Clinician's Brief Guide to the Mental Capacity Act*. RCPsych Publications.

Clarke DJ, Boer H, Whittington J, *et al* (2002) Prader–Willi syndrome, compulsive and ritualistic behaviours: the first population-based survey. *British Journal of Psychiatry*, **180**: 358–62.

Collacott RA, Cooper S-A, Branford D, *et al* (1998) Behaviour phenotype for Down's syndrome. *British Journal of Psychiatry*, **172**: 85–9.

Cooper S-A, Melville CA, Einfeld SL (2003) Psychiatric diagnosis, intellectual disabilities and Diagnostic Criteria for Psychiatric Disorders for Use with Adults with Learning Disabilities/Mental Retardation (DC–LD). *Journal of Intellectual Disability Research*, **47** (suppl 1): 3–15.

Cooper S-A, Smiley E, Morrison J, *et al* (2007) Mental ill-health in adults with intellectual disabilities: prevalence and associated factors. *British Journal of Psychiatry*, **190**: 27–35.

Cordeiro L, Ballinger E, Hagerman R, (2011) Clinical assessment of DSM-IV anxiety disorders in fragile X syndrome: prevalence and characterization. *Journal of Neurodevelopmental Disorders*, **3**: 57–67.

Cottis T (2008) *Intellectual Disability, Trauma and Psychotherapy*. Routledge.

Crocker J, Major B (1989) Social stigma and self-esteem: the self-protective properties of stigma. *Psychological Review*, **96**: 608–30.

Dagnan D, Sandhu S (1999) Social comparison, self-esteem and depression in people with disability. *Journal of Intellectual Disability Research*, **43**: 372–9.

Deb S, Thomas M, Bright C (2001) Mental disorder in adults with intellectual disability. 1: Prevalence of functional psychiatric illness among a community-based population aged between 16 and 64 years. *Journal of Intellectual Disability Research*, **45**: 495–505.

Doody GA, Johnstone EC, Sanderson TL, *et al* (1998) 'Pfropfschizophrenie' revisited. Schizophrenia in people with mild learning disability. *British Journal of Psychiatry*, **173**: 145–53.

Emerson E, Hatton C (2007) Mental health of children and adolescents with intellectual disabilities in Britain. *British Journal of Psychiatry*, **191**: 493–9.

Endicott J, Spitzer RL (1978) A diagnostic interview: the schedule for affective disorders and schizophrenia. *Archives of General Psychiatry*, **35**: 837–44.

Esbensen AJ, Benson BA (2006) A prospective analysis of life events, problem behaviours and depression in adults with intellectual disability. *Journal of Intellectual Disability Research*, **50**: 248–58.

Fletcher R, Loschen E, Stavrakaki C, *et al* (eds) (2007) *Diagnostic Manual – Intellectual Disability (DM-ID): A Clinical Guide for Diagnosis of Mental Disorders in Persons with Intellectual Disability*. NADD.

Goodman R, Ford T, Richards H, *et al* (2000) The Development and Well-Being Assessment: description and initial validation of an integrated assessment of child and adolescent psychopathology. *Journal of Child Psychology and Psychiatry*, **41**: 645–55.

Gothelf D, Frisch A, Michaelovsky E, *et al* (2009) Velo-cardio-facial syndrome. *Journal of Mental Health Research in Intellectual Disabilities*, **2**: 149–67.

Hartley SL, Maclean WE (2008) Coping strategies of adults with mild intellectual disability for stressful social interactions. *Journal of Mental Health Research in Intellectual Disabilities*, **1**: 109–27.

Hollins S, Esterhuyzen A (1997) Bereavement and grief in adults with learning disabilities. *British Journal of Psychiatry*, **170**: 497–501.

Hollins S, Sinason V (2000) Psychotherapy, learning disabilities and trauma: new perspectives. *British Journal of Psychiatry*, **176**: 32–6.

Hoppe C, Elger CE (2011) Depression in epilepsy: a critical review from a clinical perspective. *Nature Reviews, Neurology,* **7**: 462–72.

Hove O, Havik OE (2010) Developmental level and other factors associated with symptoms of mental disorders and problem behaviour in adults with intellectual disabilities living in the community. *Social Psychiatry and Psychiatric Epidemiology*, **45**: 105–13.

Jacobson JW (1982) Problem behavior and psychiatric impairment within a developmentally disabled population I: behavior frequency. *Applied Research in Mental Retardation*, **3**: 121–39.

Kraepelin E (1919) Dementia praecox and paraphrenia. In *Textbook of Psychiatry* (8th edn) (trans RM Barclay). ES Livingston.

Lhatoo SD, Sander JW (2001) The epidemiology of epilepsy and learning disability. *Epilepsia*, **42** (suppl 1): 6–9.

Lund J (1985) The prevalence of psychiatric morbidity in mentally retarded adults. *Acta Psychiatrica Scandinavica*, **72**: 563–70.

Lunsky Y (2004) Suicidality in a clinical and community sample of adults with mental retardation. *Research in Developmental Disabilities*, **25**: 231–43.

Lunsky Y (2008) The impact of stress and social support on the mental health of individuals with intellectual disabilities. *Salud Pública de México*, **50** (suppl 2): s151–3.

Lunsky Y, Benson BA (2001) Association between perceived social support and strain, and positive and negative outcome for adults with mild intellectual disability. *Journal of Intellectual Disability Research*, **45**: 106–14.

Lunsky Y, Elserafi J (2011) Life events and emergency department visits in response to crisis in individuals with intellectual disabilities. *Journal of Intellectual Disability Research*, **55**: 714–8.

Mack AH, Feldman JJ, Tsuang MT (2002) A case of 'pfropfschizophrenie': Kraepelin's bridge between neurodegenerative and neurodevelopmental conceptions of schizophrenia. *American Journal of Psychiatry*, **159**: 1104–10.

MacMahon P, Jahoda A (2008) Social comparison and depression: people with mild and moderate intellectual disabilities. *American Journal of Mental Retardation*, **113**: 307–18.

McCarthy J (2001) Post-traumatic stress disorder in young people with learning disability. *Advances in Psychiatric Treatment*, **7**: 163–9.

McGrother CW, Bhaumik S, Thorp CF, *et al* (2006) Epilepsy in adults with intellectual disabilities: prevalence, associations and service implications. *Seizure*, **15**: 376–86.

Mevissen L, de Jongh A (2010) PTSD and its treatment in people with intellectual disabilities: a review of the literature. *Clinical Psychology Review*, **30**: 308–16.

Milici P (1937) Pfropfschizophrenia: schizophrenia engrafted upon mental deficiency. *Psychiatric Quarterly*, **11**: 190–212.

Morgan VA, Leonard H, Bourke J, *et al* (2008) Intellectual disability co-occurring with schizophrenia and other psychiatric illness: population-based study. *British Journal of Psychiatry*, **193**: 364–72.

Moss S, Ibbotson B, Prosser H, *et al* (1997) Validity of the PAS-ADD for detecting psychiatric symptoms in adults with learning disability (mental retardation). *Social Psychiatry and Psychiatric Epidemiology*, **32**: 344–54.

Nyhan WL (1972) Behavioral phenotypes in organic genetic disease. Presidential address to the Society for Pediatric Research, May 1, 1971. *Pediatric Research*, **6**: 1–9.

Oliver-Africano P, Murphy D, Tyrer P (2009) Aggressive behaviour in adults with intellectual disability. *CNS Drugs*, **23**: 903–13.

Patja K, Iivanainen M, Raitasuo S, *et al* (2001) Suicide mortality in mental retardation: a 35-year follow-up study. *Acta Psychiatrica Scandinavica*, **103**: 307–11.

Reid AH (1980) Diagnosis of psychiatric disorder in the severely and profoundly retarded patient. *Journal of the Royal Society of Medicine*, **73**: 607–9.

Robins LN, Helzer JE, Croughan J, *et al* (1981) National Institute of Mental Health Diagnostic Interview Schedule. Its history, characteristics, and validity. *Archives of General Psychiatry*, **38**: 381–9.

Royal College of Psychiatrists (2001) *DC–LD [Diagnostic Criteria for Psychiatric Disorders for use with Adults with Learning Disabilities/Mental Retardation]* (Occasional Paper OP48). Gaskell.

Rutter M, Graham P, Yule W (1970) *A Neuropsychiatric Study in Childhood* (*Clinics in Developmental Medicine*, Nos 35/36). Heinemann/Spastics International Medical Publications.

Sequeira, H, Hollins, S (2003) Clinical effects of sexual abuse on people with learning disability: critical literature review. *British Journal of Psychiatry*, **182**: 13–9.

Sequeira H, Howlin P, Hollins S (2003) Psychological disturbance associated with sexual abuse in people with learning disabilities: case–control study. *British Journal of Psychiatry*, **183**: 451–6.

Shooshtari S, Martens PJ, Burchill CA, *et al* (2011) Prevalence of depression and dementia among adults with developmental disabilities in Manitoba, Canada. *International Journal of Family Medicine*, Article ID 319574.

Singhi P, Jagirdar S, Khandelwal N, *et al* (2003) Epilepsy in children with cerebral palsy. *Journal of Child Neurology*, **18**: 174–9.

Smiley E (2005) Epidemiology of mental health problems in adults with learning disability: an update. *Advances in Psychiatric Treatment*, **11**: 214–22.

Spence SJ, Schneider MT (2009) The role of epilepsy and epileptiform EEGs in autism spectrum disorders. *Pediatric Research*, **65**: 599–606.

Toone B (2000) The psychoses of epilepsy. *Journal of Neurology, Neurosurgery and Psychiatry*, **69**: 1–3.

Turk J, Robbins I, Woodhead M (2005) Post-traumatic stress disorder in young people with intellectual disability. *Journal of Intellectual Disability Research*, **49**: 872–5.

Willner P (2005) The effectiveness of psychotherapeutic interventions for people with learning disabilities: a critical overview. *Journal of Intellectual Disability Research*, **49**: 73–85.

World Health Organization (1992) *International Statistical Classification of Diseases and Related Health Problems* (10th revision) (ICD-10). WHO.

World Health Organization (2001) *International Classification of Functioning, Disability and Health: ICF*. WHO.

CHAPTER 4

Anxiety disorders

Sherva Elizabeth Cooray, Alina Bakala and Anusha Wijeratne

Anxiety is a universal human experience. It may be defined as a feeling of worry, nervousness or unease about something that has an uncertain outcome. A distressing emotion, consisting of both psychological and somatic manifestations and hyperarousal, it is frequently accompanied by behavioural reactions (Gabbard, 2014). At optimal levels, it is normal, motivational and protective and it is helpful in coping with adversity (the Yerkes–Dodson law; Yerkes & Dodson, 1906). Anxiety differs from fear, in that fear is a focused and direct response to a specific event or object that the person is consciously aware of. DSM-5 defines anxiety as: 'anticipation of future threat' and fear as 'the emotional response to real or perceived imminent threat' (American Psychiatric Association, 2013). Under 'anxiety disorders' it includes disorders that share features of excessive fear and anxiety and related behavioural disturbances, and the overlapping nature, similarities and differences between fear and anxiety are highlighted. Anxiety disorder, or pathological anxiety, occurs when the intensity or duration of anxiety is disproportionate to the potential for harm, or in the absence of recognisable threat to the individual. It involves increased levels of arousal, which has the effect of disorganising rather than facilitating an individual's performance. DSM-5 anxiety disorders include panic disorder, agoraphobia, specific phobias, generalised anxiety disorder, social phobia, obsessive–compulsive disorder (OCD), acute traumatic stress disorder and post-traumatic stress disorder (PTSD), anxiety disorder due to a general medical condition and substance-induced anxiety disorder.

Epidemiology

With a lifetime prevalence of 28.8% (Kessler, 2005), anxiety ranks among one of the most common categories of mental disorder reported in large-scale epidemiological studies in the general population (Robins & Regier, 1991; Jenkins *et al*, 1997; Kessler, 2005). In primary care in the UK, where about a third of the annual 280 million consultations relate to mental health problems (Royal College of General Practitioners, 2006), anxiety and depression account for 80% of these consultations (Cooper, 1972). Nevertheless, there is general agreement that recognition rates of these conditions in primary care could be improved (Tylee & Walters, 2007). Untreated, anxiety disorders are costly to the individual and society.

Comorbidity is significant, with 75% of individuals with an anxiety disorder satisfying criteria for at least one other psychiatric disorder (Kessler *et al*, 1994; Alonso *et al*, 2004; Kessler, 2005).

The clinical features of anxiety have psychological, cognitive, physiological and behavioural components. Psychological and cognitive elements include fearful anticipation, irritability, concentration and memory problems, repetitive worrying thoughts and fear, which when extreme leads to fully fledged panic. Physiological manifestations include dry mouth, difficulty swallowing, flushing, sweating, pallor, palpitations, tremor, hyperventilation, chest pain/tightness, headache, backache, fatigue, muscle tension, diarrhoea, increased urinary frequency, paraesthesia, heightened startle response and insomnia. Avoidance is a common behavioural manifestation of anxiety. Chronologically, anxiety can be episodic, continuous or stress related.

There is ample evidence that anxiety disorders occur in people with disorders of intellectual development (DID) (McNally & Ascher, 1987; Bailey & Andrews, 2003; Cooper *et al*, 2007); indeed, they appear to be as common as in the general population, if not more so (King *et al*, 1994; Deb *et al*, 2001*a*,*b*). Nevertheless, anxiety disorders may be underreported in this population (Reiss *et al*, 1982) and, as in the general population (Nutt *et al*, 2007), underdiagnosed by clinicians (Veerhoven & Tuinier, 1997), primarily owing to communication problems (Smiley, 2005). A Swedish 50-year cohort study reported a cumulative incidence of 11.5% for anxiety disorders in people with mild to moderate intellectual disability (Nettelbladt *et al*, 2009).

Cooper (1997) found higher rates of anxiety disorders in a sample of elderly people with DID than in younger age groups. A large-scale, population-based study of anxiety disorders in adults with DID found a point prevalence of 3.8% (Reid *et al*, 2011). Generalised anxiety disorder was the commonest (1.7%), followed by agoraphobia (0.7%). A literature review by Raghavan (1997) revealed a similar if not higher prevalence of generalised anxiety disorder in people with DID when compared with the general population. A comparative cohort study revealed significantly higher rates of phobic disorders in people with DID than in the general population (Deb *et al*, 2001*a*).

A study of a large community sample of people with DID reported that 14% had had an ICD-10 diagnosis of disabling anxiety disorder for at least 6 months (White *et al*, 2005). A cross-sectional multicentre epidemiological study (Hermans *et al*, 2013) of 990 people with DID over 50 years of age found that anxiety symptoms were prevalent in 16.3% of the sample and significantly associated with female gender and mild to moderate intellectual disability. Anxiety disorders were present in 4.4%, but there was no association with gender, age or level of intellectual disability. Significant comorbidity with depression was reported in a study by Masi *et al* (2000) in adolescents with DID.

Diagnosis and classification

Accurate diagnosis is central to the effective management of anxiety disorders. Frequently, even in the general population comorbid disorders such as depression can make the presentation and diagnosis of anxiety disorder confusing. For example, the overlap of symptoms common to both generalised anxiety disorder and depressive disorders – such as fatigue, sleep disturbance, irritability and poor concentration – may complicate recognition and diagnosis (Kessler *et al*, 2008).

The diagnosis of mental disorders overall in people with DID is challenging, with a meagre evidence base that is further weakened by difficulties in carrying out robust research (Oliver *et al*, 2003). Sovner (1986) highlighted four factors reflecting the profound biopsychosocial effects of DID that may influence the diagnostic process, to which diagnostic overshadowing (Reiss *et al*, 1982) can be added (Box 4.1).

Most studies of anxiety disorders in people with DID use some form of modified ICD or DSM criteria, with a resultant lack of consistency. The clinical utility of ICD-10 (World Health Organization, 1992) and DSM-IV–TR (American Psychiatric Association, 2000) in diagnosing anxiety disorders in people with DID is limited because these diagnostic criteria are firmly entrenched in language-based phenomenology, validated on individuals with average cognitive functioning (Ruedrich *et al*, 2001; Cooray *et al*, 2007). Overall, in people with mild to moderate DID, the ICD-10

Box 4.1 Factors that may influence the diagnostic process in disorders of development

Intellectual distortion – difficulty in eliciting the patient's emotional symptoms because of deficits in abstract thinking and in receptive and expressive language skills; for example, the phrase 'butterflies in the stomach' might not be understood

Psychosocial masking – limited social experiences can influence the content of psychiatric symptoms; for example, mania may present as a grandiose belief that the individual can drive a car

Cognitive disintegration – a decreased ability to tolerate stress can lead to anxiety-induced decompensation (sometimes misinterpreted as psychosis)

Baseline exaggeration – the severity or frequency of chronic maladaptive behaviour may increase after the onset of psychiatric illness

Diagnostic overshadowing – clinicians can overlook symptoms of mental illness, attributing them instead to the intellectual disability

(Reiss *et al*, 1982; Sovner, 1986)

---

or DSM-IV-TR criteria for anxiety disorders can be applied validly and reliably (Moss *et al*, 1997; Masi *et al*, 2002; Stavrakaki, 2002; Cooray *et al*, 2007). In individuals with severe to profound DID, psychiatric assessments must be modified within the context of limitations in cognitive function, using simple spoken language, pictures and sign language, complemented by collateral information from familiar primary carers. The interview must allow adequate time to obtain an account of events. Questions and responses may need to be repeated and rechecked. Leading questions must be avoided since people with DID can be suggestible. Matson *et al* (1997) concluded that when anxiety cannot be expressed, especially in people with more severe degrees of intellectual disability, it might manifest as a behavioural disorder.

Endeavours to address drawbacks in the current classifications include the Diagnostic Criteria for Psychiatric Disorders for Use with Adults with Learning Disabilities/Mental Retardation (DC-LD) (Royal College of Psychiatrists, 2001). This is a consensus-based Occasional Paper with operationalised diagnostic criteria reflecting expert opinion for psychiatric disorders for adults with DID. The Diagnostic Manual – Intellectual Disability (DM-ID) and companion guidelines (Fletcher *et al*, 2007) utilise DSM-IV-TR diagnostic criteria and provide a comprehensive overview of the current evidence base supported by the expert-consensus model and outlines recommendations for adaptations for people with DID. Other useful assessment tools include the Psychiatric Assessment Scale for Adults with Developmental Disability (PAS-ADD) (Moss *et al*, 1993, 1997, 2000).

Efforts to improve diagnostic practice have led to the development of guidelines (Rush & Frances, 2000; Cooray *et al*, 2007) and a number of informant and self-report assessment instruments for psychopathology (Box 4.2). However, the reliability of these instruments is variable. Moreover, Costello *et al* (1997) reported that the greatest unreliability when applying the PAS-ADD instrument related to symptoms of anxiety.

Box 4.2 Instruments for detecting psychopathology in people with disorders of intellectual development

Psychopathology Inventory for Mentally Retarded Adults (PIMRA), based on DSM-III-R (Matson *et al*, 1984)

Diagnostic Assessment for the Severely Handicapped (DASH) scale, based on DSM-III-R (Matson *et al*, 1991)

Psychiatric Assessment Scale for Adults with Developmental Disability (PAS-ADD), based on ICD-10 (Moss *et al*, 1993)

Effects of DID on the presentation of the clinical features of anxiety

Self-report of key diagnostic concepts of anxiety require an adequate level of cognitive function and linguistic skills, particularly as regards complex subjective cognitive phenomena, making subjective elements of the diagnostic criteria difficult if not impossible to apply in people with DID. Clinicians are consequently compelled to rely on signs (observed behaviours) and information gleaned from primary carers rather than self-reported distress. This has prompted interpretation of diagnostic criteria in terms of behavioural correlates (Table 4.1) that reflect verbal components of the relevant anxiety disorders (Cooray *et al*, 2007). In such instances the application of pragmatic objective equivalents in lieu of subjective criteria from DSM and ICD classificatory systems may be justifiable.

In diagnosing anxiety in people with DID, Khreim & Mikkelson (1997) emphasised phenomena such as agitation, screaming, crying, withdrawal, regressive/clingy behaviour or freezing, all of which could be interpreted as manifestations of fear. Matson *et al* (1997) concluded that where anxiety cannot be expressed, it might present as a behavioural disorder, especially in those with severe DID. However, this may be non-specific and equally reflect other triggers, such as the environment. It is hence important to distinguish between behavioural disorders and abnormal behaviours that are the consequence of an underlying mental illness. A careful history supported by collateral information from appropriate carers and a functional analysis of the behaviour could be a useful strategy. For example, manifestations of anxiety in those with poor cognitive and linguistic ability may include observed phenomena, as outlined in Table 4.1. Such issues might best be addressed via appropriate modifications to diagnostic criteria in future editions of DSM and ICD. With reference to the evidence-based assessment of anxiety in adults in the general population, see Antony & Rowa (2005).

Table 4.1 Behavioural correlates of anxiety symptoms in people with disorders of intellectual development

Anxiety symptom	Behavioural correlate
Dry mouth	Increased drinking
Sensation of shortness of breath	Hyperventilation
Sensations of anxiety	Signs of increased arousal (shortness of breath; increased pulse rate); irritability; anger; sweating; self-injurious behaviour; avoidance behaviour
Panic	Tremulousness with excessive motor activity, agitation and/or aggression (Stavrakaki, 2002)

Aetiology

Anxiety disorders appear to be caused by the impact of stressful events on individuals predisposed by a combination of genetic, neurobiological, psychological and environmental influences.

Genetic

There is substantial evidence that genetic determinants play a major role in the aetiology of anxiety (Arnold *et al*, 2004). Twin, adoption and familial studies have suggested a role for additive genetic factors in view of the high heritability of anxiety disorders (Shih *et al*, 2004). In a study of 32 monozygotic (MZ) and 53 dizygotic (DZ) adult same-sexed twins, the frequency of anxiety disorders was twice as high in MZ as in DZ co-twins (Torgersen, 1983). For a discussion of the genetics of anxiety and other neuropsychiatric disorders see, for example, Burmeister *et al* (2008).

Neurobiological

Biological vulnerability has been linked with changes in areas of the brain associated with emotional regulation and fear response. The forebrain is the area most commonly observed to have functional and anatomical abnormalities in people with anxiety disorders. The limbic system, which is involved in storing memories and creating emotions, is also thought to play a central role in processing all anxiety-related information and mediating the fear response. Both the locus coeruleus and the dorsal raphe project to the septohippocampal circuit, which in turn projects to other areas of the limbic system that mediate anxiety. The hippocampus and amygdalae are of particular importance, since they are interconnected and also project to both subcortical and cortical nuclei. Disrupted functional connectivity of the amygdalae and their processing of fear and anxiety are seen in generalised anxiety disorder (Etkin *et al*, 2009).

Abnormalities in neurotransmitter systems in the brain have been implicated in the aetiology of anxiety disorders. Evidence suggests a relative deficiency in GABA neurotransmission, which can be augmented by agents acting on different components of the GABA system (Nemeroff, 2003). Dysregulation of central serotonin (5-hydroxytryptamine, 5-HT) systems have been implicated in the pathophysiology and treatment of anxiety disorders (Heisler *et al*, 2007). Other neurotransmitters that have been implicated in anxiety disorders include corticotrophin-releasing hormone (CRH) and cholecystokinin (Coplan & Lydiard, 1998).

Dysregulation of the body's response to stress mediated via the hypothalamic–pituitary–adrenal (HPA) axis is seen in almost all anxiety disorders (Faravelli *et al*, 2012). For more detailed information on the neurobiology of anxiety see Martin *et al* (2009) and Antony & Stein (2008).

Psychological

Cognitive theories propose that anxiety disorders result from distorted beliefs focused on physical or psychological threat and an increased sense of personal vulnerability (Beck *et al*, 2005). Psychodynamic theories explain anxiety as an expression of underlying unresolved conflict (Thorn *et al*, 1999). For more detailed discussions of psychological models of anxiety see Barlow (2002).

Environmental

The role of life events in the aetiology of anxiety disorders is well recognised. In a community study in the general population, Finlay-Jones & Brown (1981) found that symptoms of anxiety were associated with events that implied some threat or harm in the future.

Risk factors in people with DID

People with DID frequently contend with lifelong adversity, inadequate social support and poor coping skills, which contribute to increased vulnerability to stressful life events that may trigger anxiety disorders.

Kessler *et al* (1994) reported that all types of mental disorder, including anxiety, decline with increasing educational level. Current psychological models of anxiety tend to incorporate the role of the individual's vulnerability, which includes both genetic (Hettema *et al*, 2001) and acquired predispositions (Coplan *et al*, 1997). Some genetic causes of DID have associations with anxiety; for example, fragile-X syndrome is associated with social anxiety disorder, Rubinstein–Taybi and Prader–Willi syndromes with OCD (Levitas & Reid, 1998) and Williams syndrome with anxiety (Einfeld *et al*, 2001) and phobias (Dykens, 2003). Hyman *et al* (2002) noted significantly high prevalence rates of compulsive behaviours in people with Cornelia de Lange syndrome.

Studies of the types of fear reported in people with DID have found similarities between children of normal intelligence and adults of equivalent mental age, highlighting the developmental perspective (Sternlicht, 1979; Duff *et al*, 1981; Pickersgill *et al*, 1994). For example, many individuals with moderate DID experience fears of animals, thunder and ghosts (preoperational thinking) and of physical injuries (concrete operational), mirroring normal Piagetian transition in children without DID. However, anxieties and phobias may also occur as transient phenomena in normal early development.

Anxiety and problem behaviour in DID

Anxiety disorders were have been found to be more prevalent in people with DID with self-injurious behaviour than in those without (Moss *et al*,

2000). Tsouris *et al* (2011) reported that anxiety was most associated with physical and verbal aggression against the self.

Treatment

There is a paucity of robust evidence-based literature on the treatment of anxiety disorders in people with DID (NICE, 2014), and so the current interventions broadly parallel those used for the rest of the population. In people with DID and anxiety disorders, a range of effective interventions is used (Stavrakaki, 1997), including medication (Kapczinski *et al*, 2003) and psychological therapies – reassurance, counselling, anxiety management (e.g. relaxation training), anger management and self-help (e.g. bibliotherapy). Desensitisation and exposure therapy are effective management strategies for OCD and social phobia.

Pharmacological therapies

The pharmacological treatment of anxiety is targeted at achieving maximum gains from the lowest effective dose and with minimum adverse effects. The guidelines from the World Federation of Societies of Biological Psychiatry (WFSBP) for the pharmacological treatment of anxiety, OCD and PTSD (Bandelow *et al*, 2008) recommend selective serotonin reuptake inhibitors (SSRIs), serotonin–noradrenaline reuptake inhibitors (SNRIs) and the calcium channel modulator pregabalin as first-line treatments for these disorders (see also NICE, 2011). Although tricyclic antidepressants (TCAs) are equally effective for some disorders, many have poorer tolerability than the SSRIs and SNRIs. Agomelatine (not licensed currently in the UK for anxiety disorders) acts on melatonergic and serotonergic receptors, and is effective and well tolerated in generalised anxiety disorder (Stein *et al*, 2008).

While the introduction of the SSRIs has significantly improved the treatment of anxiety disorders, a large proportion of patients with anxiety disorders fail to respond to first-line medication (Ipser *et al*, 2006). In a comprehensive review looking at alternative pharmacological options, Farach *et al* (2012) examined the alpha–delta calcium channel class of anticonvulsants, which reduce neuronal excitability, and concluded that pregabalin is superior to placebo in generalised anxiety disorder, is rapid in onset of action and may even reduce co-occurring depressive symptoms.

In treatment-resistant cases, benzodiazepines may be used when the patient is without a history of substance misuse (Bandelow *et al*, 2008). Benzodiazepine use should be limited to 4 weeks (because of potential adverse effects) until alternative strategies are instituted, for treatment of acute disabling anxiety resulting in significant distress. NICE guidance (2011) provides recommendations on pharmacological therapies for anxiety disorders and reiterates the association of benzodiazepines with tolerance and dependence, as well as the adverse side-effects of antipsychotics.

Consequently, they should not be used routinely to treat anxiety disorders. Healthcare professionals should be aware of circumstances in which benzodiazepines and antipsychotics may be appropriate, such as short-term care and anxiety disorder crises. NICE recommends that procedures and protocols must be in place to monitor such prescribing. Nonetheless, a few people may benefit from taking benzodiazepines long term, or from time to time. This should be carried out only by a specialist unit after other treatments have been tried and have failed (Royal College of Psychiatrists, 2013). Medications with a weaker evidence base or that are less well tolerated include buspirone (for generalised anxiety disorder and OCD) and antipsychotics (quetiapine or risperidone as antidepressant augmentation for OCD).

People with DID may not be able to report adverse effects. Consequently, impairment of cognitive and psychomotor abilities resulting from medication may have profound implications for behaviour and general functioning (Reiss & Aman, 1998). Ultimately, treatment choice should be a consequence of the assessment process and shared decision-making, with emphasis on safety, tolerability and the patient's preferences, underpinned by best available evidence.

Psychological therapy and other treatments

In patients with anxiety disorders, OCD or PTSD, cognitive–behavioural therapy (CBT) and other variants of behaviour therapy have a sufficient evidence base to support their use alone or in combination with medications (Bandelow, 2012; Bandelow et al, 2014). Systematic desensitisation is highly effective where the problem is a learned anxiety of specific objects or situations.

In people with mild or borderline DID and anxiety disorder, evidence from case studies suggests the effectiveness of CBT (Lindsay et al, 1997; Lindsay, 1999). The core principles of CBT may require modification within the context of the individual's ability. Evidence on the long-term outcome of these interventions is unavailable

Some studies in the general population suggest that optimum results are achieved by combining psychological and pharmacological interventions (Fineberg & Drummond, 1995; Kandel, 1999). The involvement of affected individuals in an effective partnership with healthcare professionals using comprehensible and clear communication has been known to improve outcomes. NICE (2011) recommendations for people with generalised anxiety disorder (GAD) who have a mild DID offer the same interventions as for other people with GAD, adjusting the method of delivery or duration of the intervention if necessary to take account of the disability or impairment. When assessing or offering an intervention to people with GAD and moderate to severe DID or moderate to severe acquired cognitive impairment, NICE (2011) recommends that consideration be given to consulting with a relevant specialist.

Training and education in relaxation techniques are also helpful for those with mild, moderate or severe DID. Martin *et al* (1998) reported successfully helping individuals with severe or profound DID to achieve states of relaxation, using multisensory stimulation ('Snoezelen environment').

A systematic review by Jayakody *et al* (2014) concluded that exercise seems to be an effective adjunctive treatment for anxiety disorders but less effective when compared with antidepressant treatment. Both aerobic and non-aerobic exercises reduce anxiety symptoms and people with social phobia may benefit from exercise combined with group CBT. Carraro & Gobbi (2012) have described the beneficial effects of exercise in a small sample of adults with DID with anxiety disorder. See also NICE (2011).

References

Alonso J, Angermeyer MC, Bernert S, *et al* (2004) 12-month comorbidity patterns and associated factors in Europe: results from the European Study of the Epidemiology of Mental Disorders (ESEMeD) project. *Acta Psychiatrica Scandinavica*, **109**: 28–37. doi: 10.1111/j.1600-0047.2004.00328.x.

American Psychiatric Association (2000) *Diagnostic and Statistical Manual of Mental Disorders* (4th edn, Text Revision) (DSM-IV-TR). APA.

American Psychiatric Association (2013) *Diagnostic and Statistical Manual of Mental Disorders* (5th edn) (DSM-5). APA.

Antony MM, Rowa K (2005) Evidence based assessment of anxiety in adults. *Psychological Assessment*, **17**: 256–266.

Antony MM, Stein MB (eds) (2008) *Oxford Handbook of Anxiety and Related Disorders*. Oxford University Press.

Arnold PD, Zai G, Richter MA (2004) Genetics of anxiety disorders. *Current Psychiatry Reports*, **6**: 243–254.

Bailey NM, Andrews TM (2003) Diagnostic criteria for psychiatric disorders for use with adults with learning disabilities/mental retardation (DC-LD) and the diagnosis of anxiety disorders. *Journal of Intellectual Disability Research*, **47** (suppl 1): 50–61.

Bandelow B (2012) Guidelines for the pharmacological treatment of anxiety disorders, obsessive–compulsive disorder and posttraumatic stress disorder in primary care. *International Journal of Psychiatry in Clinical Practice*, **16**: 77–84.

Bandelow B, Zohar J, Hollander E, *et al* (2008) World Federation of Societies of Biological Psychiatry (WFSBP) guidelines for the pharmacological treatment of anxiety, obsessive–compulsive and post-traumatic stress disorders – first revision. *World Journal of Biological Psychiatry*, **9**: 248–312.

Bandelow B, Lichte T, Rudolf S, *et al* (2014) The diagnosis of and treatment recommendations for anxiety disorders. *Deutsches Arzteblatt International*, **111**: 473–480.

Barlow DH (ed) (2002) *Anxiety and Its Disorders: The Nature and Treatment of Anxiety and Panic* (2nd edn). Guilford Press.

Beck AT, Emery G, Greenberg Rl (2005) *Anxiety Disorders and Phobias: A Cognitive Perspective* (15th edn). Basic Books.

Burmeister M, McInnis MG, Zöllner S (2008) Psychiatric genetics: progress amid controversy. *Nature Reviews: Genetics*, **9**: 527–40.

Carraro A, Gobbi E (2012) Effects of an exercise programme on anxiety in adults with intellectual disabilities. *Research in Developmental Disabilities*, **33**: 1221–6.

Cooper B (1972) Clinical and social aspects of chronic neurosis. *Proceedings of the Royal Society of Medicine*, **65**: 509–12.

Cooper SA (1997) Psychiatry of elderly compared to younger adults with intellectual disability. *Journal of Applied Research in Intellectual Disability*, **10**: 303–11.

Cooper SA, Smiley E, Morrison J, *et al* (2007) Mental ill-health in adults with intellectual disabilities: prevalence and associated factors. *British Journal of Psychiatry*, **190**: 27–35.

Cooray S, Gabriel S, Gaus V (2007) Anxiety disorders. In *Diagnostic Manual – Intellectual Disability (DM-ID): A Clinical Guide for Diagnosis of Mental Disorders in Persons with Intellectual Disability* (eds R Fletcher, E Loschen, C Stavrakaki *et al*), pp 317–48. NADD Press.

Coplan JD, Lydiard RB (1998) Brain circuits in panic disorder. *Biological Psychiatry*, **44**: 1264–76.

Coplan JD, Pine DS, Papp LA, *et al* (1997) A view on noradrenergic, hypothalamic–pituitary–adrenal axis and extrahypothalamic corticotrophin-releasing factor function in anxiety and affective disorders: the reduced growth hormone response to clonidine. *Psychopharmacology Bulletin*, **33**: 193–204.

Costello H, Moss S, Prosser H, *et al* (1997) Reliability of the ICD 10 version of the Psychiatric Assessment Schedule for Adults with Developmental Disability (PAS–ADD). *Social Psychiatry and Psychiatric Epidemiology*, **32**: 339–43.

Deb S, Thomas M, Bright C (2001a) Mental disorder in adults with intellectual disability. I: Prevalence of functional psychiatric illness among a community-based population aged between 16 and 64 years. *Journal of Intellectual Disability Research*, **45**: 495–505.

Deb S, Matthews T, Holt G, *et al* (2001b) *Practice Guidelines for the Assessment and Diagnosis of Mental Health Problems in Adults with Intellectual Disability*. Pavilion.

Duff R, La Rocca J, Lizzet A, *et al* (1981) A comparison of the fears of mildly retarded adults with children of their mental age and chronological age matched controls. *Journal of Behavior Therapy and Experimental Psychiatry*, **12**: 121–4.

Dykens EM (2003) Anxiety, fears, and phobias in persons with Williams syndrome. *Developmental Neuropsychology*, **23**: 291–316.

Einfeld SL, Tonge BJ, Rees, VW (2001) Longitudinal course of behavioural and emotional problems in Williams syndrome. *American Journal of Mental Retardation*, **106**: 73–81.

Etkin A, Prater KE, Schatzberg AF, *et al* (2009) Disrupted amygdalar subregion functional connectivity and evidence of a compensatory network in generalized anxiety disorder. *Archives of General Psychiatry*, **66**: 1361–1372.

Farach FJ, Pruitt LD, Jun JJ, *et al* (2012) Pharmacological treatment of anxiety disorders: current treatments and future directions. *Journal of Anxiety Disorders*, **26**: 833–43.

Faravelli C, Lo Sauro C, Lelli L, *et al* (2012) The role of life events and HPA axis in anxiety disorders: a review. *Current Pharmaceutical Design*, **18**: 5663–74.

Fineberg N, Drummond LM (1995) Anxiety disorders: drug treatment or behavioural cognitive psychotherapy. *CNS Drugs*, **3**: 448–66.

Finlay-Jones R, Brown GW (1981) Types of stressful life event and the onset of anxiety and depressive disorders. *Psychological Medicine*, **11**: 803–15.

Fletcher R, Loschen E, Stavrakaki C, *et al* (2007) *Diagnostic Manual – Intellectual Disability (DM-ID): A Textbook of Diagnosis of Mental Disorders in Persons with Intellectual Disability*. NADD Press.

Gabbard GO (ed) (2014) Part IV: Anxiety disorders and obsessive compulsive and related disorders. In *Treatments of Psychiatric Disorders* (5th edn). American Psychiatric Press.

Heisler LK, Zhou L, Bajwa P, *et al* (2007) Serotonin 5-HT (2C) receptors regulate anxiety-like behavior. *Genes, Brain and Behavior*, **6**: 491–6.

Hermans H, Beekman AT, Evenhuis HM (2013) Prevalence of depression and anxiety in older users of formal Dutch intellectual disability services. *Journal of Affective Disorders*, **144**: 94–100.

Hettema JM, Neale MC, Kendler KS (2001) A review and meta-analysis of the genetic epidemiology of anxiety disorders. *American Journal of Psychiatry*, **158**: 1568–78.

Hyman P, Oliver C, Hall S (2002) Self-injurious behavior, self-restraint, and compulsive behaviors in Cornelia de Lange syndrome. *American Journal on Mental Retardation*, **107**: 146–54.

Ipser JC, Carey P, Dhansay Y, *et al* (2006) Pharmacotherapy augmentation strategies in treatment-resistant anxiety disorders. *Cochrane Database of Systematic Reviews*, **4**: CD005473.

Jayakody K, Gunadasa S, Hosker C (2014) Exercise for anxiety disorders: systematic Review. *British Journal of Sports Medicine*, **48**: 187–96.

Jenkins R, Lewis G, Bebbington P, *et al* (1997) The National Psychiatric Morbidity Surveys of Great Britain – initial findings from the household survey. *Psychological Medicine*, **27**: 775–89.

Kandel ER (1999) Biology and the future of psychoanalysis: a new intellectual framework for psychiatry revisited. *American Journal of Psychiatry*, **156**: 505–24.

Kapczinski F, Lima MS, Souza JS, *et al* (2003) Antidepressants for generalized anxiety disorder. *Cochrane Database of Systematic Reviews*, **2**: CD003592.

Kessler RC (2005) Lifetime prevalence and age-of-onset distributions of DSM-IV disorders in the National Comorbidity Survey Replication (NCS-R). *Archives of General Psychiatry*, **62**: 593–602.

Kessler RC, McGonagle KA, Zhao S, *et al* (1994) Lifetime and 12-month prevalence of DSM-III-R psychiatric disorders in the United States. Results from the National Comorbidity Survey. *Archives of General Psychiatry*, **51**: 8–19.

Kessler RC, Gruber M, Hettema JM, *et al* (2008) Co-morbid major depression and generalized anxiety disorders in the National Comorbidity Survey follow-up. *Psychological Medicine*, **38**: 365–74.

Khreim I, Mikkelson E (1997) anxiety disorders in adults with mental retardation. *Psychiatric Annals*, **27**: 271–81.

King BH, DeAntonio C, McCracken JT, *et al* (1994) Psychiatric consultation in severe and profound mental retardation. *American Journal of Psychiatry*, **151**: 1802–8.

Levitas AS, Reid CS (1998) Rubinstein–Taybi syndrome and psychiatric disorders. *Journal of Intellectual Disability Research*, **42**: 284–92.

Lindsay WR (1999) Cognitive therapy. *Psychologist*, **12**: 238–41.

Lindsay WR, Neilson C, Lawrenson H (1997) Cognitive–behaviour therapy for anxiety in people with learning disabilities. In *Cognitive-Behaviour Therapy for People with Learning Disabilities* (eds B Stenfert Kroese, D Dagnan, K Loumides), pp. 124–40. Routledge.

Martin EI, Ressler KJ, Binder E, *et al* (2009) The neurobiology of anxiety disorders: brain imaging, genetics, and psychoneuroendocrinology. *Psychiatric Clinics of North America*, **32**: 549–75.

Martin NT, Gaffan EA, Williams T (1998) Behavioural effects of long-term multi-sensory stimulation. *British Journal of Clinical Psychology*, **37**: 69–82.

Masi G, Favilla L, Mucci M (2000) Generalised anxiety disorder in adolescents and young adults with mild mental retardation. *Psychiatry*, **63**: 54–64.

Masi G, Brovedani P, Mucci M, *et al* (2002) Assessment of anxiety and depression in adolescents with mental retardation. *Child Psychiatry and Human Development*, **32**: 227–37.

Matson JL, Kazdin AE, Senatore V, *et al* (1984) Psychometric properties of the Psychopathology Inventory for Mentally Retarded Adults. *Applied Research in Mental Retardation*, **5**: 881–9.

Matson JL, Gardner WI, Coe, DA, *et al* (1991) A scale for evaluating emotional disorders in severely and profoundly mentally retarded persons. Development of the Diagnostic Assessment for the Severely Handicapped (DASH) scale. *British Journal of Psychiatry*, **159**: 404–9.

Matson JL, Smiroldo BB, Hamilton M, *et al* (1997) Do anxiety disorders exist in persons with severe and profound retardation? *Research in Developmental Disabilities*, **18**: 39–44.

McNally RJ, Ascher LM (1987) Anxiety disorders in mentally retarded people. In *Anxiety and Stress Disorders: Cognitive/Behavioural Assessment and Treatment* (eds L Michelson, ML Ascher), pp 379–94. Guilford Press.

Moss S, Patel P, Prosser H, *et al* (1993) Psychiatric morbidity in older people with moderate and severe learning disability. I: Development and reliability of the patient interview (PAS–ADD). *British Journal of Psychiatry*, **163**: 471–80.

Moss S, Ibbotson B, Prosser H, *et al* (1997) Validity of the PAS–ADD for detecting psychiatric symptoms in adults with learning disability (mental retardation). *Social Psychiatry and Psychiatric Epidemiology*, **32**: 344–54.

Moss S, Emerson E, Kiernan C, *et al* (2000) Psychiatric symptoms in adults with learning disability and challenging behaviour. *British Journal of Psychiatry*, **17**: 452–6.

NICE (2011) *Generalised Anxiety Disorder and Panic Disorder (with or without Agoraphobia) in Adults: Management in Primary, Secondary and Community Care* (Clinical Guideline 113). National Institute for Health and Clinical Excellence.

NICE (2014) *Anxiety Disorders* (NICE Quality Standard 53). National Institute for Health and Care Excellence.

Nemeroff CB (2003) The role of GABA in the pathophysiology and treatment of anxiety disorders. *Psychopharmacology Bulletin*, **37**: 133–46.

Nettelbladt P, Göth M, Bogren M, *et al* (2009) Risk of mental disorders in subjects with intellectual disability in the Lundby cohort 1947–97. *Nordic Journal of Psychiatry*, **63**: 316–21.

Nutt DJ, Kessler RC, Alonso J, *et al* (2007) Consensus statement on the benefit to the community of ESEMeD (European Study of the Epidemiology of Mental Disorders) survey data on depression and anxiety. *Journal of Clinical Psychiatry*, **68** (suppl 2): 42–8.

Oliver PC, Piachaud J, Done DJ, *et al* (2003) Difficulties developing evidence-based approaches in learning disabilities. *Evidence-Based Mental Health*, **6**: 37–9.

Pickersgill MJ, Valentine JD, May R, *et al* (1994) Fears in mental retardation. Part 1. Types of fears reported by men and women with and without mental retardation. *Advances in Behaviour Research Therapy*, **16**: 277–96.

Raghavan R (1997) Anxiety disorders in people with learning disabilities: a review of the literature. *Journal of Learning Disabilities for Nursing, Health and Social Care*, **2**: 3–9.

Reid KA, Smiley E, Cooper SA. (2011) Prevalence and associations of anxiety disorders in adults with intellectual disabilities. *Journal of Intellectual Disability Research*, **55**: 172–81.

Reiss S, Aman MG (eds) (1998) *Psychotropic Medications and Developmental Disabilities: The International Consensus Handbook*. Ohio State University, Nisonger Center.

Reiss S, Levitan GW, Szyszko J (1982) Emotional disturbance and mental retardation: diagnostic overshadowing. *American Journal of Mental Deficiency*, **86**: 567–74.

Robins LN, Regier DA (1991) *Psychiatric Disorders in America: The Epidemiologic Catchment Area Study*. Free Press.

Royal College of General Practitioners (2006) *Key Demographic Statistics from UK General Practice: July 2006*. RCOGP (http://www.rcgp.org.uk/pdf/ISS_FACT_06_KeyStats.pdf, accessed 12 December 2008).

Royal College of Psychiatrists (2001) *DC-LD: Diagnostic Criteria for Psychiatric Disorders for Use with Adults with Learning Disabilities/Mental Retardation* (Occasional Paper OP48). Gaskell.

Royal College of Psychiatrists (2013) *Benzodiazepines* (Mental Health Information for all leaflet). Royal College of Psychiatrists.

Ruedrich SL, DesNoyers Hurley A (2001) Diagnostic uncertainty. *Mental Health Aspects of Developmental Disabilities*, **4**: 43–6.

Rush AJ, Frances A (eds) (2000) Expert consensus guideline series: treatment of psychiatric and behavioural problems in mental retardation. *American Journal on Mental Retardation*, **105**: 159–228.

Shih RA, Belmonte PL, Zandi PP (2004) A review of the evidence from family, twin and adoption studies for a genetic contribution to adult psychiatric disorders. *International Review of Psychiatry*, **16**: 260–83.

Smiley E (2005) Epidemiology of mental health problems in adults with learning disability: an update. *Advances in Psychiatric Treatment*, **11**: 214–22.

Sovner R (1986) Limiting factors in the use of DSM-III criteria with mentally ill/mentally retarded persons. *Psychopharmacology Bulletin*, **22**: 1055–9.

Stavrakaki C (1997) Anxiety disorders in persons with mental retardation: diagnostic, clinical and treatment issues. *Psychiatric Annals*, **27**: 182–9.

Stavrakaki C (2002) The DSM-IV and how it applies to persons with developmental disabilities. In *Dual Diagnosis: An Introduction to the Mental Health Needs of Persons with Developmental Disabilities* (eds D Griffiths, C Stavrakaki, J Summers), pp 115–49. Habilitative Mental Health Resource Network.

Stein DJ, Ahokas AA, de Bodinat C (2008) Efficacy of agomelatine in generalized anxiety disorder: a randomized, double-blind, placebo-controlled study. *Journal of Clinical Psychopharmacology*, **28**: 561–6.

Sternlicht M (1979) Fears of institutionalised mentally retarded adults. *Journal of Psychology*, **101**: 57–71.

Thorn GR, Chosak A, Baker SL, *et al* (1999) Psychological theories of panic disorder. In *Panic Disorder: Clinical Diagnosis, Management and Mechanisms* (eds DJ Nutt, JC Ballenger, JP Lépine), pp 93–108. Martin Dunitz.

Torgersen S (1983) Genetic factors in anxiety disorders. *Archives of General Psychiatry*, **40**: 1085–9.

Tsouris JA, Kim SY, Brown WT, *et al* (2011) Association of aggressive behaviours with psychiatric disorders, age, sex and degree of intellectual disability: a large-scale survey. *Journal of Intellectual Disability Research*, **55**: 636–49.

Tylee A, Walters P (2007) Underrecognition of anxiety and mood disorders in primary care: why does the problem exist and what can be done? *Journal of Clinical Psychiatry*, **68** (suppl 2): 27–30.

Veerhoven WMA, Tuinier S (1997) Neuropsychiatric consultation in mentally retarded patients. *European Psychiatry*, **12**: 242–8.

White P, Chant D, Edwards N, *et al* (2005) Prevalence of intellectual disability and comorbid mental illness in an Australian community sample. *Australian and New Zealand Journal of Psychiatry*, **39**: 395–400.

World Health Organization (1992) *International Statistical Classification of Diseases and Related Health Problems* (10th revision) (ICD-10). WHO.

Yerkes RM, Dodson JD (1906) The relation of strength of stimulus to rapidity of habit formation. *Journal of Comparative Neurology and Psychology*, **18**: 459–82.

CHAPTER 5

Behaviour problems

Elspeth Bradley and Marika Korossy

Preamble

Problem or challenging behaviours are the terms most frequently used to describe the behaviours under review here. Both terms direct attention to the fact that these behaviours are particularly problematic to care providers and the public; neither, however, speaks adequately to the co-constructed nature of these behaviours, nor to the personal distress individuals engaging in these behaviours may be experiencing. People with disorders of intellectual development (PWDID) in this context are communicating their needs, desires, medical conditions and mental distress as best they can. When asked to evaluate these behaviours, it is this communication we need to analyse and understand.

In this chapter, the abbreviation PB will be used when reporting previously published literature on problem and challenging behaviours. Depending on the focus of concern, we use the terms 'distress behaviours' and 'socially unacceptable behaviours' respectively to denote more precisely behaviours individuals are engaging in because they are distressed and behaviours that are distressing to care providers and the public but not necessarily to the individual.

Introduction

Thus, 'PB' refers to a broad class of behaviours shown by PWDID. They include aggression to self (e.g. self-injury), to others (e.g. hitting, biting) and to the environment (e.g. destructiveness), stereotyped mannerisms and a range of other behaviours which may be either harmful to the individual (e.g. eating inedible substances), challenging for care providers (e.g. persistent screaming, disturbed sleep patterns, overactivity, non-compliance) and/or objectionable to members of the public (e.g. smearing of faeces or saliva on self and others, regurgitation of food) (Emerson & Einfeld, 2011). These behaviours prevent full integration of some PWDID into mainstream life and impoverish quality of life for them and their care providers.

Prevalence estimates of PB range widely from a 'best estimate' of 15–17.5% in general populations of PWDID (Koritsas & Iacono, 2012a) to 42–82% in those with profound intellectual and multiple disabilities

(Poppes *et al*, 2010). Differences in rates are associated with: ascertainment methodology; type of PB; individual characteristics such as gender, age, severity of disability, associated impairments, other developmental and medical conditions; and living arrangement.

A review of the causes of PB identified three perspectives that have dominated the literature (Koritsas & Iacono, 2012*b*): (1) applied behavioural analysis (ABA), which includes the impact of biological events (e.g. menses, otitis media, constipation); (2) biological factors (e.g. medical conditions, behavioural phenotypes and neurochemical transmitters); and (3) psychiatric disorders. The focus has been on single causes without exploration of possible interactions between various causes. These reviewers and others (Benson & Brooks, 2008), on the other hand, support biopsychosocial approaches that reveal more complex explanations of the determinants of the concerning behaviours. Dosen (2007) proposes the addition of a developmental perspective, while Banks *et al* (2007) recommend a framework of 'enabling environments', shifting the concept of PB from an attribution of the individual to a circumstance that is co-constructed between an individual with unique needs and the environment of supports. From this perspective, the assessment of PB should include assessment of the environment and supports available, while treatment should include making necessary accommodations.

In assessing PB, clinicians often make inferences about individual behaviour, without the individual being able to attribute subjective meaning to these behaviours. Crucially, emotional and lived experiences are embedded in behavioural expression; as such, while some PB may be socially unacceptable, they may nevertheless be understandable from individual personal perspectives, developmental and historical contexts.

In the absence of identifying single causes and the pressure to eliminate PB because of their socially unacceptable nature, interventions used have not always been optimal for PWDID. Understanding and embracing the aetiological complexity of these behaviours are key considerations in the provision of effective treatments and bespoke interventions.

The current authors recently participated in developing healthcare guidelines for family practitioners treating PWDID and tools to implement these guidelines (Developmental Disabilities Primary Care Initiative, 2011; Sullivan *et al*, 2011). Here we build on one of these tools to understand, assess and treat PB within a shared-care family medicine/psychiatry specialist model. This 'HELP' framework (Fig. 5.1), considers the aetiologies of PB within four main conceptual themes: (1) **H**ealth; (2) **E**nvironments and supports; (3) **L**ived experience and emotional well-being; and (4) **P**sychiatric concerns. The evidence base related to these themes is explored below, while suggestions for clinical practice, along with additional resources and tools, are documented in Tables 5.1–5.4. The Social Care Institute for Excellence presents films on challenging behaviour in PWDID at http://www.scie.org.uk/socialcaretv/topic.asp?t=challengingbehaviourandlearningdisabilities.

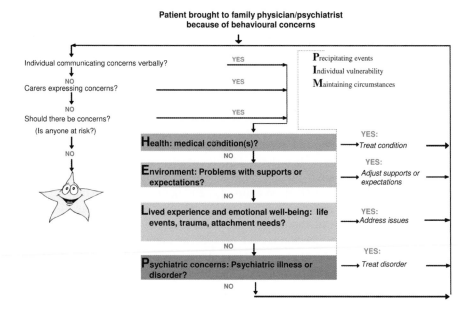

Fig 5.1 Diagnostic formulation of problem behaviours: an approach to assessment and treatment – HELP. © Elspeth Bradley 2013. The colour original of the figure (used by the authors when teaching) has the 'Health' box in blue and then a traffic light system for the next three boxes: 'Environment' in a green box to indicate optimal environments and supports; the 'Lived experience and emotional well-being' box in orange and the 'Psychiatric concerns' box in red.

(1) Health

Medical conditions give rise to PB. These PB are distress behaviours communicating physical discomfort and pain.

Compared with the general population, physical and mental health concerns are greater in the PWDID (Beange *et al*, 1995; Kwok & Cheung, 2007; McDermott *et al*, 2008; O'Hara *et al*, 2010; Emerson & Baines, 2011); they experience greater health inequalities (Ouellette-Kuntz, 2005) and have poorer health outcomes (McCarthy & O'Hara, 2011) and greater mortality at a younger age (Hollins *et al*, 1998). Difficulties in recognising medical conditions, inadequate investigation and incorrect diagnoses generally increase with greater severity of the DID and coexisting disabilities. This gives rise to untreated medical conditions that cause discomfort and pain which PWDID may communicate atypically. Recognition of unmet health needs has prompted several jurisdictions to develop guidelines recommending systematic annual health checks to minimise missed diagnoses of treatable medical conditions and propose vigorous advocacy for equity in healthcare for this population (Lennox & Developmental Disability Steering Group, 2005; Lennox *et al*, 2011; Sullivan *et al*, 2011).

Physical and mental health

Several studies found high rates of previously unidentified medical conditions in PWDID referred for psychiatric assessment or receiving psychiatric services (Beange et al, 1995; Ryan & Sunada, 1997; Kastner et al, 2001; Lehotkay et al, 2009; Charlot et al, 2011). Prevalence of a physical (medical) condition is greater in those with severe and profound DID (Lehotkay et al, 2009) and comorbidity of more than one physical condition or psychiatric disorder is common and increases with greater severity of IDD (Kwok & Cheung, 2007; Lehotkay et al, 2009).

Medical conditions

Ryan & Sunada (1997) suggest that a common mechanism by which medical problems influence behaviour is through conferring a non-specific stress (general 'unwellness') on the person's system, which interferes with the effectiveness of other treatments and programmes the person is receiving. For example, frequency and intensity of PB have been reported to be greater on 'sick' days than on 'well' days (Carr & Owen-DeSchryver, 2007). Bosch et al (1997) describe how medical conditions, even when not the cause of PB, may exacerbate them; treatment of these medical conditions was followed by reduction in the PB. They note that, when working with PWDID and impaired communication skills, obtaining accurate and detailed medical histories can be difficult and medical pain-related conditions must be considered in determining the aetiology of the PB.

Pain

Pain is a universal biological experience alerting us to danger and as such essential to promoting health. It is associated with tremendous suffering that compromises quality of life when underrecognised or poorly treated (Oberlander & Symons, 2006). Our expression of pain is both verbal and non-verbal (by gestures or body language); both may be compromised in PWDID. Pain may not be recognised if it presents atypically and is seen as a PB. Despite the formidable difficulties in assessing pain in some PWDID, there is no evidence that they suffer any less from a noxious experience.

An audit of residential staff's beliefs about pain thresholds and strategies they adopt to recognise and manage pain in PWDID suggested that pain is not effectively recognised or managed (Beacroft & Dodd, 2010), that staff beliefs may be influencing care of residents who experience pain and that use of structured communication aids and additional training may be helpful (Beacroft & Dodd, 2011; Rose, 2011).

Pain may be a setting event for PB resulting in greater frequency and intensity. Carr & Owen-DeSchryver (2007) used a threefold strategy to address pain-related PB associated with menstrual discomfort (Carr et al, 2003): (1) mitigate the pain (e.g. symptomatic relief with pain medication and non-drug interventions, depending on the nature of the pain); (2) redesign the environment (e.g. postpone a difficult task until the client is better); and (3) teach coping skills to manage the task (e.g. more frequent rest breaks).

Self-injurious behaviour (SIB)

Past assumptions were that PWDID who self-injure continued to do so because they had lower sensitivity to pain consequent to opioid receptors being upregulated resulting in raised pain thresholds. While aberrant pain mechanisms in some specific DID (e.g. altered pain sensation in fragile-X and Rett syndromes) have been reported (Peebles & Price, 2012), in the population as a whole evidence is accumulating of generally intact pain systems and possibly greater expression of pain experience (Oberlander & Symons, 2006; Symons et al, 2009; Courtemanche et al, 2012). It is known that pain can lead to self-injurious behaviour (SIB), but as Symons (2011) eloquently points out, little is known about whether SIB leads to pain and the resulting neuron–immune cascade of effects. He notes that SIB and altered pain experiences are also associated with a wide spectrum of neurological (e.g. acquired sensory neuropathies), psychiatric (e.g. borderline personality disorder) and developmental (e.g. autistic spectrum) disorders. He proposes that in response to repeated tissue damage associated with SIB, a cascade of neuron–immune activity occurs that acts on the brain to cause sickness-like behaviour (e.g. disrupted exploratory behaviour, disrupted social behaviour, disrupted sleep) and sensitises primary sensory nerve afferents, contributing to pain hypersensitivity (i.e. hyperalgesia and altered sensory and pain thresholds, reactivity and expressivity).

There is greater prevalence of SIB in individuals with autism spectrum disorder (ASD) and the presence of ASD phenomenology increases the risk of self-injury in individuals with known genetic disorders but without a diagnosis of idiopathic autism (Richards et al, 2012). Characteristics associated with self-injury in ASD indicate a role for impaired behavioural inhibition (greater impulsivity and hyperactivity), low levels of ability (and speech) and negative affect (Richards et al, 2012). Oliver et al (2013) describe three types of SIB in children and adults with ASD: (1) pain-related SIB (see Table 5.1), (2) SIB as a learned behaviour and (3) SIB and behaviour dysregulation. They also note that children and adults with ASD may have an unusual experience of pain and/or unusual responses to pain and may not be able to communicate their experience to others.

Genetic syndromes

Particular genetic syndromes are associated with specific medical risks and pain-related conditions (Cassidy & Allanson, 2010). Additionally, some PB are associated with specific syndromes, for example self-biting with fragile-X syndrome, skin picking with Prader–Willi syndrome and eye poking with Lowe syndrome and visual impairment. In one study, a range of distinctive SIB topographies was associated with each of Smith–Magenis, cri du chat and Cornelia de Lange syndromes (Arron et al, 2011). Self-injury in Cornelia de Lange, fragile-X, Lowe and Prader–Willi syndromes were associated with repetitive behaviour, overactivity and impulsivity. On the other hand, overactivity or impulsivity, but not repetitive behavior, was associated with physical aggression in all participants regardless of syndrome group. The prevalence of aggression was significantly heightened in Angelman syndrome and Smith–Magenis syndrome. Aggression and SIB are two of the most concerning PB seen in PWDID; their different topographies in specific syndromes highlight the causal complexities of at least some PB and the need to consider both personal characteristics (including those of genetic origin) and environmental factors.

In different genetic syndromes, PB have been found to serve different functions: participants with Smith–Magenis syndrome were significantly more likely to display PB related to physical discomfort, while those with fragile-X syndrome were less likely to display attention-maintaining PB than escape or tangible maintained PB (Langthorne & McGill, 2012). Chronic sleep disturbance, thought to be related to an inversion in the circadian melatonin sleep cycle, is considered characteristic of Smith–Magenis syndrome; targeting sleep disturbance has resulted in improvements in other PB (De Leersnyder et al, 2001a, 2001b). These studies further highlight not only the aetiological complexities of PB but also the consequent nuances of effective interventions.

Medication

Psychotropic medications have been a frequent intervention for PWDID engaging in PB (Matson & Dempsey, 2008; Matson & Neal, 2009; Matson & Hess, 2011) and, despite lack of evidence of efficacy, antipsychotics continue to be used to treat aggression and other PB in the absence of a diagnosis of psychotic disorder (Tsiouris, 2010; Lunsky & Elserafi, 2012). Evidence from a multicentre controlled trial demonstrated no greater benefits of antipsychotics than for placebo in reducing aggression in PWDID (Tyrer et al, 2008). Polypharmacy is common and overall rates of medication use are higher than rates of behaviour therapy or counselling (Tsiouris, 2010; Lunsky & Elserafi, 2012). Those with ASD are even more heavily medicated (Lake et al, 2012) and over time are 11 times more likely to remain on medication than to stop (Esbensen et al, 2009).

Medication side-effects may also cause PB. In one study, PB were directly linked to medication side-effects in 9% of patients referred for psychiatric and behavioural treatment (Kastner et al, 2001). PB have been found to be significantly correlated with the number of daily prescribed medications (Beange et al, 1995; de Kuijper et al, 2010). Absence of documentation of regular monitoring and medication side-effects remains problematic (Griffiths et al, 2012).

Any medication runs the risk of producing side-effects, which can be minimised with optimum benefit by careful drug selection and appropriate monitoring, with specific patient vulnerabilities in mind.

Table 5.1 A pragmatic guide to understanding problem behaviours: Health (elaboration of the first of the four aetiological conceptual themes in Fig. 5.1)

Comments and clinical tips	Resources and tools
Preparation by the doctor and of the client for the clinical encounter will result in more effective outcomes Scenarios typically seen in clinical practice (Ryan & Sunada, 1997): <ul><li>initial presentation (of the medical condition) may be a change in behaviour</li><li>common conditions present atypically</li><li>conditions considered uncommon may occur more frequently</li><li>findings on abbreviated history or examination may be minimal and more tests than usual may be needed</li></ul>	Online resources to aid client and doctor: http://www.easyhealth.org.uk (accessible health information that uses easy words and pictures) http://www.intellectualdisability.info (a learning resource for medical, nursing and other healthcare professionals and students) http://www.surreyplace.on.ca/Primary-Care/Pages/Home.aspx Guidelines http://www.cfp.ca/content/57/5/541.full.pdf+html http://www.surreyplace.on.ca/Primary-Care/Pages/Tools-for-primary-care-providers.aspx (tools to help primary care providers follow best practices) http://www.booksbeyondwords.co.uk/ (stories in pictures help clients to explore and understand how to cope with difficult life and health issues)
Physical health and medical conditions Common medical conditions often go unrecognised They may present as 'psychiatric' Multiple comorbidities are common (Charlot *et al*, 2011) Medical conditions may present as problem behaviours Comorbid medical conditions may give rise to more behavioural difficulties (De Winter *et al*, 2011)	Screen routinely for: <ul><li>dysphagia, gastro-oesophageal reflux disease and *H. pylori* (all frequent in rumination behaviours), constipation</li><li>menstrual cycle phases; urinary tract infections; urinary incontinence</li><li>otitis; dental</li><li>dementia; specific subtypes of epilepsy (e.g. people with generalised epileptic activity, more severe or frequent seizures); chronic sleep problems</li><li>medication side-effects</li><li>physical disability and pain related to cerebral palsy</li><li>visual impairment</li></ul>
Pain (and sleep) Chronic pain and sleep problems are common (Van de Wouw *et al*, 2012) Sleep, anxiety and PB are common in children with DID (Stores & Wiggs, 2001; Rzepecka *et al*, 2011) Pain disrupts sleep (night waking, parasomnias, sleep-disordered breathing) in children with DID. Even when this is being managed pharmacologically, pain treatment may not always be effective. Pain should be considered routinely during evaluation and management of sleep problems (Breau & Camfield, 2011)	Each individual's unique behavioural responses to pain should be identified and documented Screen for pain-related medical conditions using tools such as DisDat (http://disdattool.wordpress.com/about)

Comments and clinical tips	Resources and tools
Self-injurious behaviour (SIB)	
SIB is associated with visual impairment (De Winter *et al*, 2011) and ASD (Richards *et al*, 2012)	Screen for visual impairment and ASD ASD NICE guidelines: children, http://www.nice.org.uk/CG128; adults, http://www.nice.org.uk/CG142
Syndromes associated with SIB include Cornelia de Lange, *cri du chat*, fragile X, Lowe, Prader–Willi, Smith–Magenis	Consider SIB-related genetic syndrome and refer for genetics assessment as indicated
In pain-related SIB, there may be periods of SIB unrelated to environmental events, accompanied by changes in: vocalisations; facial expression (furrowed brow); sociability (withdrawal, irritable); activity (especially overactive, restless);body movements (flinching, protecting); eating and sleeping (Oliver *et al*, 2013: pp. 5–6)	Screen for SIB-related medical conditions, such as: ear infection, tooth decay, untreated gastrointestinal problems (especially reflux) In concert with someone with experience of behavioural recording methods and with appropriate medical surveillance, consider a brief trial of a strong analgesic; monitor target pain behaviours and use an ABAB design
Genetic syndromes and other established aetiologies	
Confirmed genetic disorders (e.g. Down syndrome) or anomalies of environmental origin (e.g. fetal alcohol spectrum disorder) provide opportunities to screen for associated health conditions, implement specific treatments and anticipate future medical risks (Ryan & Sunada, 1997; Lopez-Rangel *et al*, 2008; Cassidy & Allanson, 2010)	Society for the Study of Behavioural Phenotypes – syndrome updates at http://www.ssbp.org.uk and http://www.ssbpconference.org/docs/new_york_conference_book_2014.pdf 'Unique – Understanding chromosome disorders', at http://www.rarechromo.org/html/home.asp GeneReviews: expert-authored disease descriptions (including fetal alcohol spectrum disorder) at http://www.ncbi.nlm.nih.gov/books/NBK1116/
Medication	
PWDID are overmedicated yet undertreated	International guide for prescribing psychotropic medication in intellectual
Side-effects may increase the PB, resulting in higher medication doses and polypharmacy	disabilities at http://www.ncbi.nlm.nih.gov/pmc/articles/PMC2758582/ 'Using medication to manage behavioural
DID-associated coexisting disabilities, medical and syndrome-specific conditions and polypharmacy confer greater risk	problems in adults with learning disabilities' (includes an easy read version) at http://www.birmingham.ac.uk/research/activity/ld-medication-guide/index.aspx
PWDID are less able to communicate discomforts they may be experiencing other than through their behaviour	
Use of medications in this population should be judicious and carefully monitored. Baseline behaviours and target symptoms should be monitored prior to starting any medication and side-effects proactively looked for given the side-effect profile of the medication and the behavioural repertoire of the individual	

ASD, autism spectrum disorders; PB, problem behaviours; DID, disorders of intellectual development; PWDID, people with DID.

Medication usage for PB appears linked to the availability of formal training in DID medicine for practitioners and to whether or not services are crisis-oriented or more proactive and preventive (Bradley & Cheetham, 2010). In jurisdictions where prescribing practices are more consistent with recognised standards, misuse of antipsychotics is less evident (Paton *et al*, 2011). Guidelines on the use of psychotropic medication for the management of PB in PWDID are available (Reiss & Aman, 1998; Rush & Frances, 2000; Bhaumik & Branford, 2008; Deb *et al*, 2009; Bradley & Developmental Disabilities Primary Care Initiative Co-editors, 2011).

(2) Environments and supports

Here PB may arise around personal preferences or where there is a mismatch between needs and accommodations to meet these needs. These PB, while socially unacceptable, may or may not be distressing to the individual.

Across the Western world, the history of DID services is peppered with inquiries into abuses, such as Willowbrook in North America (Rivera, 1972), and Cornwall (Healthcare Commission, 2006), Sutton (Commission for Healthcare Audit and Inspection, 2007) and Winterbourne (Department of Health, 2012) in the UK. PWDID and coexisting ASD are especially vulnerable and even more so when they develop PB (Wing, 1989). Conclusions from these inquiries describe recurring themes: overcrowding, isolation, impoverished environments of care, lack of meaningful activities aligned with poor staffing levels, low staff morale and poor practices. A paradigm shift from 'one size fits all' to genuine, robust person-centred care in the context of a well-thought-out, coordinated and long-term strategy is needed (Cooper, 2012). As Cooper comments, the frameworks are available (Banks *et al*, 2007; Department of Health, 2007; Mansell, 1993, 2012); what is needed now is the 'compulsion to deliver' (Cooper, 2012: p. 234).

Individual needs

PWDID have unique circumstances and capacities associated with the origins of their disabilities. While in earlier decades their general support needs were viewed in terms of functioning level (mild, moderate, severe and profound), the current view recognises unique differences across several domains (e.g. cognitive, adaptive and emotional functioning, receptive and expressive communication, autism spectrum, including associated sensory hypersensitivities, and other perceptual–motor atypicalities, specific syndromes, and medical conditions and other disabilities such as cerebral palsy and sensory impairments). In addition, superimposed on these is the heterogeneity seen in the general population related to age, stage and gender (Maslow, 1954; Chapman, 2001–07; AAIDD Ad Hoc Committee on Terminology and Classification, 2010).

Person-centred, comprehensive, multidisciplinary assessment (Craft *et al*, 1985; Summers *et al*, 2002) repeated at key life stages (e.g. when the DID diagnosis is first made, times of transition such as first entering school, transitioning to secondary school and to adult services) should be undertaken to optimise functioning capacities, health and well-being across the life span (Drew & Hardman, 2007; AAIDD Ad Hoc Committee on Terminology and Classification, 2010). These approaches help to minimise behavioural distress arising from these recognised and predictable psychosocial crises (Levitas & Gilson, 2001).

Developmental, psychological and other unique needs

These refer to the individual's profile of mental and emotional development that include cognitive capacities, memory, learning styles, adaptive skills and emotional responses. We now understand that some DID are associated with differences in neurobiological functioning, giving rise to unique needs such as the hypersensitivities and proprioceptive deficits seen in ASD. These unique needs in turn will dictate the nature of required supports and accommodations (Bradley & Caldwell, 2013).

Misunderstanding the capacities of service users contributes to PB and subsequent placement breakdown (Phillips & Rose, 2010); for example, failure to appreciate sensory and perceptual experiences of people with ASD may result in misinterpretation of coping behaviours as PB and negative attributions (e.g. manipulative, attention seeking, non-compliant) (Bogdashina, 2003; Caldwell & Horwood, 2008; Bradley *et al*, 2013).

Communication

Communicating and interacting with others is a basic need and crucial to mental and physical well-being. Communication is also about supporting the input of PWDID into decisions that affect their lives, promoting their greater independence in everyday life and supporting their full participation in their communities. Most importantly, it is about allowing PWDID to express their feelings (Goldbart & Caton, 2010). Communication occurs through verbal (e.g. spoken words and conversations) and non-verbal (e.g. visual materials, gestures, body language) means. Non-verbal communication becomes increasingly important for those with more severe DID. The onus is on care providers to learn the communicative language of each individual, adopting any alternative communication system they may be using, such as the Picture Exchange Communication System (PECS), a picture-based strategy (Bondy & Frost, 2011), or non-verbal approaches such as Intensive Interaction (Box 5.1).

Individuals with ASD also communicate needs by engaging in PB (Chiang, 2008; Matson *et al*, 2013); PECS used in this context has shown some positive effect on social communicative behaviours and PB (Preston & Carter, 2009; Hart & Banda, 2010). Two reviews support functional communication training (FCT) as a treatment for PB (Mancil, 2006; Kurtz *et al*, 2011).

The emotional milieu

Individuals with more severe DID and ASD may escalate in response to emotional expression such as anxiety and aggression in others and to the emotional tone of their surroundings. Promoting low-stress emotional environments, teaching clients everyday skills to manage stress and anger, involving clients in activities to lower arousal, training care staff to recognise potential anxiety-provoking situations proactively and preparing clients for these are all ways to enhance emotional well-being and prevent PB (McDonnell, 2010; Woodcock & Page, 2010). Exploring emotional responses by using aids such as Books Beyond Words (Hollins, 1989–2012), will empower the more able with emotional resilience. For those with little or no language, approaches now available include Intensive Interaction (Caldwell, 2013) and Intensive Therapy for Attachment and Behaviour (ITAB) (Sterkenburg, 2008; Schuengel *et al*, 2009*a*, 2009*b*) (see Box 5.1). Emotional needs are covered more fully in section 3 of this chapter ('Lived experience and emotional well-being').

Behavioural

In a comprehensive review of PB, Emerson & Einfeld (2011) conclude that behavioural approaches (specifically ABA, which has evolved into positive behavioural support) can result in significant and widespread reductions in severely challenging behaviours that (1) may be associated with a range of positive side-effects, (2) may generalise to new settings and (3) may be maintained over long periods.

Behavioural approaches conceptualise PB as contingent on environmental events and therefore changes in environmental contingencies in response to behaviour will change the behaviour (Embregts *et al*, 2009). However, examination of SIB, aggressive and other PB in several DID-associated genetic syndromes identified different prevalences, indicating that an exclusively operant account of PB cannot explain differences in personal characteristics between those with SIB and aggression and those without (Arron *et al*, 2011). In addition, this behavioural conceptualisation may not take account of emotional needs or triggers, meaningful only to the individual in the context of past traumas (see section 3).

Along with ABA and positive behavioural support, medication has been the mainstay of managing PB and crises that arise from these. Unfortunately, in the absence of opportunities for full multidisciplinary assessment, medication may become part of chronic crisis management. Use of medication for PB partly arises from the mistaken belief that they constitute a disorder to be treated like any other medical condition, rather than a co-constructed circumstance related to needs and supports.

The physical environment

Apart from a limited literature on ASD and sensory hypersensitivities, there is a paucity of published evidence on the impact of the physical environment on the presence of PB in PWDID. Day-to-day practice, however, reminds us that PWDID frequently live in relatively impoverished environments and in arrangements not of their choice. High rates of obesity (Bhaumik *et al*, 2008) attest to limited access to physical activity (Howie *et al*, 2012). Not infrequently, PWDID live with people not of their choice and are often subjected to the disruption and annoyance of the PB of their peers.

Snoezelen rooms

Reviews support the use of multisensory therapy (a Snoezelen room) to enhance feelings of pleasure and well-being in PWDID (Chan *et al*, 2010), but the limited evidence suggests the benefits may not generalise beyond the therapy itself, and no superior effects compared with other therapies such as outdoor or activity therapy have been established. For adults with profound DID, a Snoezelen intervention decreased disruptive behaviour (aggressive and stereotyped) but only for those with coexisting ASD; here the effects did carry over to the living room and Snoezelen exposure had to be intense and frequent to be effective (Fava & Strauss, 2010). Cuvo *et al* (2001) found stereotyped behaviours reduced and engagement (interaction with people and objects) increased when PWDID were involved in outdoor activities (the most positive impact) compared with being in the Snoezelan room (an intermediate impact) or living room (the least favourable impact).

Physical exercise

Lang *et al* (2010) reviewed 18 studies meeting predetermined inclusion criteria involving physical exercise and individuals with ASD. Decreases in stereotypies, aggression, off-task behaviours and elopement followed exercise interventions, supporting a conclusion that regular and specific types of exercise may be beneficial. In contrast, Kasner *et al* (2012) reviewed 12 research studies exploring the effects of antecedent exercise on self-stimulatory behaviours and concluded that the evidence for the beneficial effects of exercise was inconclusive. The possible benefits of exercise may need to be examined in more aetiologically homogeneous groups, as the aetiology of the PB may be different (e.g. aggression associated with hyperarousal states in ASD). In addition, different types of exercise may have different effects on different PB topographies.

Services

Staff and care provider supports

The prevalence of PB is positively linked to living with paid carers and the level of restrictiveness in residential settings (Emerson & Einfeld, 2011). However, it remains unclear whether this is because both are also related to the severity of the DID.

Several studies report a mismatch between clients' level of understanding and staff interaction, with staff (1) showing an overreliance of verbal communication, even when working with predominantly non-verbal clients,

(2) underestimating their own use of verbal communication, and (3) failing to adapt their communication to the skills of the service user (McConkey *et al*, 1999; Bradshaw, 2001). Communication training for support staff and training in working with people with ASD increases staff communication efficacy and confidence and is effective in reducing PB (Smidt *et al*, 2007; Caldwell & Horwood, 2008; Kyle *et al*, 2010; McDonnell, 2010).

Rose (2011) reviewed studies addressing staff psychological factors on outcomes for PWDID under their care. Attributions staff make concerning PB can influence their willingness to offer help and support. While the correlations between staff stress and burnout and PB in PWIDD are inconsistent, some studies found that the characteristics of the organisation were more influential in eliciting staff stress than the behaviours of the PWDID (Thomas & Rose, 2010).

Acceptance-based interventions with staff have been shown to have positive outcomes for residents. Such interventions include changing the psychological perceptions of staff using a PACT (promotion of acceptance in carers and teachers) approach, which has been shown to help reduce staff stress even when their work remains the same (Noone & Hastings, 2010). The use of restraints and medications for PB and staff injuries diminished after mindfulness interventions (Singh *et al*, 2009). Negative attitudes and emotions are reported in general hospital staff towards PWIDD; changing attitudes in this setting may result in better physical healthcare (Rose, 2011). Staff training was shown to increase staff confidence in the management of aggression in people with ASD (McDonnell *et al*, 2008).

Crisis services

PB may escalate to crisis levels and emergency services (e.g. police, medical services) may be called in to assist. Sometimes this is a crisis resulting from a client issue such as an unrecognised medical condition. However, not infrequently the escalation is the result of unmet or unrecognised needs and inadequate supports. Ideally, a visit to a hospital emergency department should draw attention to any medical concerns and lead to triage to developmental services for more comprehensive assessment and treatment of the PB (Bradley & Lofchy, 2005). Unfortunately, in the absence of these options, interventions with medication may start in the emergency department, with the individual discharged to the residential setting without resolution of the issues giving rise to the PB and now with the addition of medication with all attendant side-effects. Client, families and emergency medical staff have shared their negative experience of the 'revolving door' approach (Lunsky & Gracey, 2009; Lunsky *et al*, 2008; Weiss *et al*, 2009). Several tools have been developed to assist care providers to manage behavioural crises (Developmental Disabilities Primary Care Initiative, 2011).

Specialist services

Specialist interdisciplinary teams are recognised as good practice in the support of PWDID and PB (Benson & Brooks, 2008).

Table 5.2 A pragmatic guide to understanding problem behaviours: Environments and supports (elaboration of the second of the four aetiological conceptual themes in Fig. 5.1)

Comments and clinical tips	Resources and tools
Individual needs are related to age and stage, as well as the specific DID and its aetiology. PB arising from developmental needs are illuminated by medical, genetic, developmental, psychological, occupational therapy/sensory, communication, emotional, behavioural and other assessments contributing to a multiperspective diagnostic understanding	Disciplines that may contribute to multi- and interdisciplinary work are outlined by Craft *et al* (1985), Summers *et al* (2002) and Bradley *et al* (2009)
Communication	
Communication is crucial to mental well-being across the range of developmental capacities and across the life span. In general terms, communication using gestures and body language and other visual aids requires less processing than word-based communication; as such, the former is preferred in those with greater severity of disability, where ASD coexists, and for more able individuals when in distress, at which time functioning capacity may diminish significantly	Talking Mats® is an evidence-based communication framework that enables people who have difficulty communicating to express their views, at http://www.talkingmats.com/ PECS (Picture Exchange Communication System) at http://www.pecs-canada.com/ Brochures/Bondy-TPRVOL62No4.pdf FCT (Functional Communication Training) at http://www.ncbi.nlm.nih.gov/pmc/articles/PMC2846575/ Engaging the individual emotionally is facilitated by: • Books Beyond Words, at http://www.booksbeyondwords.co.uk • Intensive Interaction, at http://www.phoebecaldwell.co.uk/work.asp • Integrative Therapy for Attachment and Behaviour, at http://dare.ubvu.vu.nl/bitstream/handle/1871/15813/8494.pdf?sequence=5 See also Box 5.1
Meeting with individuals in their own familiar places: • permits environments and supports to be observed at first hand • contributes to the clinical psychiatric evaluation (in this context there is greater opportunity to build on client initiatives, thus enhancing emotional engagement and the mental state examination) • provides the opportunity to experience at first hand the emotional milieu and the impact of others and the social environment	Easy-read information, at http://www.bild.org.uk/easy-read/easy-read-information/health-easy-read-links/

Table continues over

Comments and clinical tips	Resources and tools
Behavioural approaches provide: • structure and consistency for both PWDID and care providers • robust data from which a better understanding of the cause and function of the PB may emerge • a context within which to evaluate intervention outcomes Important components of the behavioural approach include: • ABC (antecedent–behaviour–consequences) monitoring; • assessment of the function of the behaviour, the latter now being seen as part of best practice in the field of DID (Tasse, 2006) • at times of crises, an escalation continuum, which provides clear direction for staff responses.	Consultation with behavioural therapist/psychologist Behavioural and mental health tools at http://www.surreyplace.on.ca/Primary-Care/Pages/Tools-for-primary-care-providers.aspx including: • initial management of behavioural crises in family medicine • risk assessment tool for adults with DID in behavioural crises • a guide to understanding PB and emotional concerns • ABC (antecedent–behaviour–consequences) chart • crisis prevention and management plan • essential information for emergency department • guidance about emergencies of caregivers
Physical environment Special adaptations may be required for those with motor (e.g. CP) or sensory (e.g. hearing, vision) impairments, sensory hypersensitivities and proprioceptive needs (e.g. ASD)	Consultation with occupational/sensory integration therapist
Snoezelen rooms May be particularly helpful in ASD and lower-functioning individuals through impact on affect regulation	http://www.youtube.com/watch?v=8doQvPjBiQg
Physical exercise May be particularly helpful in ASD through impact on arousal and affect regulation	Health matters: the exercise, nutrition, and health education curriculum for people with developmental disabilities (Marks *et al*, 2010) http://www.youtube.com/watch?v=zTBBVJsksal Exercise intervention research on persons with disabilities: what we know and where we need to go (Rimmer *et al*, 2010)
Services Note importance of service structure, service availability, service access (promoting crises reactive or crises preventive activities; multidisciplinary approaches)	The Greenlight Toolkit is about planning good services for people with mental health problems and intellectual disabilities, at http://www.learningdisabilities.org.uk/content/assets/pdf/publications/green-light.pdf?view=Standard

Comments and clinical tips	Resources and tools
	Hospital passports aim to assist PWDID by providing hospital staff with important information about them and their health, at http://www.easyhealth.org.uk/listing/hospital-passports-(leaflets)
	General issues section in the Care of Adults with Developmental Disabilities at http://www.surreyplace.on.ca/Primary-Care/Pages/Tools-for-primary-care-providers.aspx
Staff and care-provider supports	
Note importance of: (1) staff training about DID, communication and crises management; (2) role of negative attitudes and emotions; (3) emerging practices (e.g. training in acceptance-based interventions, mindfulness, low-arousal approaches)	Primary care of adults with developmental disabilities, at http://www.cfp.ca/content/57/5/541.full.pdf+html
	Advocacy, at http://www.surreyplace.on.ca/Documents/Advocacy%20Role%20of%20Family%20Physician.pdf

ASD, autism spectrum disorders; CP, cerebral palsy; DID, disorders of intellectual development; PB, problem behaviours; PWDID, people with DID.
Copyright © Elspeth Bradley, 2013.

Box 5.1 Reducing problem behaviour (PB) through communication and connection with others

Books Beyond Words (BBW)

> 'It is a penny dropping moment – both for you and the person themselves – you because you understand the power of pictures to explain and for them – because a new experience has been opened up and they feel better prepared, better able to cope.' (From Hollins, http://www.booksbeyondwords.co.uk)

Books Beyond Words are stories told in pictures to:

- check for understanding
- explore feelings
- share experience
- support decision-making.

The pictures are in colour and are designed particularly for adults. The books are the outcome of the Beyond Words method of putting people with intellectual disabilities and others who struggle with words at the centre of the communication exchange. The Beyond Words method has developed as a partnership involving self-advocates with intellectual disabilities and those who provide everyday and professional supports (Bradley & Hollins, 2013).

Box continues over

Box 5.1 *Continued*

Intensive Interaction (Int Int)

> 'in this population, who have been lacking approaches sensitive to their emotional needs, Intensive Interaction is a practical route into understanding how an individual with idiosyncratic, perhaps pre-intentional communication, is feeling.' (Nind, 2012: p. 34)

Intensive Interaction is an approach based on the mother–infant imitation dialogue, where the infant initiates a sound or movement, which is confirmed by the mother. It uses the individual's own body language to build up emotional engagement (Caldwell, 2012*b*, 2013). The approach is helpful in engaging both children and adults with severe DID and/or autism, who do not have language, or find it difficult. Using an Intensive Interaction approach, communication becomes mutually adaptive and responsive for both client and care provider, thereby sustaining interaction, feelings of efficacy and well-being for both (Barber, 2008; Hewett, 2012). Evaluations of effectiveness have been directed to the enjoyable interactions that develop between those with these complex communication needs and significant others in their lives; any gains in communication or reduction in ritualistic, stereotyped or other PB are seen as secondary. However, significant reductions in PB are documented by many Intensive Interaction practitioners (Caldwell, 2006; Caldwell *et al*, 2009; Hewett, 1998; Nind & Hewett, 2005; Nind, 2006; Nind & Kellett, 2002).

Intensive Interaction is used most extensively in the UK but now is also used in Australia and several countries in Europe. It has been demonstrated that practitioners can be trained in the basics quickly and at low cost (Zeedyk *et al*, 2009).

Intensive Therapy for Attachment and Behaviour (ITAB)

> 'Relational therapy is provided by caregivers who, from within a relationship based on trust, create a basic feeling of safety within a relationship, get the child to calm down, stimulate social-emotional development and teach new desirable behaviour.' (Dosen, 1983; in guidebook to DVD, Sterkenburg & IJzerman, 2007)

ITAB is an integrative psychotherapeutic treatment for children with complex needs (multiple disabilities) for whom other treatments have failed. Developed by Sterkenburg (2008), it focuses on promoting care providers' interactive skills. The treatment, based partly on Dosen's (2001) developmental–dynamic relationship therapy, combines an attachment-based approach with a behavioural intervention in order to replace maladaptive with more adaptive behaviours. Sterkenburg proposes that caregivers, in the context of a caring relationship providing comfort and safety, are important as stress regulators and as such indirectly reduce the likelihood of PB.

Damen *et al* (2011) used video feedback interaction training (sometimes also referred to as 'sensitive responsiveness') with children and adults with visual and intellectual disabilities. Significant reductions in PB and improvement in affective mutuality were reported (see also Janssen *et al*, 2002).

(3) Lived experience and emotional well-being

Emotional concerns give rise to PB. These PB are distress behaviours communicating personal distress.

Stress

PWDID are more vulnerable to stress and use less effective coping strategies (Janssen et al, 2002). When events exceed what an individual can handle, psychological stress is experienced. Such threat to the organism's homeostasis and survival activates the body's autonomic and endocrine control systems, resulting initially in hyperarousal (sympathetic nervous system activation), mobilising the individual to run away or fight off the threat. In the absence of adequate coping strategies, threat that is perceived as too overwhelming to fight or flee from may result in immobilisation and dissociated states (body shutdown, involving the parasympathetic nervous system) (Porges, 2011).

Activation of the fight (hitting out) – flight (withdrawing) – freeze (catatonic-like behaviours) and 'shutdown' responses can be observed in people with ASD or DID in response to environments that are experienced as overwhelming (Wing & Shah, 2000; Hare & Malone, 2004; Loos & Loos Miller, 2004; Loos Miller & Loos, 2004). These responses may be mistakenly viewed as PB in the absence of understanding that their origins may be embedded in sensory hypersensitivities, processing problems and other neurobiological differences associated with ASD (Bradley et al, 2013). Aggressive and self-injurious PB are conceptualised in the behavioural tradition as being motivated by attention and escape (Embregts et al, 2009; Matson et al, 2011; Rojahn et al, 2012), rather than the consequence of autonomic nervous system survival responses in distressed individuals unable to process what is going on (Bradley & Caldwell, 2013).

Physiological signs of stress (changes in heart and respiration rate, body temperature and blood pressure) in a sample of institutionalised individuals with profound DID were found to be associated with their history of stress diseases, changes in surroundings and events not considered threatening by others, and PB (e.g. resistiveness, hyperactivity and aggression). Reactions occurred to both pleasant and unpleasant stimuli and were greatest at clinical examinations and being stared at (Chaney, 1996). Several studies have indicated that cumulative psychosocial stress is positively associated with PB and that adaptive competence in coping is negatively associated with PB. Medication directed at reducing arousal (mediated by the cortisol-dependent stress homeostasis mechanism) has for some resulted in reduced PB (Ratey et al, 1987; Verhoeven & Tuinier, 1996; Lovallo & Thomas, 2000).

Attachment

PWDID are also at risk of developing insecure attachment patterns (especially disorganised type) with primary care providers (Hollins &

Sinason, 2000; Janssen *et al*, 2002; Schuengel *et al*, 2009*a*, 2013) as well as reactive attachment disorders in response to social deprivation such as institutionalisation (Gleason *et al*, 2011) and maltreatment (Minnis *et al*, 2010). Attachment patterns emerge from early infancy and contribute to differences in susceptibility to stress. Secure attachments facilitate successful regulation of behaviour and affective arousal (De Schipper & Schuengel, 2010). Disorganised attachment may interfere with the early development of the right brain's stress-coping system (Bradley, 2000; Schore, 2003), contributing to difficulties in affect regulation. Meta-analysis of attachment styles showed fewer secure attachments for individuals with neurological abnormalities, including ASD, Down syndrome and cerebral palsy, with more having a disorganised type of attachment (van Ijzendoorn *et al*, 1992). ASD alone is not associated with insecure or disorganised attachment; however, the majority of children studied with the combination ASD and DID showed disorganised attachment (Willemsen-Swinkels *et al*, 2000).

The support of an attachment figure may be especially important for PWDID because they are less able to deal with stressful situations on their own (De Schipper & Schuengel, 2010). Young people living in group care who showed more secure attachment behaviour towards professional caregivers were found to be less irritable, less lethargic and less stereotypical in their behaviour, even after controlling for developmental age and ASD. Each relationship with a member of the care staff was found to bear uniquely on their PB (De Schipper & Schuengel, 2010).

The combination of stress, less effective coping strategies, greater rates of insecure or disorganised attachment, reactive attachment disorders and consequent difficulties in affect regulation likely contributes to the increased prevalence of mental ill health and PB in PWDID (Clegg & Sheard, 2002; Schuengel *et al*, 2009*a*, 2013; Larson *et al*, 2011).

Emotional engagement

Opportunities for PWDID to share their inner worlds and subjective experiences may be limited unless facilitated by care providers. The greater the disabilities, the greater the likelihood PWDID will be excluded from reciprocal emotional exchanges (Goldbart & Caton, 2010). Instead, emotional responses may be restricted or unpredictable and out of control; this distress may be interpreted as PB. Caldwell, using an Intensive Interaction approach (Box 5.1), has sensitively demonstrated that deep and meaningful emotional connection can occur in the absence of verbal language and in the context of severe cognitive and communication disabilities in individuals presenting with extreme PB (Caldwell, 2006, 2012*a*). Intimate communication exchanges not previously seen by care providers, between individuals with long histories of PB and the therapist, are captured on videotape and occur after relatively short periods of engagement of the two communicating partners. Significant reductions in PB and improvement in affective mutuality are also reported using an interactive approach (Intensive Therapy for Attachment and Behaviour – ITAB, Box 5.1), based on a stress/attachment model of support (Janssen *et al*, 2002; Damen *et al*, 2011). Both Intensive Interaction and ITAB are best offered as a total-communication approach in all environments where individuals spend time.

Social relationships and networks

Social isolation is a recognised reality for many PWDID (Department of Health, 2001); they need supports to enable them to develop a range of friendships, activities and relationships (Department of Health, 2001: p. 127). The perception PWDID have of their supports and relationships and not just that observed and reported by others, is a predictor of subsequent mental and physical health (Lunsky & Benson, 2001). PWDID report well-being and satisfaction with their lives as being associated with meaningful social interactions (Miller & Chan, 2008) and social relationships (Emerson & Hatton, 2008). Relationships with friends who also have intellectual disabilities appear to be protective against feeling helpless (Emerson & Hatton, 2008). On the other hand, a great deal of stress is also reported from negatively perceived interpersonal relationships with peers and others (Bender *et al*, 1999; Bramston *et al*, 1999; Hartley & MacLean Jr, 2009). The availability of supportive therapy may help to reduce stress and enhance resilience.

Life events and traumatic experiences

Life events contribute to stress and are clearly established as impacting on mental health in the general population. In a comprehensive review of PB, Emerson & Enfield (2011) report current evidence suggesting that PB or mental health problems in PWDID may be associated with (1) cumulative exposure to acute life stresses or adverse life events, (2) exposure to specific life events such as abuse, parental death and placement outside the home, (3) poorer family functioning and (4) being brought up by a single parent. Exposure to all these events is significantly more likely among people in lower socioeconomic circumstances.

Totsika & Hastings (2009) note the absence of evidence that systematically points to personal characteristics in the persistence of PB and they highlight instead the importance of life events as a factor that may influence the course of these behaviours.

Martorell & Tsakanikos (2008) distinguish between life events and traumatic experiences and note the 'thin red line' between the two insofar as events that would be viewed as non-traumatic from the general population perspective may become traumatic in PWDID owing to their difficulties in understanding; additionally, with greater severity of disability a 'bearable' life event may become 'unbearable'. They report how traumatic experiences may play a more significant role in pathology than life events *per se*. In their group of 177 participants with DID, 75% had experienced at least one traumatic life event and 51% of trauma experiences were related to learning of the sudden death or serious injury of a spouse, child, parent, close relative or friend. The authors suggest that, in a diathesis trauma model, traumatic experiences across the life span would count as predisposing factors, whereas life events would be precipitating ones (see Fig. 5.1). Others also report lower levels of cognitive ability as a risk factor for post-traumatic stress disorder (Macklin *et al*, 1998) and trauma symptoms as being significantly underrecognised in PWDID (Hollins & Sinason, 2000).

Abuse

Abuse is the most frequently studied trauma in PWDID (Tsakanikos *et al*, 2006; Martorell & Tsakanikos, 2008). PWDID experience greater physical, sexual and emotional abuse, victimisation and repeated victimisation more frequently than peers. The abuse often goes unreported or when reported is disregarded (Reiter *et al*, 2007) and few cases reach criminal court; it is common for the victim to be moved following abuse and therapeutic services are rarely offered. Behaviours consequent to sexual abuse and abuse at school (which was subsequently the focus of an inquiry) are described in Table 5.3; reports by parents of the abuse at school showed, contrary to expectations, considerable consistency in behavioural changes described (Howlin & Clements, 1995).

Neglect – institutional, emotional, social and physical

A poignant description of the emotional distress of male individuals considered to have the most severe PB and living, many since childhood, in a locked ward of a hospital is provided by Hubert & Hollins (2006). These men had lost their individual and social identity, which complicated the presentation of their PB and mental ill health.

Different neurobiology and physical–sensory–psychological frames of reference

It is not known whether there are differences in the stress response and coping strategies associated with the different genetic DID. While not considered a behavioural phenotype, ASD is underpinned by a different neurobiology and consequent differences in neuropsychological functioning, such as sensory hypersensitivities and processing difficulties (Bradley *et al*, 2013). Environments normally tolerated without a problem by most may, for people with ASD, be inherently stressful and directly contribute to at least some of the PB seen in those with DID and ASD. Narratives by those with ASD (some of whom refer to themselves as 'neuro-atypical') have alerted

Table 5.3 A pragmatic guide to understanding problem behaviours: Lived experience and emotional well-being (elaboration of the third of the four aetiological conceptual themes in Fig. 5.1)

Comments and clinical tips	Resources and tools
PWDID are vulnerable to emotional distress but much can be done to prevent this at the individual, support and system levels Emotional coping and emotional concerns can be explored routinely, and adverse life experiences and atypical arousal states screened for, in the clinical psychiatric evaluation	Strategies for emotional engagement – see Box 5.1

Stress

Stress arises from: • physical ill health • when events exceed what the individual can handle • unidentified and unmet developmental and other needs • insufficient or inadequate supports • over- or underestimation of capacities Stress results in anxiety and changes in ANS activity, giving rise to: • hyperarousal resulting in acute (e.g. panic) and chronic (e.g. increased basal heart rate) states and 'fight/flight' reactions • being overwhelmed, resulting in shutdown states (including catatonic behaviours and dissociative responses) Reducing stress reduces anxiety	Stress management includes: • physical activities/exercise (walking, running, swimming) (Marks *et al*, 2010) • mindfulness and meditation practices (help modulate ANS arousal) • affect-regulation approaches and practices • sensory diet (http://www.pearsonassessments.com/HAIWEB/Cultures/en-us/Productdetail.htm?Pid=076-1638-008) • decreasing environmental contributors e.g., Promoting Autism faVourable Environments (PAVE) (Bradley & Caldwell, 2013) • low-stress approaches (http://lowarousal.com/) • increasing supports • enhancing coping strategies • medication (e.g. beta-blocker) acting on the ANS to help decrease arousal

Attachment

Precursors of insecure attachment may include parental stress, ineffective parenting, the individual's limited cognitive skill (e.g. deficits in object permanence will lead to an almost permanent state of separation anxiety) and institutionalisation (Janssen *et al*, 2002) Frightening parental/care provider behaviour or abuse is found to predict disorganised attachment (Janssen *et al*, 2002)	Attachment styles include: secure, insecure-avoidant, ambivalent-resistant, disorganised Attachment disorders include reactive attachment disorder (DSM-IV-TR and ICD-10) (American Psychiatric Association, 2000; World Health Organization, 1992) and disinhibited attachment disorder (ICD-10)

Table continues over

Comments and clinical tips	Resources and tools
Negative attachment experiences leave PWDID more vulnerable throughout the life span to losses, abuses and fragile attachment relationships	Psychotherapeutic approaches (Box 5.1)
Relationships of PWDID with individual care staff bears uniquely on PB (De Schipper & Schuengel, 2010)	
Service systems may inadvertently mirror poor attachment figures	
Emotional engagement protects against stress and promotes learning	Psychotherapeutic approaches (Box 5.1)
Social relationships and networks	
Opportunities for inclusion, acceptance, positive regard, with appropriate accommodations and sensitivity to specific disabilities (e.g. ASD, cerebral palsy)	Special Olympics, at http://www. specialolympics.org Buddy schemes The Specials, at http://www.the-specials.com
Life events and traumatic experiences	
• Placement out of the parental home and parental death have been found to be predictors of change in functional abilities and change in health (Esbensen *et al*, 2008) • Depression, personality disorder and adjustment reaction (any of which may manifest as PB) are reliability associated with life events (the most common being moving place of residence) • Bereavement is associated with mixed psychopathology (Tsakanikos *et al*, 2006; Dodd & Guerin, 2009). Hollins & Esterhuyzen (1997) report PB and pathological grief following significant losses • Exposure to bullying is associated with the development of hyperactivity and emotional problems, while family- and school-related adverse events predicted the development of PB (Gunther *et al*, 2007; Martorell & Tsakanikos, 2008) • Two or more life events increased the odds of emotional and conduct disorder in children (Hatton & Emerson, 2004)	Screen for significant adverse events, including: • abuse (physical, sexual, emotional) • parental death and loss of significant others • placement out of the parental home • changing place of residence • family- and school-related adverse events • bullying Screen for specific life events that most frequently resulted in crisis visits to emergency department (Lunsky & Elserafi, 2011): • move of house or residence • serious problem with family, friend or caregiver • problems with police or other authority • unemployed for more than 1 month • recent trauma/abuse • drug or alcohol problem
Consequences of sexual abuse include PTSD (under-recognised in PWDID) and PB such as self-harm, stereotypical and sexualised behaviours (Peckham *et al*, 2007)	
The most noticeable change in children with ASD abused in school was in fears of, and resistance in, going to school; several developed a new type of eating problem that consisted of grabbing and bolting food and drink (Howlin & Clements, 1995)	

Comments and clinical tips	Resources and tools
	Interventions Provision of safe and predictable environments • specialist support for victims of abuse (http://www.respond.org.uk/watch-listen-learn) • individual and group psychological supports • trauma therapies such as eye movement desensitisation reprocessing (EMDR) appropriately modified to embrace developmental needs (Mevissen *et al*, 2010)
Different neurobiology and physical–sensory–psychological frames of reference Unrecognised by others these may give rise to physical and emotional distress such as unrecognised hypersensitivities in ASD	Personal accounts by people with DID/ASD now available providing the DID/ASD perspective that can inform services and supports and accommodations (Bradley & Caldwell, 2013)

ANS, autonomic nervous system; ASD, autism spectrum disorders; DID, disorders of intellectual development PB, problem behaviours; PTSD, post-traumatic stress disorder; PWDID, people with DID.
Copyright © Elspeth Bradley, 2013.

the 'neuro-typical' world to the problematic daily realities of ASD, and the possibility that those with ASD and DID may be frequently experiencing traumatising events unrecognised by their neuro-typical care providers. It is apparent that, as health professionals and care providers, we must try as best we can to step outside of our neuro-typical worlds and enter into the physical, sensory, perceptual and psychological frame of reference of our DID–ASD clients so as to ensure the environments in which they are living are, from their perspective, nurturing rather than toxic.

(4) Psychiatric concerns:

PB may signal psychiatric disorder. These PB are communicating mental distress.

While there is an increasing evidence base on the relationships between mental disorders and PB (Hemmings *et al*, 2008; Grey *et al*, 2010), these relationships have yet to be adequately explored (Allen & Davies, 2007; Thakker *et al*, 2012). PB and the behaviours and symptoms of mental disorders overlap; the challenge is to determine whether these arise from the same or different aetiologies (Allen *et al*, 2012). PB have historically been included in many studies of the wider concept of mental ill health in PWDID but most have not sought to clarify whether these behaviours are underpinned by specific psychiatric illness. In an exception to this, Hemmings *et al* (2008) found schizophrenia spectrum disorders and personality disorders independently predicted the presence of severe PB, while anxiety disorder independently predicted their absence.

Emerson *et al* (1999) have suggested three ways in which psychiatric illness and PB may interact: (1) the PB are an atypical presentation of mental disorder (a 'behavioural equivalent'); (2) the PB occur as a secondary feature, such as mood-related aggression; or (3) the PB provide a motivational basis (e.g. depression related to unwillingness to participate). Consideration that PB and mental health problems are conceptually and clinically distinct conditions has also been proposed (Whitaker & Read, 2006; Bouras, 2011).

In summary, there remains a lack of clarity as to the conceptual basis, aetiological determinants and clinical presentation between PB and psychiatric disorders in PWDID. In recent years, however, greater understanding has emerged concerning issues that need to be considered to identify correctly those PB that may be underpinned by psychiatric disorder. These are discussed below.

Mental state examination

The mental state examination is core to the psychiatric assessment. Special accommodations are required when interviewing PWDID (Deb *et al*, 2001; Royal College of Psychiatrists, 2001). For those with more severe disabilities and coexisting ASD, a verbal exchange to access mental content and subjective experience may not be helpful. However, using visual materials, stories such as Books Beyond Words (Hollins, 2003) and non-verbal communication approaches (see Box 5.1), meaningful emotional engagement with lower-functioning individuals with severe ASD and PB is possible. Using these visual and empathetic strategies as part of the mental state examination is therapeutic as well as informing the diagnostic assessment; for instance, a previously withdrawn individual engaged in SIB may resonate warmly to the examiner's response to non-verbal behaviours, thus dispelling immediate concerns of psychosis.

Diagnostic criteria

DSM-5 (American Psychiatric Association, 2013), or earlier iterations, and ICD-10 (World Health Organization, 1992), do not recognise PB in PWDID as a diagnostic category. While DM-ID (Diagnostic Manual – Intellectual Disability; Fletcher *et al*, 2007) makes criteria adaptations so as to increase diagnostic accuracy for psychiatric disorder in lower-functioning individuals, there is no separate category for PB. DC-LD (*Diagnostic Criteria for Psychiatric Disorders for Use with Adults with Learning Disabilities/Mental*

Retardation) is an adaptation of ICD (Royal College of Psychiatrists, 2001) and includes a category 'Problem Behaviours' (Axis III, level D).

Point prevalences of clinical diagnoses of PB made by DID psychiatry specialists were found to be greater (at 22.5%) than for any of the formal diagnostic systems (DC-LD at 18.7%; ICD at 0.1%; DSM at 0.1%) (Smiley *et al*, 2007; Jones *et al*, 2008; Cooper *et al*, 2009a, 2009b; Tully *et al*, 2012). This finding is likely related to specialists being able to provide a developmental and historical context for the individual's behaviours.

Missed and problematic diagnoses

As reported in the previous section, PWDID have a high prevalence of exposure to abuse and traumatic events. PTSD is increasingly being recognised as a missed diagnosis in people presenting with PB (Hollins & Sinason, 2000; Hubert & Hollins, 2006; Fletcher *et al*, 2007). To date, PTSD has not been specifically looked for, nor included, as a potential diagnosis in any epidemiological studies of mental ill health in PWDID. Symptoms and behaviours associated with trauma and PTSD overlap with psychotic disorder and schizophrenia; the latter diagnoses are particularly problematic in PWDID, especially in those with more severe disorders and coexisting ASD (Myers, 2010; Bradley *et al*, 2011a). Behaviours associated with triggers from past trauma may be seen as PB if the significance of these triggers is not recognised. Personality disorder is also problematic in DID if not appropriately embedded in an understanding of the individual's developmental history and attachment needs.

Multiple diagnoses

Concurrent psychiatric and somatic conditions

The number of concurrent somatic and psychiatric diagnoses increases with increasing severity of DID. Lehotkay *et al* (2009) suggest that correct identification of symptoms resulting in a correct diagnostic decision would be enhanced by the use of the medical record.

Concurrent psychiatric conditions

Detailed psychiatric examination of teenagers with DID in the Niagara region of Ontario, Canada (Niagara population-based studies) identified concurrent episodic psychiatric disorders – such as adjustment and mood disorders – and non-episodic psychiatric disorders – for instance related to attention-deficit hyperactivity disorder (ADHD), tics, stereotypic, phobic disorders (Bradley & Bolton 2006; Bradley & Isaacs, 2006; Bradley *et al*, 2011b). Episodic disorders were relapsing and remitting and non-episodic disorders typically started more insidiously in childhood; greater prevalence of both types was found in those with coexisting ASD. In the absence of an account from some individuals about their symptoms

Table 5.4 A pragmatic guide to understanding problem behaviours: **P**sychiatric concerns (elaboration of the fourth of the four aetiological conceptual themes in Fig. 5.1)

Comments and clinical tips	Resources and tools
The overlap between PB and psychiatric disorder remains aetiologically and clinically complex; ongoing comprehensive psychiatric evaluations and multiperspective diagnostic formulations are essential; robust person-centred clinical supports will provide a context within which intervention trials can be implemented and any provisional psychiatric diagnoses confirmed	
Mental state examination (MSE) enhanced by: • communicating with individuals in a way meaningful to them (Boardman *et al*, 2014) • emotional engagement with client established over time • informant-based information • behavioural data • appreciating the impact of different levels of functioning on client presentation	Int Int; ITAB; BBW (see Box 5.1) Informant who knows client well DC-LD (Royal College of Psychiatrists, 2001); DM-ID (Fletcher *et al*, 2007); practice guidelines for the assessment and diagnosis of mental health problems in adults with DID (Deb *et al*, 2001); mental health problems and related issues for people with developmental disability and DID (Bouras, 2011) Functional analysis, target behaviours (Tasse, 2006)
Psychiatric diagnoses and diagnostic criteria PB may or may not underpin psychiatric illness. Caution: psychotic disorders are overdiagnosed, while anxiety is underdiagnosed (including PTSD, adjustment and mood disorders) Cautionary note from DM-ID: 'Mental ill health can be positively misdiagnosed when the individual with ID or ASD is under stress' Using DC-LD (Jones *et al*, 2008; Cooper *et al*, 2009*a*, 2009*b*): • all PB were independently associated with lower ability, living arrangement and not having Down syndrome • some PB were independently associated with other medical conditions (e.g. urinary incontinence, visual impairment, physical disabilities) and psychiatric conditions (e.g. attention-deficit hyperactivity disorder)	DSM and ICD criteria should be applied according to developmental and functioning capacities – taking note of other handicaps (e.g. sensory impairments) and other developmental conditions (e.g. ASD) No diagnostic criteria for PB in DSM and ICD DC-LD and DM-ID adaptations are available DC-LD has criteria for PB Special chapter on PTSD in DM-ID

Comments and clinical tips	Resources and tools

ASD, DID and mental ill health

Atypical presentations of mental ill health greater where ASD and DID coexist (ASD present in up to one-third of PWDID)

Unrecognised and problematic psychiatric diagnoses

Personality disorder, psychotic disorder, schizophrenia and PTSD are disorders that are at high risk of being missed, overdiagnosed and underdiagnosed if patients are not evaluated systematically and symptoms and behaviours embedded in an understanding of the patient's developmental, medical and life history context

Multiple diagnoses

i. Concurrent psychiatric and somatic conditions:
• coexisting physical and mental ill health conditions frequently occur and these may manifest as PB
• correct diagnosis enhanced by reference to medical record

ii. Concurrent psychiatric conditions:
• coexisting psychiatric disorders frequently occur and these may manifest as PB
• correct diagnosis enhanced by careful evaluation, looking for episodic as well as non-episodic psychiatric conditions

Specific aetiological (e.g. genetic syndrome) associated PB and psychiatric disorders occur

Screen for ASD (see http://www.nice.org.uk/CG142)
Promote Autism faVourable Environments (PAVE (Bradley & Caldwell, 2013); once PAVE is established reassess PB and repeat psychiatric evaluation

Steps to determine psychiatric diagnosis in PWDID and ASD (SAPPA criteria – see below)

• Establish baseline behaviours prior to onset of PB
• Determine whether there is a significant change from baseline behaviours
• Does change meet criteria for psychiatric illness?

Rigorous medical reviews required until aetiology of PB identified

SAPPA criteria (Bolton & Rutter 1994, outlined in Bradley & Bolton, 2006)
1 Episode of illness: (a) either psychotic symptoms (delusions, hallucinations, catatonia, etc.) lasting at least 3 days; (b) or a change in behaviour outside the range of normal variation for the individual, lasting at least 1 week; (c) and definite diminution in level of social functioning as shown by at least two of: (i) loss of interest in play, (ii) loss of self-care, (iii) loss of social involvements, (iv) loss of initiative, (v) need for change in supervision and/or placement.
2 Episodes of changed behaviour are explored further to obtain systematic standardised information on symptoms. A symptom is deemed clinically significant if: (a) it is outside the range of normal behaviour for that individual; (b) it intrudes into, or disrupts, the individual's ordinary activities; (c) it is of a degree that is not readily controlled by the individual or caregivers; (d) it is sufficiently pervasive to extend into at least two activities.

Identify aetiology of DID, including any syndrome present (Lopez-Rangel *et al*, 2008)

ASD, autism spectrum disorders; DID, disorders of intellectual development; PB, problem behaviours; PTSD, post-traumatic stress disorder; PWDID, people with DID.
Copyright © Elspeth Bradley, 2013.

(because of the severity of their DID) some of the significant episodes of psychiatric disturbance remained 'probable' rather than 'definite'. For these individuals, meeting full ICD diagnostic criteria was impossible. Many individuals, especially those with ASD, had concurrent and multiple episodic and non-episodic disorders (with adjustment, mood, compulsive and ADHD-type behaviours, stereotypies as well as specific manifestations of anxiety, fears and phobias behaviours being greater in the ASD group); the aetiology of the overlapping behaviours giving rise to these episodic and non-episodic diagnoses could be correctly identified only after careful clinical evaluation of premorbid baseline behaviours. Identifying separately episodic and non-episodic mental ill health (e.g. differentiating an increase in impulsive behaviours associated with ADHD from a manic episode or increase in tic behaviours from side-effects of medication) has implications for effective treatment. Typically, different PB also coexist; some of these may start in childhood and may also be relapsing and remitting (Cooper *et al*, 2009*b*). In clinical practice, separating out episodic from background psychiatric and behavioural disorders, and the patterns over time of these symptoms and behaviours, requires a person-centred, historical account, embedded in the individual's unique life circumstances.

ASD and IDD

As previously noted, the population of PWDID is heterogeneous in terms of the cause of each individual's DID. ASD, present in up to a third of PWDID, is specifically associated with PB (Brereton *et al*, 2006; Cooper *et al*, 2009*a*, 2009*b*; McCarthy *et al*, 2010; Rojahn *et al*, 2010), as is greater severity of the DID. PB in PWDID and ASD (as in other aetiologically distinct groups) may have different as well as overlapping aetiologies compared with PWDID without ASD. When DID-ASD and DID-only groups of adults are matched on other variables associated with mental ill health and PB (age, gender, functioning), no difference in prevalence of psychiatric disorder was found (McCarthy *et al*, 2010); only severity of DID and presence of ASD predicted PB. This is in contrast to children and teenagers, where a greater number of psychiatric disorders is seen in ASD groups (Bradley & Bolton, 2006; Leyfer *et al*, 2006; Bradley *et al*, 2011*b*). Similarly, in an epidemiological study of mental ill health in PWDID, the adults with autism had a higher point prevalence of PB compared with the whole population with DID, but when individually matched these differences disappeared (Melville *et al*, 2008); the adults with autism were, however, less likely to recover over a 2-year period than the matched controls. Only a handful of studies have so far separated out DID-ASD from IDD-only when considering PB and other mental ill health.

Summary

Determining whether PB are underpinned by psychiatric disorder is very problematic. From the clinical perspective, several steps may enhance greater understanding: (1) attending to PB arising from medical conditions or from problems in the environment or system of supports (see sections 1–3); (2) optimising the mental state examination so that the emotional responsiveness of clients at all functioning levels can be evaluated directly; (3) generating a multi-perspective diagnostic formulation, including provisional psychiatric diagnosis where indicated; and (4) robustly evaluating this formulation through interventions appropriate to the psychiatric diagnosis.

Conclusion

This chapter has described a multi-perspective multidimensional framework to understanding PB in PWDID. We have redefined PB as those that originate from distress associated with physical, emotional and mental ill health and those that may not necessarily be distressing to the individual but are socially unacceptable. Not infrequently, PB are adaptive responses by PWDID, in the context of the repertoire of responses available to them when in difficult or distressing circumstances. Historically, treatment has focused on the PB; the review here, however, suggests that greater attention to individual physical health, emotional well-being, developmental circumstances, responsive supports and needed accommodations may prevent many PB from developing. In this context, advocacy is a crucial role for the clinician working with PWDID and PB.

Acknowledgements

Dr Phoebe Caldwell generously contributed to discussions that clarified the need to consider separately distress and socially unacceptable PB. The authors have also appreciated the assistance provided by Heidi Diepstra (literature searches), Dr Marie Challita and Kim Ankers (Fig. 5.1).

References

AAIDD Ad Hoc Committee on Terminology and Classification (2010) *Intellectual Disability: Definition, Classification, and Systems of Supports* (11th edn). American Association on Intellectual and Developmental Disabilities.

Allen D, Davies D (2007) Challenging behaviour and psychiatric disorder in intellectual disability. *Current Opinion in Psychiatry,* **20**: 450–5.

Allen D, Lowe K, Matthews H, *et al* (2012) Screening for psychiatric disorders in a total population of adults with intellectual disability and challenging behaviour using the PAS-ADD checklist. *Journal of Applied Research in Intellectual Disabilities,* **25**: 342–9.

American Psychiatric Association (2000) *Diagnostic and Statistical Manual of Mental Disorders* (4th edn, Text Revision) (DSM-IV-TR). APA.

American Psychiatric Association (2013) *Diagnostic and Statistical Manual of Mental Disorders* (5th edn) (DSM-5). APA.

Arron K, Oliver C, Moss J, *et al* (2011) The prevalence and phenomenology of self-injurious and aggressive behaviour in genetic syndromes. *Journal of Intellectual Disability Research,* **55**: 109–20.

Banks R, Bush A, Baker P, *et al* (2007) *Challenging Behaviour: A Unified Approach* (College Report CR144). Royal College of Psychiatrists, British Psychological Society and Royal College of Speech and Language Therapists. Available from http://www.rcpsych.ac.uk/files/pdfversion/cr144.pdf (accessed April 2013).

Barber M (2008) Using intensive interaction to add to the palette of interactive possibilities in teacher–pupil communication. *European Journal of Special Needs Education,* **23**: 393–402.

Beacroft M, Dodd K (2010) Pain in people with learning disabilities in residential settings – the need for change. *British Journal of Learning Disabilities,* **38**: 201–9.

Beacroft M, Dodd K (2011) 'I feel pain' – audit of communication skills and understanding of pain and health needs with people with learning disabilities. *British Journal of Learning Disabilities,* **39**: 139–47.

Beange H, McElduff A, Baker W (1995) Medical disorders of adults with mental retardation: a population study. *American Journal on Mental Retardation,* **99**: 595–604.

Bender WN, Rosenkrans CB, Crane M (1999) Stress, depression, and suicide among students with learning disabilities: assessing the risk. *Learning Disability Quarterly,* **22**: 143–56.

Benson BA, Brooks WT (2008) Aggressive challenging behaviour and intellectual disability. *Current Opinion in Psychiatry,* **21**: 454–8.

Bhaumik S, Branford D (2008) *The Frith Prescribing Guidelines for Adults with Learning Disability* (2nd edn). HealthComm UK.

Bhaumik S, Watson JM, Thorp CF, *et al* (2008) Body mass index in adults with intellectual disability: distribution, associations and service implications. A population-based prevalence study. *Journal of Intellectual Disability Research,* **52**: 287–98.

Boardman L, Bernal J, Hollins S (2014) Communicating with people with intellectual disabilities: a guide for general psychiatrists. *Advances in Psychiatric Treatment,* **20**: 27–36.

Bogdashina O (2003) *Sensory Perceptual Issues in Autism and Asperger Syndrome: Different Sensory Experiences – Different Perceptual Worlds.* Jessica Kingsley.

Bolton PF, Rutter M (1994) *Schedule for Assessment of Psychiatric Problems Associated with Autism (and Other Developmental Disorders) (SAPPA): Informant Version.* Developmental Psychiatry Section, University of Cambridge & Child Psychiatry Department, Institute of Psychiatry.

Bondy A, Frost L (2011) *A Picture's Worth: PECS and Other Visual Communication Strategies in Autism* (2nd edn). Woodbine House.

Bosch J, Van Dyke DC, Smith SM, *et al* (1997) Role of medical conditions in the exacerbation of self-injurious behavior: an exploratory study. *Mental Retardation,* **35**: 124–30.

Bouras N (2011) Mental health problems and related issues for people with developmental and intellectual disability. *Current Opinion in Psychiatry,* **24**: 365–6.

Bradley E, Bolton P (2006) Episodic psychiatric disorders in teenagers with learning disabilities with and without autism. *British Journal of Psychiatry,* **189**: 361–6.

Bradley E, Caldwell P (2013) Mental health and autism: Promoting Autism FaVourable Environments (PAVE). *Journal on Developmental Disabilities,* **19**(1): 1–23. Also available from http://www.oadd.org/docs/41015_JoDD_19-1_8-23_Bradley_and_Caldwell.pdf (accessed November 2013).

Bradley E, Cheetham T (2010) The use of psychotropic medication for the management of problem behaviours in adults with intellectual disabilities living in Canada. *Advances in Mental Health and Intellectual Disabilities,* **4**: 12–26.

Bradley E, Developmental Disabilities Primary Care Initiative Co-editors (2011) Auditing psychotropic medication therapy. In *Tools for the Primary Care of People with Developmental Disabilities.* Available from http://www.surreyplace.on.ca/Documents/Auditing%20Psychotropic%20Medication%20Therapy.pdf (accessed November 2012).

Bradley E, Hollins S (2013) Books beyond Words: using pictures to communicate. *Journal on Developmental Disabilities,* **19**(1): 24–32. Also available from http://www.oadd.org/docs/41015_JoDD_19-1_24-32_Bradley_and_Hollins.pdf (accessed November 2013).

Bradley EA, Isaacs BJ (2006) Inattention, hyperactivity, and impulsivity in teenagers with intellectual disabilities, with and without autism. *Canadian Journal of Psychiatry*, **51**(9): 598–606.

Bradley E, Lofchy J (2005) Learning disability in the accident and emergency department. *Advances in Psychiatric Treatment*, **11**: 45–57.

Bradley E, Goody R, McMillan S (2009) A to Z of disciplines that may contribute to the multi- and interdisciplinary work as applied to mood and anxiety disorders. In *Intellectual Disability Psychiatry: A Practical Handbook* (eds A Hassiotis, DA Barron, IP Hall), pp. 257–63. Wiley-Blackwell.

Bradley E, Lunsky Y, Palucka A, *et al* (2011a) Recognition of intellectual disabilities and autism in psychiatric inpatients diagnosed with schizophrenia and other psychotic disorders. *Advances in Mental Health*, **5**: 4–18.

Bradley E, Ames CS, Bolton PF (2011b) Psychiatric conditions and behavioural problems in adolescents with intellectual disabilities: correlates with autism. *Canadian Journal of Psychiatry*, **56**: 102–9.

Bradley E, Caldwell P, Underwood L (2013) Autism spectrum disorder. In *Handbook of Psychopathology in Intellectual Disability* (eds J McCarthy, E Tsakanikos), pp. 237–64. Springer.

Bradley SJ (2000) *Affect Regulation and the Development of Psychopathology*. Guilford Press.

Bradshaw J (2001) Complexity of staff communication and reported level of understanding skills in adults with intellectual disability. *Journal of Intellectual Disability Research*, **45**: 233–43.

Bramston P, Fogarty G, Cummins RA (1999) The nature of stressors reported by people with an intellectual disability. *Journal of Applied Research in Intellectual Disabilities*, **12**: 1–10.

Breau LM, Camfield CS (2011) Pain disrupts sleep in children and youth with intellectual and developmental disabilities. *Research in Developmental Disabilities*, **32**: 2829–40.

Brereton AV, Tonge BJ, Einfeld SL (2006) Psychopathology in children and adolescents with autism compared to young people with intellectual disability. *Journal of Autism and Developmental Disorders*, **36**: 863–70.

Caldwell P (2006) *Finding You Finding Me: Using Intensive Interaction to Get in Touch with People Whose Severe Learning Disabilities are Combined with Autistic Spectrum Disorder*. Jessica Kingsley.

Caldwell P (2012a) *Autism and Intensive Interaction – Films*. Available from http://www.phoebecaldwell.co.uk/films.asp (accessed November 2012).

Caldwell P (2012b) *Delicious Conversations: Reflections on Autism, Intimacy and Communication*. Pavilion Press.

Caldwell P (2013) Intensive interaction: using body language to communicate. *Journal on Developmental Disabilities*, **19**(1): 33–39. Also available from http://www.oadd.org/docs/41015_JoDD_19-1_33-39_Caldwell.pdf (assessed November 2013).

Caldwell P, Horwood J (2008) *Using Intensive Interaction and Sensory Integration: A Handbook for Those Who Support People with Severe Autistic Spectrum Disorder*. Jessica Kingsley.

Caldwell P, Hoghton M, Mytton P (2009) *Autism and Intensive Interaction: Using Body Language to Get in Touch with Children on the Autistic Spectrum*. Jessica Kingsley.

Carr EG, Owen-DeSchryver J (2007) Physical illness, pain, and problem behavior in minimally verbal people with developmental disabilities. *Journal of Autism and Developmental Disorders*, **37**: 413–24.

Carr EG, Smith CE, Giacin TA, *et al* (2003) Menstrual discomfort as a biological setting event for severe problem behavior: assessment and intervention. *American Journal of Mental Retardation*, **108**: 117–33.

Cassidy SB, Allanson JE (2010) *Management of Genetic Syndromes* (3rd edn). Wiley-Blackwell.

Chan SW, Thompson DR, Chau JPC, *et al* (2010) The effects of multisensory therapy on behaviour of adult clients with developmental disabilities – a systematic review. *International Journal of Nursing Studies*, **47**: 108–22.

Chaney RH (1996) Psychological stress in people with profound mental retardation. *Journal of Intellectual Disability Research*, **40**: 305–10.

Chapman A (2001–07) *Maslow's Hierarchy of Needs*. Available from http://www.businessballs.com/maslowhierarchyofneeds5.pdf (accessed December 2012).

Charlot L, Abend S, Ravin P, *et al* (2011) Non-psychiatric health problems among psychiatric inpatients with intellectual disabilities. *Journal of Intellectual Disability Research*, **55**: 199–209.

Chiang HM (2008) Expressive communication of children with autism: the use of challenging behaviour. *Journal of Intellectual Disability Research*, **52**: 966–72.

Clegg J, Sheard C (2002) Challenging behaviour and insecure attachment. *Journal of Intellectual Disability Research*, **46**: 503–6.

Commission for Healthcare Audit and Inspection (2007) *Investigation into the Service for People with Learning Disabilities Provided by Sutton and Merton Primary Care Trust*. Available from http://webarchive.nationalarchives.gov.uk/20060502043818/http://healthcarecommission.org.uk/_db/_documents/Sutton_and_Merton_inv_Main_Tag.pdf (accessed March 2013).

Cooper SA, Smiley E, Allan LM, *et al* (2009*a*) Adults with intellectual disabilities: Prevalence, incidence and remission of self-injurious behaviour, and related factors. *Journal of Intellectual Disability Research*, **53**: 200–16.

Cooper SA, Smiley E, Jackson A, *et al* (2009*b*) Adults with intellectual disabilities: prevalence, incidence and remission of aggressive behaviour and related factors. *Journal of Intellectual Disability Research*, **53**: 217–32.

Cooper V (2012) Support and services for individuals with intellectual disabilities whose behaviour is described as challenging, and the impact of recent inquiries. *Advances in Mental Health and Intellectual Disabilities*, **6**: 229–35.

Courtemanche A, Schroeder S, Sheldon J, *et al* (2012) Observing signs of pain in relation to self-injurious behaviour among individuals with intellectual and developmental disabilities. *Journal of Intellectual Disability Research*, **56**: 501–15.

Craft MJ, Bicknell DJ, Hollins S (1985) *Mental Handicap: A Multi-disciplinary Approach*. Baillière Tindall.

Cuvo AJ, May ME, Post TM (2001) Effects of living room, Snoezelen room, and outdoor activities on stereotypic behavior and engagement by adults with profound mental retardation. *Research in Developmental Disabilities*, **22**: 183–204.

Damen S, Kef S, Worm M, *et al* (2011) Effects of video-feedback interaction training for professional caregivers of children and adults with visual and intellectual disabilities. *Journal of Intellectual Disability Research*, **55**: 581–95.

de Kuijper G, Hoekstra P, Visser F, *et al* (2010) Use of antipsychotic drugs in individuals with intellectual disability (ID) in the Netherlands: prevalence and reasons for prescription. *Journal of Intellectual Disability Research*, **54**: 659–67.

De Leersnyder H, De Blois M, Claustrat B, *et al* (2001*a*) Inversion of the circadian rhythm of melatonin in the Smith–Magenis syndrome. *Journal of Pediatrics*, **139**: 111–16.

De Leersnyder H, De Blois MC, Vekemans M, *et al* (2001*b*) Beta(1)-adrenergic antagonists improve sleep and behavioural disturbances in a circadian disorder, Smith–Magenis syndrome. *Journal of Medical Genetics*, **38**: 586–90.

De Schipper JC, Schuengel C (2010) Attachment behaviour towards support staff in young people with intellectual disabilities: associations with challenging behaviour. *Journal of Intellectual Disability Research*, **54**: 584–96.

De Winter CF, Jansen AAC, Evenhuis HM (2011) Physical conditions and challenging behaviour in people with intellectual disability: a systematic review. *Journal of Intellectual Disability Research*, **55**: 675–98.

Deb S, Matthews T, Holt G, *et al* (2001) *Practice Guidelines for the Assessment and Diagnosis of Mental Health Problems in Adults with Intellectual Disabilities*. Pavilion Press.

Deb S, Kwok H, Bertelli M, *et al* (2009) International guide to prescribing psychotropic medication for the management of problem behaviours in adults with intellectual disabilities. *World Psychiatry*, **8**: 181–6.

Department of Health (2001) *Valuing People: A New Strategy for Learning Disability for the 21st Century*. Department of health. Available from http://www.archive.official-documents. co.uk/document/cm50/5086/5086.pdf (accessed November 2012).

Department of Health (2007) *Services for People with Learning Disabilities and Challenging Behaviour or Mental Health Needs* (revised edn). Department of Health.

Department of Health (2012) *Transforming Care: A National Response to Winterbourne View Hospital Department of Health Review: Final Report*. Department of Health.

Developmental Disabilities Primary Care Initiative (ed) (2011) *Tools for the Primary Care of People with Developmental Disabilities* (1st edn). MUMS Guideline Clearing House. Also available from http://www.surreyplace.on.ca/Primary-Care/Pages/Home.aspx (accessed March 2013).

Dodd PC, Guerin S (2009) Grief and bereavement in people with intellectual disabilities. *Current Opinion in Psychiatry*, **22**: 442–6.

Dosen A (1983) *Psychische Stoornissen Bij Zwakzinnige Kinderen*. Swets & Zeitlinger.

Dosen A (2001) Developmental–dynamic relationship therapy: an approach to more severely mentally retarded children. In *Treating Mental Illness and Behavior Disorders in Children and Adults with Mental Retardation* (eds A Dosen, K Day), pp. 415–27. American Psychiatric Publishing.

Dosen A (2007) Integrative treatment in persons with intellectual disability and mental health problems. *Journal of Intellectual Disability Research*, **51**: 66–74.

Drew CJ, Hardman ML (2007) *Intellectual Disabilities Across the Lifespan* (9th edn). Pearson Merril Prentice Hall.

Embregts PJCM, Didden R, Schreuder N, *et al* (2009) Aggressive behavior in individuals with moderate to borderline intellectual disabilities who live in a residential facility: an evaluation of functional variables. *Research in Developmental Disabilities*, **30**: 682–8.

Emerson E, Baines S (2011) Health inequalities and people with learning disabilities in the UK. *Tizard Learning Disability Review*, **16**: 42–8.

Emerson E, Einfeld SL (2011) *Challenging Behaviour* (3rd edn). Cambridge University Press.

Emerson E, Hatton C (2008) Self-reported well-being of women and men with intellectual disabilities in England. *American Journal on Mental Retardation*, **113**: 143–55.

Emerson E, Moss S, Kiernan C (1999) The relationship between challenging behaviour and psychiatric disorders. In *Psychiatric and Behavioural Disorders in Developmental Disabilities and Mental Retardation* (ed N Bouras), pp. 38–48. Cambridge University Press.

Esbensen AJ, Seltzer MM, Krauss MW (2008) Stability and change in health, functional abilities, and behavior problems among adults with and without Down syndrome. *American Journal on Mental Retardation*, **113**: 263–77.

Esbensen AJ, Greenberg JS, Seltzer MM, *et al* (2009) A longitudinal investigation of psychotropic and non-psychotropic medication use among adolescents and adults with autism spectrum disorders. *Journal of Autism and Developmental Disorders*, **39**: 1339–49.

Fava L, Strauss K (2010) Multi-sensory rooms: comparing effects of the Snoezelen and the stimulus preference environment on the behavior of adults with profound mental retardation. *Research in Developmental Disabilities*, **31**: 160–71.

Fletcher R, Loschen E, Stavrakaki C, *et al* (eds) (2007) *DM-ID: Diagnostic Manual – Intellectual Disability. A Textbook of Diagnosis of Mental Disorders in Persons with Intellectual Disability*. NADD Press.

Gleason MM, Fox NA, Drury S, *et al* (2011) Validity of evidence-derived criteria for reactive attachment disorder: indiscriminately social/disinhibited and emotionally withdrawn/inhibited types. *Journal of the American Academy of Child and Adolescent Psychiatry*, **50**: 216–31.

Goldbart J, Caton S (2010) *Communication and People with the Most Complex Needs: What Works and Why This Is Essential*. Available from http://www.mencap.org.uk/Communication_complex_needs (accessed November 2012).

Grey I, Pollard J, McClean B, *et al* (2010) Prevalence of psychiatric diagnoses and challenging behaviors in a community-based population of adults with intellectual disability. *Journal of Mental Health Research in Intellectual Disabilities*, **3**: 210–22.

Griffiths H, Halder N, Chaudhry N (2012) Antipsychotic prescribing in people with intellectual disabilities: a clinical audit. *Advances in Mental Health and Intellectual Disabilities*, **6**: 215–22.

Gunther N, Drukker M, Feron F, *et al* (2007) No ecological effect modification of the association between negative life experiences and later psychopathology in adolescence: a longitudinal community study in adolescents. *European Psychiatry*, **22**: 296–304.

Hare DJ, Malone C (2004) Catatonia and autistic spectrum disorders. *Autism*, **8**: 183–95.

Hart SL, Banda DR (2010) Picture exchange communication system with individuals with developmental disabilities: a meta-analysis of single subject studies. *Remedial and Special Education*, **31**: 476–88.

Hartley SL, MacLean WE Jr (2009) Stressful social interactions experienced by adults with mild intellectual disability. *American Journal on Intellectual and Developmental Disabilities*, **114**: 71–84.

Hatton C, Emerson E (2004) The relationship between life events and psychopathology amongst children with intellectual disabilities. *Journal of Applied Research in Intellectual Disabilities*, **17**: 109–17.

Healthcare Commission (2006) *Joint Investigation into the Provision of Services for People with Learning Disabilities at Cornwall Partnership NHS Trust*. Commission for Healthcare Audit and Inspection.

Hemmings CP, Tsakanikos E, Underwood L, *et al* (2008) Clinical predictors of severe behavioural problems in people with intellectual disabilities referred to a specialist mental health service. *Social Psychiatry and Psychiatric Epidemiology*, **43**: 824–30.

Hewett D (1998) *Challenging Behaviour: Principles and Practices*. D. Fulton.

Hewett D (ed) (2012) *Intensive Interaction: Theoretical Perspectives*. SAGE.

Hollins S (1989–2012) *Books Beyond Words – 40 Titles*. Available from http://www.booksbeyondwords.co.uk/welcome (accessed July 2012).

Hollins S (2003) *Books Beyond Words: Telling the Whole Story in Pictures @ Understanding Intellectual Disability and Health*. Available from http://www.intellectualdisability.info/how-to../books-beyond-words-telling-the-whole-story-in-pictures/?searchterm=books (accessed August 2012).

Hollins S, Esterhuyzen A (1997) Bereavement and grief in adults with learning disabilities. *British Journal of Psychiatry*, **170**: 497–501.

Hollins S, Sinason V (2000) Psychotherapy, learning disabilities and trauma: new perspectives. *British Journal of Psychiatry*, **176**: 32–6.

Hollins S, Attard MT, von Fraunhofer N, *et al* (1998) Mortality in people with learning disability: risks, causes, and death certification findings in London. *Developmental Medicine and Child Neurology*, **40**: 50–6.

Howie EK, Barnes TL, McDermott S, *et al* (2012) Availability of physical activity resources in the environment for adults with intellectual disabilities. *Disability and Health Journal*, **5**: 41–8.

Howlin P, Clements J (1995) Is it possible to assess the impact of abuse on children with pervasive developmental disorders. *Journal of Autism and Developmental Disorders*, **25**: 337–54.

Hubert J, Hollins S (2006) Men with severe learning disabilities and challenging behaviour in long-stay hospital care: qualitative study. *British Journal of Psychiatry*, **188**: 70–4.

Janssen CG, Schuengel C, Stolk J (2002) Understanding challenging behaviour in people with severe and profound intellectual disability: a stress–attachment model. *Journal of Intellectual Disability Research*, **46**: 445–53.

Jones S, Cooper SA, Smiley E, *et al* (2008) Prevalence of, and factors associated with, problem behaviors in adults with intellectual disabilities. *Journal of Nervous and Mental Disease*, **196**: 678–86.

Kasner M, Reid G, MacDonald C (2012) Evidence-based practice: quality indicator analysis of antecedent exercise in autism spectrum disorders. *Research in Autism Spectrum Disorders*, **6**: 1418–25.

Kastner T, Walsh KK, Fraser M (2001) Undiagnosed medical conditions and medication side effects presenting as behavioral/psychiatric problems in people with mental retardation. *Mental Health Aspects of Developmental Disabilities*, 4: 101–7.

Koritsas S, Iacono T (2012*a*) Challenging behaviour and associated risk factors: an overview (part I). *Advances in Mental Health and Intellectual Disabilities*, 6: 199–214.

Koritsas S, Iacono T (2012*b*) Challenging behaviour: the causes (part II). *Advances in Mental Health and Intellectual Disabilities*, 6: 236–48.

Kurtz PF, Boelter EW, Jarmolowicz DP, *et al* (2011) An analysis of functional communication training as an empirically supported treatment for problem behavior displayed by individuals with intellectual disabilities. *Research in Developmental Disabilities*, 32: 2935–42.

Kwok H, Cheung PW (2007) Co-morbidity of psychiatric disorder and medical illness in people with intellectual disabilities. *Current Opinion in Psychiatry*, 20: 443–9.

Kyle S, Melville CA, Jones A (2010) Effective communication training interventions for paid carers supporting adults with learning disabilities. *British Journal of Learning Disabilities*, 38: 210–16.

Lake JK, Balogh R, Lunsky Y (2012) Polypharmacy profiles and predictors among adults with autism spectrum disorders. *Research in Autism Spectrum Disorders*, 6: 1142–9.

Lang R, Koegel LK, Ashbaugh K, *et al* (2010) Physical exercise and individuals with autism spectrum disorders: a systematic review. *Research in Autism Spectrum Disorders*, 4: 565–76.

Langthorne P, McGill P (2012) An indirect examination of the function of problem behavior associated with fragile X syndrome and Smith–Magenis syndrome. *Journal of Autism and Developmental Disorders*, 42: 201–9.

Larson FV, Alim N, Tsakanikos E (2011) Attachment style and mental health in adults with intellectual disability: self-reports and reports by carers. *Advances in Mental Health and Intellectual Disabilities*, 5: 15–23.

Lehotkay R, Varisco S, Deriaz N, *et al* (2009) Intellectual disability and psychiatric disorder: more than a dual diagnosis. *Schweizer Archiv für Neurologie und Psychiatrie*, 160: 105–15.

Lennox N, Developmental Disability Steering Group (2005) *Management Guidelines: Developmental Disability* (version 2 edn). Therapeutic Guidelines.

Lennox N, Ware R, Bain C, *et al* (2011) Effects of health screening for adults with intellectual disability: a pooled analysis. *British Journal of General Practice*, 61: 193–6.

Levitas AS, Gilson SF (2001) Predictable crises in the lives of people with mental retardation. *Mental Health Aspects of Developmental Disabilities*, 4: 89–100.

Leyfer OT, Folstein SE, Bacalman S, *et al* (2006) Comorbid psychiatric disorders in children with autism: interview development and rates of disorders. *Journal of Autism and Developmental Disorders*, 36: 849–61.

Loos HG, Loos Miller IM (2004) Shutdown states and stress instability in autism. Available from http://www.de-poort.be/cgi-bin/Document.pl?id=374 (accessed May 2015).

Loos Miller IM, Loos HG (2004) *Shutdowns and Stress in Autism*. Available from http://autismawarenesscentre.com/shutdowns-stress-autism (accessed December 1 2011).

Lopez-Rangel E, Mickelson ECR, Lewis MES (2008) The value of a genetic diagnosis for individuals with intellectual disabilities: optimising healthcare and function across the lifespan. *British Journal of Developmental Disabilities*, 54: 69–82.

Lovallo WR, Thomas TL (2000) Stress hormones in psychophysiological research. In *Handbook of Psychophysiology* (2nd edn) (eds JT Cacioppo, LG Tassinary, GG Berntson), pp. 342–67. Cambridge University Press.

Lunsky Y, Benson BA (2001) Association between perceived social support and strain, and positive and negative outcome for adults with mild intellectual disability. *Journal of Intellectual Disability Research*, 45: 106–14.

Lunsky Y, Elserafi J (2011) Life events and emergency department visits in response to crisis in individuals with intellectual disabilities. *Journal of Intellectual Disability Research*, 55: 714–18.

Lunsky Y, Elserafi J (2012) Antipsychotic medication prescription patterns in adults with developmental disabilities who have experienced psychiatric crisis. *Research in Developmental Disabilities*, **33**: 32–8.

Lunsky Y, Gracey C (2009) The reported experience of four women with intellectual disabilities receiving emergency psychiatric services in Canada: a qualitative study. *Journal of Intellectual Disabilities*, **13**: 87–98.

Lunsky Y, Gracey C, Gelfand S (2008) Emergency psychiatric services for individuals with intellectual disabilities: perspectives of hospital staff. *Intellectual and Developmental Disabilities*, **46**: 446–55.

Macklin ML, Metzger LJ, McNally RJ, *et al* (1998) Lower precombat intelligence is a risk factor for posttraumatic stress disorder. *Journal of Consulting and Clinical Psychology*, **66**: 323–6.

Mancil GR (2006) Functional communication training: a review of the literature related to children with autism. *Education and Training in Developmental Disabilities*, **41**: 213–24.

Mansell J (1993) *Services for People with Learning Disabilities and Challenging Behaviour or Mental Health Needs: Report of a Project Group*. HMSO.

Mansell J (2012) *Active Support: Enabling and Empowering People with Intellectual Disabilities*. Jessica Kingsley.

Marks B, Sisirak J, Heller T (2010) *Health Matters: The Exercise, Nutrition, and Health Education Curriculum for People with Developmental Disabilities* (CD-ROM with instructor references and participant handouts edn). Paul H Brookes.

Martorell A, Tsakanikos E (2008) Traumatic experiences and life events in people with intellectual disability. *Current Opinion in Psychiatry*, **21**: 445–8.

Maslow AH (1954) *Motivation and Personality* (1st edn). Harper.

Matson JL, Dempsey T (2008) Autism spectrum disorders: pharmacotherapy for challenging behaviors. *Journal of Developmental and Physical Disabilities*, **20**: 175–91.

Matson JL, Hess JA (2011) Psychotropic drug efficacy and side effects for persons with autism spectrum disorders. *Research in Autism Spectrum Disorders*, **5**: 230–6.

Matson JL, Neal D (2009) Psychotropic medication use for challenging behaviors in persons with intellectual disabilities: an overview. *Research in Developmental Disabilities*, **30**: 572–86.

Matson JL, Kozlowski AM, Worley JA, *et al* (2011) What is the evidence for environmental causes of challenging behaviors in persons with intellectual disabilities and autism spectrum disorders? *Research in Developmental Disabilities*, **32**: 693–8.

Matson JL, Hess JA, Mahan S (2013) Moderating effects of challenging behaviors and communication deficits on social skills in children diagnosed with an autism spectrum disorder. *Research in Autism Spectrum Disorders*, **7**: 23–8.

McCarthy J, O'Hara J (2011) Ill-health and intellectual disabilities. *Current Opinion in Psychiatry*, **24**: 382–6.

McCarthy J, Hemmings C, Kravariti E, *et al* (2010) Challenging behavior and co-morbid psychopathology in adults with intellectual disability and autism spectrum disorders. *Research in Developmental Disabilities*, **31**: 362–6.

McConkey R, Morris I, Purcell M (1999) Communications between staff and adults with intellectual disabilities in naturally occurring settings. *Journal of Intellectual Disability Research*, **43**(3): 194–205.

McDermott S, Moran RR, Platt T (2008) *The Epidemiology of Common Health Conditions Among Adults with Developmental Disabilities in Primary Care*. Nova Biomedical Books.

McDonnell AM (2010) *Managing Aggressive Behaviour in Care Settings: Understanding and Applying Low Arousal Approaches*. John Wiley.

McDonnell AM, Sturmey P, Oliver C, *et al* (2008) The effects of staff training on staff confidence and challenging behavior in services for people with autism spectrum disorders. *Research in Autism Spectrum Disorders*, **2**: 311–19.

Melville CA, Cooper SA, Morrison J, *et al* (2008) The prevalence and incidence of mental ill-health in adults with autism and intellectual disabilities. *Journal of Autism and Developmental Disorders*, **38**: 1676–88.

Mevissen L, Lievegoed R, de Jongh A (2010) EMDR treatment in people with mild ID and PTSD: 4 cases. *Psychiatric Quarterly*, **82**: 1–15.

Miller SM, Chan F (2008) Predictors of life satisfaction in individuals with intellectual disabilities. *Journal of Intellectual Disability Research*, **52**: 1039–47.

Minnis H, Fleming G, Cooper SA (2010) Reactive attachment disorder symptoms in adults with intellectual disabilities. *Journal of Applied Research in Intellectual Disabilities*, **23**: 398–403.

Myers R (2010) *Recognizing Psychosis in Persons with Intellectual Disabilities Who Do Not Use Speech*. Available from http://www.intellectualdisability.info/diagnosis/recognizing-psychosis-in-nonverbal-patients-with-developmental-disabilities?searchterm=psychosis (accessed March 2013).

Nind M (2006) Stereotyped behaviour: resistance by people with profound learning disabilities. In *Exploring Experiences of Advocacy by People with Learning Disabilities: Testimonies of Resistance* (ed D Mitchell), pp.. 202–11. Jessica Kingsley.

Nind M (2012) Intensive interaction, emotional development and emotional well-being, In *Intensive Interaction: Theoretical Perspectives* (ed D Hewett), pp. 22–39. SAGE.

Nind M, Hewett D (2005) *Access to Communication: Developing the Basics of Communication with People with Severe Learning Difficulties through Intensive Interaction*. D. Fulton.

Nind M, Kellett M (2002) Responding to individuals with severe learning difficulties and stereotyped behaviour: challenges for an inclusive era. *European Journal of Special Needs Education*, **17**: 265–82.

Noone SJ, Hastings RP (2010) Using acceptance and mindfulness-based workshops with support staff caring for adults with intellectual disabilities. *Mindfulness*, **1**: 67–73.

Oberlander TF, Symons FJ (2006) An introduction to the problem of pain in developmental disability. In *Pain in Children and Adults with Developmental Disabilities*. (eds TF Oberlander, FJ Symons), pp. 1–4. Paul H. Brookes.

O'Hara J, McCarthy JM, Bouras N (2010) *Intellectual Disability and Ill Health: A Review of the Evidence*. Cambridge University Press.

Oliver C, Davies L, Richards C (2013) *Self-injurious Behaviour in Children with Intellectual Disability*. Cerebra Centre for Neurodevelopmental Disorders, University of Birmingham. Available from http://w3.cerebra.org.uk/research/research-papers/self-injurious-behaviour-in-children-with-intellectual-disability (accessed May 2015).

Ouellette-Kuntz H (2005) Understanding health disparities and inequities faced by individuals with intellectual disabilities. *Journal of Applied Research in Intellectual Disabilities*, **18**: 113–21.

Paton C, Flynn A, Shingleton-Smith A, *et al* (2011) Nature and quality of antipsychotic prescribing practice in UK psychiatry of intellectual disability services. *Journal of Intellectual Disability Research*, **55**:, 665–74.

Peckham NG, Howlett S, Corbett A (2007) Evaluating a survivors group pilot for women with significant intellectual disabilities who have been sexually abused. *Journal of Applied Research in Intellectual Disabilities*, **20**: 308–22.

Peebles KA, Price TJ (2012) Self-injurious behaviour in intellectual disability syndromes: evidence for aberrant pain signalling as a contributing factor. *Journal of Intellectual Disability Research*, **56**: 441–52.

Phillips N, Rose J (2010) Predicting placement breakdown: individual and environmental factors associated with the success or failure of community residential placements for adults with intellectual disabilities. *Journal of Applied Research in Intellectual Disabilities*, **23**: 201–13.

Poppes P, van der Putten AJ, Vlaskamp C (2010) Frequency and severity of challenging behaviour in people with profound intellectual and multiple disabilities. *Research in Developmental Disabilities*, **31**: 1269–75.

Porges SW (2011) *The Polyvagal Theory: Neurophysiological Foundations of Emotions, Attachment, Communication, and Self-Regulation*. WW Norton.

Preston D, Carter M (2009) A review of the efficacy of the picture exchange communication system intervention. *Journal of Autism and Developmental Disorders*, **39**: 1471–86.

Ratey JJ, Mikkelsen E, Sorgi P, *et al* (1987) Autism: the treatment of aggressive behaviors. *Journal of Clinical Psychopharmacology*, **7**: 35–41.

Reiss S, Aman MG (1998) *Psychotropic Medications and Developmental Disabilities: The International Consensus Handbook*. Ohio State University Nisonger Center.

Reiter S, Bryen DN, Shachar I (2007) Adolescents with intellectual disabilities as victims of abuse. *Journal of Intellectual Disabilities*, **11**: 371–87.

Richards C, Oliver C, Nelson L, *et al* (2012) Self-injurious behaviour in individuals with autism spectrum disorder and intellectual disability. *Journal of Intellectual Disability Research*, **56**: 476–89.

Rimmer JH, Chen MD, McCubbin JA, *et al* (2010) Exercise intervention research on persons with disabilities: what we know and where we need to go. *American Journal of Physical Medicine and Rehabilitation*, **89**: 249–63.

Rivera G (1972) *Willowbrook: The Last Great Disgrace*. WABC-TV, New York, USA. Available from http://www.ovguide.com/willowbrook-the-last-great-disgrace-9202a8c04000641f800000000ba061e6 (accessed December 2012).

Rojahn J, Wilkins J, Matson JL, *et al* (2010) A comparison of adults with intellectual disabilities with and without ASD on parallel measures of challenging behaviour: the Behavior Problems Inventory-01 (BPI-01) and Autism Spectrum Disorders–Behavior Problems for intellectually disabled adults (ASD-BPA). *Journal of Applied Research in Intellectual Disabilities*, **23**: 179–85.

Rojahn J, Zaja RH, Turygin N, *et al* (2012) Functions of maladaptive behavior in intellectual and developmental disabilities: behavior categories and topographies. *Research in Developmental Disabilities*, **33**: 2020–7.

Rose J (2011) How do staff psychological factors influence outcomes for people with developmental and intellectual disability in residential services? *Current Opinion in Psychiatry*, **24**: 403–7.

Royal College of Psychiatrists (2001) *DC-LD: Diagnostic Criteria for Psychiatric Disorders for Use with Adults with Learning Disabilities/Mental Retardation*. Gaskell.

Rush AJ, Frances A (2000) Expert consensus guideline series: treatment of psychiatric and behavioral problems in mental retardation. *American Journal on Mental Retardation*, **105**: 165–88.

Ryan R, Sunada K (1997) Medical evaluation of persons with mental retardation referred for psychiatric assessment. *General Hospital Psychiatry*, **19**: 274–80.

Rzepecka H, Mckenzie K, McClure I, *et al* (2011) Sleep, anxiety and challenging behaviour in children with intellectual disability and/or autism spectrum disorder. *Research in Developmental Disabilities*, **32**: 2758–66.

Schore AN (2003) *Affect Regulation and the Repair of the Self*. WW Norton.

Schuengel C, Oosterman M, Sterkenburg PS (2009*a*) Children with disrupted attachment histories: interventions and psychophysiological indices of effects. *Child and Adolescent Psychiatry and Mental Health*, **3**: 26. Also available from http://www.ncbi.nlm.nih.gov/pmc/articles/PMC2749813/pdf/1753-2000-3-26.pdf (accessed April 2015).

Schuengel C, Sterkenburg PS, Jeczynski P, *et al* (2009*b*) Supporting affect regulation in children with multiple disabilities during psychotherapy: a multiple case design study of therapeutic attachment. *Journal of Consulting and Clinical Psychology*, **77**: 291–301.

Schuengel C, de Schipper JC, Sterkenburg PS, *et al* (2013) Attachment, intellectual disabilities and mental health: research, assessment and intervention. *Journal of Applied Research in Intellectual Disabilities*, **26**: 34–46.

Singh NN, Lancioni GE, Winton ASW, *et al* (2009) Mindful staff can reduce the use of physical restraints when providing care to individuals with intellectual disabilities. *Journal of Applied Research in Intellectual Disabilities*, **22**: 194–202.

Smidt A, Balandin S, Reed V, *et al* (2007) A communication training programme for residential staff working with adults with challenging behaviour: pilot data on intervention effects. *Journal of Applied Research in Intellectual Disabilities*, **20**: 16–29.

Smiley E, Cooper SA, Finlayson J, *et al* (2007) Incidence and predictors of mental ill-health in adults with intellectual disabilities. Prospective study. *British Journal of Psychiatry*, **191**: 313–19.

Sterkenburg PS (2008) *Intervening in Stress, Attachment and Challenging Behaviour: Effects in Children with Multiple Disabilities*. Available from http://dare.ubvu.vu.nl/bitstream/handle/1871/15813/8494.pdf?sequence=5 (accessed January 2013).

Sterkenburg PS, IJzerman J (2007) *Attachment: A Psychotherapeutic Treatment* [DVD; Guidebook]. Bartimeus Reeks.

Stores G, Wiggs L (2001) *Sleep Disturbance in Children and Adolescents with Disorders of Development: Its Significance and Management*. MacKeith.

Sullivan WF, Berg JM, Bradley E, *et al* (2011) Primary care of adults with developmental disabilities: Canadian consensus guidelines. *Canadian Family Physician*, **57**: 541–53, e154–68.

Summers J, Boyd K, Reid J, *et al* (2002) The interdisciplinary mental health team. In *Dual Diagnosis: An Introduction to the Mental Health Needs of Persons with Developmental Disabilities* (eds DM Griffiths, C Stavrakaki, J Summers), pp. 325–57. Habilitative Mental Health Resource Network. Also available at http://www.naddontario.net/pdf/EnglishPublication/Chapter10.pdf (accessed November 2013).

Symons FJ (2011) Self-injurious behavior in neurodevelopmental disorders: relevance of nociceptive and immune mechanisms. *Neuroscience and Biobehavioral Reviews*, **35**: 1266–74.

Symons FJ, Harper VN, McGrath PJ, *et al* (2009) Evidence of increased non-verbal behavioral signs of pain in adults with neurodevelopmental disorders and chronic self-injury. *Research in Developmental Disabilities*, **30**: 521–8.

Tasse MJ (2006) Functional behavioural assessment in people with intellectual disabilities. *Current Opinion in Psychiatry*, **19**: 475–80.

Thakker Y, Bamidele K, Ali A, *et al* (2012) Mental health and challenging behaviour: an overview of research and practice. *Advances in Mental Health and Intellectual Disabilities*, **6**: 249–57.

Thomas C, Rose J (2010) The relationship between reciprocity and the emotional and behavioural responses of staff. *Journal of Applied Research in Intellectual Disabilities*, **23**: 167–78.

Totsika V, Hastings RP (2009) Persistent challenging behaviour in people with an intellectual disability. *Current Opinion in Psychiatry*, **22**: 437–41.

Tsakanikos E, Costello H, Holt G, *et al* (2006) Psychopathology in adults with autism and intellectual disability. *Journal of Autism and Developmental Disorders*, **36**: 1123–9.

Tsiouris JA (2010) Pharmacotherapy for aggressive behaviours in persons with intellectual disabilities: treatment or mistreatment? *Journal of Intellectual Disability Research*, **54**: 1–16.

Tully J, Schirliu D, Moran M (2012) Application of DC-LD to an intellectual disability population. *Advances in Mental Health and Intellectual Disabilities*, **6**: 259–64.

Tyrer P, Oliver-Africano PC, Ahmed Z, *et al* (2008) Risperidone, haloperidol, and placebo in the treatment of aggressive challenging behaviour in patients with intellectual disability: a randomised controlled trial. *Lancet*, **371**: 57–63.

Van de Wouw E, Evenhuis HM, Echteld MA (2012) Prevalence, associated factors and treatment of sleep problems in adults with intellectual disability: a systematic review. *Research in Developmental Disabilities*, **33**: 1310–32.

van Ijzendoorn MH, Goldberg S, Kroonenberg PM, *et al* (1992) The relative effects of maternal and child problems on the quality of attachment: a meta-analysis of attachment in clinical samples. *Child Development*, **63**: 840–58.

Verhoeven WM, Tuinier S (1996) The effect of buspirone on challenging behaviour in mentally retarded patients: an open prospective multiple-case study. *Journal of Intellectual Disability Research*, **40**: 502–8.

Weiss JA, Lunsky Y, Gracey C, *et al* (2009) Emergency psychiatric services for individuals with intellectual disabilities: Caregivers' perspectives. *Journal of Applied Research in Intellectual Disabilities*, **22**: 354–62.

Whitaker S, Read S (2006) The prevalence of psychiatric disorders among people with intellectual disabilities: an analysis of the literature. *Journal of Applied Research in Intellectual Disabilities*, **19**: 330–45.

Willemsen-Swinkels S, Bakermans-Kranenburg M, Buitelaar JK, *et al* (2000) Insecure and disorganised attachment in children with a pervasive developmental disorder: relationship with social interaction and heart rate. *Journal of Child Psychology and Psychiatry and Allied Disciplines*, **41**: 759–67.

Wing L (1989) *Hospital Closure and the Resettlement of Residents: The Case of Darenth Park Mental Handicap Hospital*. Avebury.

Wing L, Shah A (2000) Catatonia in autistic spectrum disorders. *British Journal of Psychiatry*, **176**: 357–62.

Woodcock L, Page A (2010) *Managing Family Meltdown: The Low Arousal Approach and Autism*. Jessica Kingsley.

World Health Organization (1992) *International Statistical Classification of Diseases and Related Health Problems* (10th revision) (ICD-10). WHO.

Zeedyk MS, Caldwell P, Davies CE (2009) How rapidly does intensive interaction promote social engagement for adults with profound learning disabilities? *European Journal of Special Needs Education*, **24**: 119–37.

CHAPTER 6

Epilepsy

Marc Woodbury-Smith and Howard Ring

Epilepsy is a common, often chronic neuropsychiatric disorder that sits firmly between the disciplines of neurology and psychiatry. A detailed lexicon has evolved to capture the phenomenology of seizures, and there is increasing understanding of the complex relationship between seizures and associated psychological and behavioural manifestations, as well as frank psychiatric comorbidity. This has facilitated their earlier management. Moreover, research has continued to make significant progress in identifying genetic and metabolic factors that contribute to the aetiology of epilepsy.

Epilepsy is notably more prevalent among individuals with disorders of intellectual development (DID). Disproportionate severity in all the neuropsychiatric characteristics of epilepsy, compounded by unique challenges in diagnosis and management, occur in this population. In this chapter, those aspects of epilepsy that are most relevant to this population will be discussed.

Epidemiology

Epilepsy is a common neuropsychiatric disorder characterised by episodic disturbances of consciousness, sensorimotor function, behaviour and emotion resulting from paroxysmal abnormalities of the electrical activity of the brain. While the seizure itself is described by the symptomatic disturbance, the term 'epilepsy' is used when seizures become recurrent, more specifically when there are two unprovoked seizures more than 24 hours apart. The prevalence of epilepsy in the general population is 0.5–1.0% (Banerjee et al, 2009), and the lifetime prevalence is 1.5–5.0%. Among those with DID, however, this prevalence is increased several-fold. For example, among those with severe DID (IQ<50), a prevalence of 30% has been reported, and even among those with milder DID (IQ≥50), the prevalence is still relatively high, at 15% or more (Hannah & Brodie, 1998; Lhatoo & Sander, 2001; McGrother et al, 2006). The risk appears to be higher among those with additional neurological diagnoses, such as cerebral palsy (Singhi et al, 2003), and among those with autism spectrum disorder (ASD) (Spence & Schneider, 2009). As will be discussed below, the prevalence is also higher in association with particular genetic intellectual disability syndromes. Also of note is that the prevalence of the psychological, behavioural and psychiatric manifestations associated with epilepsy are more frequent among those with DID. There is very little difference in prevalence according to gender, and little bias in prevalence is seen according to class, ethnicity or geographical location (Banerjee *et al*, 2009).

Classification

The consensus classification of the International League Against Epilepsy (ILAE) published in 1981 and 1989 continues to be used to this day (Fisher *et al*, 2005), although new recommendations have recently been made to modify existing terms and concepts to incorporate the vast advances that have been made in neurobiology in recent decades (Berg & Scheffer, 2011). The system in current use is set out in Box 6.1. In short, seizures are classified according to whether the onset is localised to a specific hemisphere (focal, also termed partial), arises within bilateral networks (generalised), or is unclassifiable in such terms (unclassifiable). Generalised seizures are further classified according to their motor manifestations (as summarised in Box 6.1), while focal seizures are classified according to whether there is loss of consciousness (complex focal) or not (simple focal). It has been suggested by the ILAE, though at the time of writing this remains a matter of debate, that this distinction of simple versus complex is artificial, and rather than being divided as such, focal seizures should instead be described according to the exact manifestation (in terms of the nature of the aura, sensorimotor manifestations and so forth). Similarly, suggestions have been put forward to attempt to better describe the aetiology of the seizure disorder in genetic and structural–metabolic terms, taking advantage of the unprecedented advances in scientific discovery (classification is discussed further by Berg & Scheffer, 2011).

Box 6.1 Outline of the International League Against Epilepsy (ILAE) classification of epilepsy

Generalised epilepsies
- Tonic–clonic
- Atonic
- Absence
- Tonic
- Clonic
- Myoclonic

Focal (partial) epilepsies
- Simple
- Complex

Unclassifiable

Aetiology

The causes of seizures are many and varied, and are summarised in Box 6.2. In early life, factors such as birth injury and anoxia, infections and metabolic disturbance (e.g. hypoglycaemia, hypocalcaemia or hyponatraemia) may all result in seizures. Through childhood, infections and head trauma are the

---

Box 6.2 Aetiology of seizures

Genetic
- Mendelian/single-gene disorders
  - fragile-X syndrome
  - Angelman syndrome
  - Down syndrome
  - tuberous sclerosis
  - Rett syndrome
- Polygenic:
  - microdeletions of 16p11

Perinatal brain injury
- Birth trauma

Infections
- Prenatal: toxoplasmosis, cytomegalovirus
- Postnatal: viral encephalitis, meningitis

Other developmental
- Cerebral palsy
- Autism spectrum disorder

Space-occupying lesions
- Hydrocephalus
- Tumour

Metabolic:
- Uraemia
- Hypoglycaemia
- Hypocalcaemia

Drug-related
- Alcohol withdrawal
- Benzodiazepine withdrawal
- Antipsychotics

Neurodegenerative
- Alzheimer's disease

Specific epilepsy syndromes
- West syndrome
- Lennox–Gastaut syndrome

---

commonest causes of seizures. In adulthood, the new onset of seizures raises the suspicion of a tumour or neurodegenerative disorder. In later life, seizures are most commonly seen in association with neurodegenerative disorders or cerebrovascular disease.

In recent years, the focus has been on elucidating the genetic risk factors underlying epilepsy. Twin studies have shown concordance rates of 50–60% in monozygotic twins and 15% in dizygotic twins (Berkovic *et al*, 1998), translating into heritability of approximately 53%. Certain Mendelian disorders are associated with both DID and epilepsy, and such associations continue to be identified in the scientific literature. However, individually and collectively rare, these disorders will account for only a small proportion of epilepsy's genetic aetiology.

The explosion of genetic studies secondary to the increased availability of affordable high-throughput technologies has identified new mutations that confer susceptibility to particular genetic syndromes. Most mutations uncovered so far occur in genes encoding ion channels, the so-called 'channelopathies', and most are inherited in an autosomal dominant fashion (Pandolfo, 2011). Mutations in the voltage-gated K-channel resulting in benign familial neonatal seizures are an example. Other Mendelian inherited genetic abnormalities can result in progressive myoclonic forms of epilepsy, such as the neuronal ceroid lipofuscinoses.

In contrast to the association between epilepsy and rare Mendelian forms of DID, identifying polygenic risk factors in the general population has met with limited success. In short, no specific 'common genetic variants' of epilepsy have been identified consistently, although specific forms of epilepsy have been found to be associated with particular single-nucleotide polymorphisms (SNPs) (e.g. juvenile myoclonic epilepsy and the BRD2 gene – see Pal *et al*, 2003). The more recent recognition that copy number variants (CNVs) are important in human phenotypic variability has led to further investigation of the association of CNVs with complex diseases. Although individually rare, collectively these microduplications and deletions may begin to explain a growing proportion of epilepsy's 'missing' genetic aetiology (see e.g. Helbig *et al*, 2009; Striano *et al*, 2012).

The specific association between DID and epilepsy

The specific association between DID and epilepsy can be understood in terms of the aetiological factors set out above. In addition, epilepsy is also a characteristic of certain genetic DID syndromes. For example, seizures occur in 80% or more of individuals with tuberous sclerosis and Sturge–Weber syndrome, and 25% of people with fragile-X syndrome also have epilepsy. Epilepsy also occurs in Down syndrome, with a bimodal age of onset clustered around childhood and during the middle years. The later peak represents the neurodegenerative aspect of the disorder. In terms of seizure morphology, no specific type of seizure seems to be associated with any one syndrome, with the exception of late-onset myoclonic epilepsy in Down syndrome (De Simone *et al*, 2010).

Autism spectrum disorder (ASD, described in Chapter 8) is also associated with both DID and epilepsy, and the conjunction of ASD and epilepsy is relatively common. Between 15% and 20% of individuals with classically defined ASD also have epilepsy (Fombonne, 1999), although different studies have reported prevalence rates as low as 5% and as high as 40%, depending on the sample considered. A meta-analysis revealed that the prevalence of epilepsy was 21.5% in those who had ASD together with DID, compared with 8% in those without DID (Amiet *et al*, 2008).

It has been reported that ASD as it occurs in people with epilepsy is associated with earlier age at first recognition, high rates of repetitive object use, unusual sensory interests and clumsiness (Turk *et al*, 2009; Cuccaro *et al*, 2012). All seizure types have been described in association with ASD (for reviews of epilepsy in association with ASD see e.g. Tuchman & Rapin, 2002; Filipek, 2005), with the most commonly observed including focal seizures with altered awareness, atypical absences and generalised tonic–clonic seizures. In relation to the management of seizures in ASD, there is no evidence of different patterns of epilepsy's responsiveness to anti-epileptic agents compared with epilepsy without ASD. Possible aetiological mechanisms linking ASD and epilepsy have to be defined, although, in general terms, Brooks-Kayal (2010), reviewing the topic, suggested that involved processes may include abnormal neuronal excitability with disrupted synaptic plasticity and impaired integration and control of neural activity in circuits across the cortex.

Neuropsychiatric manifestations of epilepsy

Mood disorders

Estimates of the prevalence rates of depressive disorder among individuals with epilepsy vary considerably. For example, among the larger community-based studies, rates of between 13% and 26% are reported (Hoppe & Elger, 2011). In contrast, in highly selected groups attending a tertiary clinic, the rate has been reported to be nearer 50% (Hoppe & Elger, 2011). In the general population, the 12-month prevalence rate is 12% in the USA, and somewhat lower in other Western countries, indicating that the rates among those with epilepsy are higher than in the general population. Such differences are not well understood, but over and above the background risk factors, a number of different biological (neurotransmitter abnormalities), psychological (coping with chronic illness) and social factors (stigmatisation, impact on employment and independence) are likely to play their respective roles (Mula & Schmitz, 2009; Hoppe & Elger, 2011).

Psychosis

Psychosis is reported more frequently in people with epilepsy than in the general population (for a review see Toone, 2000). Individuals with epilepsy who experience psychotic symptoms include those whose symptoms are transient, and appear in close association with their seizures, either ictally or post-ictally, and those whose seizures have no such relationship, and whose psychotic symptoms occur inter-ictally. Further, among some individuals the psychotic symptoms are chronic in nature, and are consistent with a diagnosis of schizophrenia (for a more detailed discussion see Toone, 2000). Clinical studies over the years have highlighted a tendency for more preservation of affect in epileptic psychoses than is often the case in schizophrenia. The interaction between family history of psychosis as a risk factor for post-ictal psychosis is complex, with, for instance, Adachi et al (2012) reporting that those with a family history are more likely to have a longer duration of post-ictal psychotic episodes, while in an earlier paper Adachi and colleagues reported that the presence of a family history of psychosis predicted an increased risk of inter-ictal psychosis (Adachi et al, 2000).

The most common phenomenon seen is post-ictal psychosis, which itself occurs most commonly among those with focal (partial) seizures. For example, post-ictal psychosis is seen among 7% of individuals with a diagnosis of temporal lobe epilepsy (Cleary et al, 2013). The psychotic symptoms are usually florid, including a combination of delusions, which may be persecutory or grandiose in nature, and the onset is often after a cluster of particularly severe seizures. Affective symptoms such as elevated mood are common, as are 'organic' symptoms, such as altered level of consciousness (see Kanemoto et al, 1996). The symptoms are generally relatively short-lived, lasting from hours or days, and in the great majority of cases will have resolved within a month. They generally resolve gradually and spontaneously. In some circumstances medication may be required, however, which could include benzodiazepines to help reduce levels of agitated behaviour, or antipsychotics if florid psychotic symptoms require amelioration. Importantly, depending on the antipsychotic selected, the potential lowering of the seizure threshold needs to be considered. However, although clozapine, for example, is known to lower the seizure threshold, an increase in seizure frequency is not necessarily seen in clinical practice (Langosch & Trimble, 2002). Therefore, treatment decisions need to weigh risk against the morbidity of failing to treat the psychosis. Some individuals experience recurrent post-ictal psychosis, and a relatively small proportion of patients experience both post-ictal and inter-ictal psychoses (Adachi et al, 2002).

Ictal psychosis has also been described, occurring in the context of a non-convulsive status lasting several hours or even, in some cases, several days (Mula & Monaco, 2011). However, the exact prevalence of this phenomenon has not been well described. The symptoms are generally organic in nature, and include, for example, automatisms, simple repetitive movements and altered level of consciousness and responsiveness of fluctuating severity.

Temporal lobe non-convulsive status epilepticus has been associated with episodes of ictal psychosis lasting for hours to days and occasionally longer. An electroencephalogram (EEG) is usually diagnostic in cases of ictal psychosis, and treatment should be aimed at the underlying seizure (Mula & Monaco, 2011). However, it is an uncommon diagnosis and the frequency with which such diagnoses are missed is unknown.

In inter-ictal psychosis the onset of the psychotic symptoms is not directly related to the occurrence of seizures, and when chronic, the symptoms themselves are often indistinguishable phenomenologically from schizophrenia. As such, the common presentation is with first-rank paranoid-hallucinatory symptoms, including formal thought disorder, although affect is generally preserved. Studies have generally described little differentiation from schizophrenia in the absence of epilepsy, although negative symptoms are uncommonly reported in the epilepsy group. Although it is generally believed that the course is more benign than schizophrenia in the absence of epilepsy, at least two studies have indicated that in approximately two-thirds of cases the course is chronic, similar to figures for schizophrenia more generally. In perhaps the largest population-based cohort study of inter-ictal psychosis in epilepsy, a median relative risk of 2.48 was found for schizophrenia in epilepsy compared with the general population (Qin et al, 2005). There was no sex bias in prevalence and the risk increased with age. Family history of psychosis increased significantly the risk for schizophrenia in epilepsy, while a family history of epilepsy also increased the risk, but only marginally so.

The aetiology of psychotic symptoms in association with epilepsy is not well understood, particularly for the chronic inter-ictal cases. The concept of 'forced normalisation' needs special attention in this regard. Landolt first described a group of patients among whom an improvement in their seizure control, as evidenced by clinical symptoms and normalisation of their EEGs, was associated with a deterioration of their mental well-being, with the onset of frank psychotic symptoms. This concept has continued to receive attention since, and among a number of individuals with epilepsy such an association appears to be present, independent of any psychotic symptoms that may be precipitated by anti-epileptic medication. Moreover, this association does appear to be more common among both those with a severe seizure disorder and those with an associated DID (for a more detailed discussion see Krishnamoorthy et al, 2002). It is also worth noting that not just features of psychosis but also affective symptoms and behavioural disturbances may be manifest in the context of a period of relative reduction or complete absence of seizures, remitting when regular seizures re-establish themselves. These sequences of events may occur spontaneously but have also been reported to occur in conjunction with the development of improved seizure control associated with an anti-epileptic drug or surgical intervention.

Immune-mediated epilepsy syndromes may also be associated with psychiatric and behavioural manifestations. The concept of antibody-mediated disorders of the central nervous system is a recent development, with the identification of autoimmune forms of encephalitis with antibodies directed against, for example, voltage-gated potassium channels (VGKC) (McKnight *et al*, 2005) or the N-methyl-D-aspartate (NMDA) glutamate receptor (Wandinger *et al*, 2011). Such disorders may have seizure and other neuropsychiatric manifestations, and in general the treatment is likely to be very different from traditional anti-epileptic or antipsychotic medications. To date, both anti-VGKC and anti-NMDA syndromes have both been described, and both have cognitive, seizure, psychiatric and behavioural manifestations. In addition, seizures are a well recognised feature of systemic lupus erythematosus and may be the presenting feature of cerebral involvement in that condition.

Behaviour disorders

Challenging behaviours, defined as behaviours that challenge the delivery of care (see e.g. Emerson, 2001; Banks *et al*, 2007), are commonly described in individuals with DID. Although the frequency and nature of behavioural disorders in DID does not seem to be increased among those with associated seizure disorders, a number of epilepsy-related factors have been linked to increased rates of behavioural disturbance. These factors include high seizure frequency, presence of tonic–clonic seizures, and polypharmacy (Kerr *et al*, 2013). These factors represent potentially modifiable risk factors for behaviour disorders in this population and therefore demand special attention.

Anti-epileptic medication can also result in behavioural disturbance. In particular, a number of anti-epileptics, such as vigabatrin and levetiracetam, have been reported to result in agitation, aggression and mood changes. However, the quality of the published literature concerning such associations has been questioned (Besag, 2001). Individuals with DID appear to be more susceptible to the adverse behavioural effects of anti-epileptic medication, implying that clinicians should place particular emphasis on warning patients, parents and carers to report these promptly.

Behavioural changes may be coincidental and unrelated to the seizures. Of note, a number of genetic syndromes associated with both epilepsy and DID are also associated with specific patterns of behaviour. Cornelia da Lange syndrome, which is associated with self-injurious behavior, is one such example from among many well characterised 'behavioural phenotypes' (see e.g. Finegan, 1998; and see Chapter 2 of the present volume for a discussion of behavioural phenotypes).

Cognitive function

The emphasis, so far, has been on epilepsy and global intellectual disability. However, there is also evidence of a specific association between certain epilepsy syndromes and more specific cognitive abnormalities. The relationship is complex, and many factors are relevant. Information processing is directly impacted during the ictal and immediate post-ictal phases of a seizure, but evidence suggests that even 30 days beyond a seizure residual cognitive impairments may exist (Aldenkamp, 1997). Seizure type is important, as this relationship holds strongest for tonic–clonic seizures. Frequency of seizures may also impact on cognition, with evidence that, over time, those individuals with frequent seizures have gradual cognitive decline, as evidenced by performance on standardised intelligence tests (Lodhi & Agrawal, 2012). Other factors, such as anti-epileptic medication and comorbid diagnoses, may confound this relationship.

Certainly, one factor that impacts on the nature of the cognitive impairments is the epileptogenic focus. For example, left temporal lobe epilepsy can impact on verbal memory, while right temporal lobe epilepsy can impact on visual memory. Long-term memory decline has also been reported in association with temporal lobe epilepsy. Similarly, frontal lobe epilepsy can be associated with dysexecutive features (discussed by Lodhi & Agrawal, 2012).

Assessment and diagnosis

The diagnosis of epilepsy depends principally on a detailed history provided by an informant who has witnessed the episodes, together with a description of the sequence of events as recalled by the individual. Diagnosis may be confounded for a number of reasons. First, it is not unusual for an untrained staff member to accompany the patient to out-patient appointments, but that staff member may not have witnessed the event. However, because the description by a witness is so crucial in establishing a diagnosis, the diagnosing clinician should insist that the patient be accompanied by such a person. Furthermore, descriptions offered by different carers may be contradictory. Finally, among individuals with DID there is a high comorbidity with psychiatric disorders, ASD and behavioural symptoms, all of which may be confused with different manifestations of seizures (such as the prodrome, aura or seizure itself).

The history should focus on obtaining information about the characteristics of the episode and its context, including information about coexisting medical and neuropsychiatric symptoms and the relationship between these various items. A detailed medical history will include eliciting information about any of the possible aetiological factors described above, including any history of brain trauma or acute illness, such as encephalitis or meningitis. The history should include an account of all medications taken, both prescribed and over-the-counter preparations. Any possible interactions between the medications should be noted and managed appropriately. A history focusing on neuropsychiatric disorders may provide additional insight into possible comorbidity or diagnoses to consider in differential diagnosis. Finally, if there is a family history of epilepsy, this points towards one of the autosomal dominant forms of the disorder, or familial polygenic risk that may require further investigation (by, for example, micro-array). It may also be helpful if an example of the patient's typical seizure(s) is video-recorded and brought to the consultation. Before performing video-recording, any relevant ethical and safety considerations must be taken into account.

If possible, blood and urine should be collected if a metabolic cause of seizures is suspected. Testing blood for amino acids and urine for organic acids may assist in identifying a considerable number of these. If familial genetic risk is present, karyotyping and micro-array may also be warranted. An EEG will not usually enable the diagnosis of epilepsy to be made, with certain notable exceptions, but it may help to support the diagnosis. Furthermore, an EEG may be difficult to perform in someone who has DID. The exceptional cases in which an EEG is particularly helpful in the diagnosis include infantile spasms, in which the EEG is characterised by the grossly disorganised high-voltage, slow-wave pattern of hypsarrhythmia, or the three-per-second spike-wave discharges that are usually induced by overbreathing for 3–4 minutes in absence seizures. Nocturnal EEG recordings, preferably accompanied by video-monitoring, can sometimes be helpful in identifying odd night-time episodes, such as frequent tonic seizures, although it is again important to emphasise that a normal EEG does not necessarily exclude a seizure or epilepsy diagnosis. Prolonged EEG monitoring may be indicated in some cases, but there are practical difficulties and so the individual may not tolerate the equipment. EEG video-telemetry can also be helpful, particularly if the individual is being considered for resective epilepsy surgery.

It is important to realise that EEG abnormalities will be recorded in 0.5% of healthy adults and 2% of healthy children (Smith, 2005). Moreover, among individuals with known cerebral pathology, 10–30% of EEGs will be characterised by abnormalities in the absence of clinical seizure activity (Smith, 2005). Therefore, in general terms, there is not a clear correlation between EEG activity and clinical seizure manifestation. However, one large study indicated that 51% of individuals with seizure activity within 24 hours of an EEG demonstrated EEG abnormalities; that proportion fell to 34% beyond this 24-hour window (King *et al*, 1998). Antiepileptic medication will decrease the proportion of patients in whom EEG abnormalities are present after a seizure. Yield may be improved, however, by repeating the recording several times. Indeed, the combination of 'wake' and 'sleep' EEG increases the yield significantly (for a discussion of the merits of performing EEG in the diagnosis of epilepsy see Smith, 2005).

Neuropsychological testing may be useful, particularly if the seizure is deemed to be focal and associated with particular neuropsychological impairments. In general, cognitive testing may provide patients and those supporting them with a useful account of patterns of cognitive strengths and weaknesses, which can inform approaches to cognitive remediation or optimisation of functioning. Detailed neuropsychological testing can be helpful in pointing to the possible location of an epileptic focus.

Finally, neuroimaging is another investigative procedure often requested in the context of suspected epilepsy. An account of the roles of neuroimaging in the diagnosis and management of epilepsy in the presence of developmental disorder is outside the scope of this chapter. In reality, this investigation may yield results only if there is a focal nature to the seizure and there is a suspicion of a space-occupying lesion, or a neurodegenerative disorder. It does, however, have a valuable role in evaluating patients as part of pre-surgical evaluation (see e.g. Pittau *et al*, 2014). Given the difficulty that many with DID have in coping with the demands of magnetic resonance imaging, computerised tomography or positron emission tomography, leading to the need for imaging to be undertaken under a general anaesthetic, it is important to consider the balance between risks and benefits before undertaking such imaging.

Management

Pharmacological management

The pharmacological management of epilepsy is no different from that in the population without DID, apart from particular vigilance to monitor for adverse effects. A number of different anti-epileptics are available: some indicated for monotherapy (e.g. carbamazepine, valproic acid and lamotrigine); others as 'add-ons' (e.g. pregabalin and levetiraceptam); some for specific seizure types (e.g. ethosuximide for absence seizures); and others for specific seizure syndromes (e.g. vigabatrin in West syndrome).

In general terms, the clinician should strive for monotherapy, or, where more than one agent is required, for the fewest possible, using the lowest effective dose that achieves adequate seizure control yet avoids unacceptable adverse effects. Achieving this balance is often difficult, for many reasons. First, individuals with DID often have refractory epilepsy, sometimes despite polypharmacy. Second, people with DID are often more susceptible to the adverse effects of the medication. Third, individuals with DID are often on antipsychotics that may lower the seizure threshold. And fourth, it is often difficult to obtain an objective history of the seizures, particularly in instances where the patient lives in a group home with a high turnover of minimally trained staff. A pragmatic approach is therefore required, in which the outcome may be more focused on quality of life than simply seizure control.

It is important to note that there is a wide range of drug–drug interactions between anti-epileptic agents and other drugs and between the different anti-epileptic agents themselves, although the newer agents tend to have fewer. For an account of interactions between anti-epileptic drugs see, for instance, Patsalos (2013).

The Cochrane Collaboration has reviewed the evidence concerning the use of anti-epileptic medication in individuals with DID (Beavis *et al*, 2007*a*). A number of randomised placebo-controlled trials are discussed, along with their inherent limitations and conclusions that can be drawn regarding their use (Beavis *et al*, 2007*a*). Twelve studies were reviewed, with a total study population of 761 participants and eight different anti-epileptics. The studies comprised five cross-over trials, six parallel trials and one open-label trial. The main source of possible bias in the studies related to methods of randomisation not being clearly stated. It is also noteworthy that several of the studies had very small sample sizes. Although four studies had over 90 participants each (range 92–169), in each the study population was identified as having Lennox–Gastaut syndrome, so the results cannot be generalised to the wider population of individuals with DID and epilepsy. Drugs studied in these trials include lamotrigine, topiramate, rufinamide and clobazam, each compared, in terms of efficacy and safety, to placebo. Each of these studies identified a reduction in seizure frequency (relative to baseline) in the treatment group. Of note, in the topiramate study (Glauser *et al*, 1999) this was true only of 'drop attacks'. Moreover, in a study of modest sample size ($n = 72$; Kerr *et al*, 2005), the authors failed to find any evidence of any improvement in seizures with topiramate. Some of the smaller studies included in the review are also noteworthy. For example, a reasonably sized study ($n = 71$) of felbamate in Lennox–Gastaut syndrome recorded three individuals achieving complete seizure remission. It should be noted, however, that while reportedly effective, felbamate has been associated with two potential idiosyncratic serious side-effects: aplastic anaemia and liver failure (Pellock *et al*, 2006). None of the trials was particularly notable for the frequency of adverse effects reported.

These same studies also describe the range and frequency of adverse effects in the study populations. No one drug appears to have a particular propensity to cause side-effects in the DID population over and above the risk of side-effects in the general population. Topiramate, lamotrigine and gabapentin have each been studied in the DID population in double-blind placebo-controlled trials, and the frequency of drug-related adverse effects has been reported to be between 25 and 33% (Beavis *et al*, 2007*a*). However, among individuals with DID, certain side-effects may have a greater impact. For example, valproic acid often causes weight gain, which may be particularly problematic in a population that is less active and may be on other weight-enhancing medications (such as the atypical antipsychotics).

For women with DID who may be or become pregnant, just as for females across the population, the teratogenic risks of anti-epileptic agents should be carefully considered. Becoming pregnant should be considered as part of the risk–benefit considerations that underlie anti-epileptic treatment selection and this may indicate changing treatment. Of the agents currently used more frequently, sodium valproate has been associated with higher rates of congenital malformations and ASD in the offspring of mothers taking this drug (Campbell *et al*, 2013; Christensen *et al*, 2013).

In general terms, the anti-epileptics with known safety and efficacy in the general population can also be used in those with DID, and the same indications apply (in terms of seizure type, add-on versus monotherapy and so forth).

Non-pharmacological management

A variety of non-pharmacological interventions are available, many of which have been investigated for efficacy and safety in this population. For example, surgical intervention continues to be used for refractory epilepsy, with one study indicating favourable outcomes in a small (*n* = 16) population with borderline DID, including 14 patients who became completely free of seizures (Gleissner *et al*, 1999). In a register-based study in Sweden (Malmgren *et al*, 2008), of 72 individuals with DID (IQ<70) who had undergone resective surgery for epilepsy, 24 were seizure free 2 years later, although this number was much less than the 61% seizure free in the comparison group (people with no developmental disorder). Low IQ should not preclude the consideration of surgery for those with refractory epilepsy. However, when considering issues around capacity to consent to surgery, which is likely to be limited or absent in many of those with DID, the required approach and legal structures in the relevant jurisdiction should be consulted.

Vagus nerve stimulation may be used in people with DID. The indications for its use are generally similar to those employed in the rest of the population. Consideration does, however, need to be given to whether a potential recipient will be able to cooperate with the demands of surgery, but anecdotally many do cope well (see e.g. Buoni *et al*, 2004; Cersósimo *et al*, 2011). Ketogenic diets are also considered to have a place in the management of some people, mostly children, with refractory epilepsy. However, they can be challenging to deliver and accept. Currently, it is not possible to predict which patients are most likely to benefit from this intervention (Schoeler *et al*, 2013).

A variety of psychological interventions have also been described in the literature with apparent seizure-reducing effects. These include relaxation therapy, biofeedback and cognitive–behavioural therapy. While it is well established that stress, anxiety and high levels of emotional arousal can precipitate seizures, there is little evidence supporting the efficacy of any of these psychological treatments. Several studies have investigated efficacy, but methodological issues confound data interpretation: most notably, little information is given in studies of concomitant seizure medication, and changes made to seizure medication during the course of the study. In short, more robust data are required before conclusions can be drawn and recommendations made (Beavis *et al*, 2007*b*).

Management of the neuropsychiatric manifestations of epilepsy

The management of the neuropsychiatric manifestations of the disorder should accord with the latest evidence-based literature (Farooq & Sherin, 2008). There is no indication that any of the psychiatric manifestations require any specific treatment beyond these generic recommendations. However, the use of psychotropic medication among those with DID needs to be cautious, with slow and careful titration. The propensity of certain medications to lower the seizure threshold also needs to be borne in mind when making a decision about which medication to use and at which dose.

Service issues

People with DID who have associated epilepsy should be as able as anyone else to access specialist healthcare for the management of their epilepsy (Department of Health, 2001). Such specialist services may be available through regular learning disability services, through regular epilepsy services or through specialist tertiary care. There also appears to be a role for specialist epilepsy nurses in supporting people with DID and epilepsy and those who care for them (Christodoulou, 2012). A person may also require access to different types of management resource at different phases of their epilepsy care, depending on the clinical issues arising: for instance if their seizures are poorly controlled, if they have been seizure free for a prolonged period of time with no changes to their mediation and no ongoing risk factors, or if the individual is on polypharmacy and medication needs to be rationalised. There appears to be no particular pattern in terms of who accesses which service (Ring *et al*, 2009). For example, in the observational survey reported by Ring *et al*, degree of DID, duration of epilepsy or severity of epilepsy did not differ between patients attending different services. There appears to be no apparent consistency as to whether or why a psychiatrist specialising in DID or a general neurologist manages epilepsy among those with DID in the UK. The impact this may have on patients in terms of their illness is unclear and further research is needed to advise policy makers and commissioners of healthcare to plan for the healthcare needs of this population.

Conclusion

Epilepsy is commonly seen in association with DID, introducing new levels of complexity in the healthcare of this population. A significant amount is known about the aetiology and diagnosis, but there is a dearth of evidence-based literature on the use of anti-epileptics and non-pharmacological management strategies for individuals with DID and comorbid epilepsy. Moreover, there is a need for careful consideration of the planning and implementation of services at a national level, with clearly defined pathways of primary, secondary and tertiary care, to ensure that all individuals with DID have access to high-quality services.

Acknowledgements

MWS acknowledges the support of the Canadian Institutes of Health Research (CIHR) and Scottish Rite (Canada) Charitable Foundation during the preparation of this manuscript. During the time that this manuscript was prepared, HR received support from the NIHR (UK) CLAHRC for Cambridgeshire and Peterborough.

References

Adachi N, Matsuura M, Okubo Y, *et al* (2000) Predictive variables of interictal psychosis in epilepsy. *Neurology*, **55**: 1310–4.

Adachi, N, Matsuura M, Hara, T, *et al* (2002) Psychoses and epilepsy: are interictal and postictal psychoses distinct clinical entities? *Epilepsia*, **43**: 1574–82.

Adachi N, Akanuma N, Ito M, *et al* (2012) Interictal psychotic episodes in epilepsy: duration and associated clinical factors. *Epilepsia*, **53**: 1088–94.

Aldenkamp AP (1997) Effect of seizures and epileptiform discharges on cognitive function. *Epilepsia*, **38** (suppl 1): S52–5.

Amiet C, Gourfinkel-An I, Bouzamondo A, *et al* (2008) Epilepsy in autism is associated with intellectual disability and gender: evidence from a meta-analysis. *Biological Psychiatry*, **64**: 577–82.

Banerjee PN, Filippi D, Allen Hauser W (2009) The descriptive epidemiology of epilepsy – a review. *Epilepsy Research*, **85**: 31–45.

Banks R, Bush A, Baker P, *et al* (2007) *Challenging Behaviour: A Unified Approach*. Royal College of Psychiatrists, British Psychological Society and Royal College of Speech and Language Therapists.

Beavis J, Kerr M, Marson AG (2007*a*) Pharmacological interventions for epilepsy in people with intellectual disabilities. *Cochrane Database of Systematic Reviews*, CD005399.

Beavis J, Kerr M, Marson AG (2007*b*) Non-pharmacological interventions for epilepsy in people with intellectual disabilities. *Cochrane Database of Systematic Reviews*, CD005502.

Berg AT, Scheffer IE (2011) New concepts in classification of the epilepsies: entering the 21st century. *Epilepsia*, **52**: 1058–62.

Berkovic SF, Howell RA, Hay DA, *et al* (1998) Epilepsies in twins: genetics of the major epilepsy syndromes. *Annals of Neurology*, **43**: 435–45.

Besag FM (2001) Behavioural effects of the new antiepileptics. *Drug Safety*, **24**: 513–36.

Brooks-Kayal A (2010) Epilepsy and autism spectrum disorders: are there common developmental mechanisms? *Brain Development*, **32**: 731–8.

Buoni S, Mariottini A, Pieri S, *et al* (2004) Vagus nerve stimulation for drug-resistant epilepsy in children and young adults. *Brain Development*, **26**: 158–63.

Campbell E, Kennedy F, Irwin B, *et al* (2013) Malformation risks of antiepileptic drug monotherapies in pregnancy. *Journal of Neurology, Neurosurgery and Psychiatry*, **84**: e2.

Cersósimo RO, Bartuluchi M, Fortini S, *et al* (2011) Vagus nerve stimulation: effectiveness and tolerability in 64 paediatric patients with refractory epilepsies. *Epileptic Disorders*, **13**: 382–8.

Christensen J, Grønborg TK, Sørensen MJ, *et al* (2013) Prenatal valproate exposure and risk of autism spectrum disorders and childhood autism. *JAMA*, **309**: 1696–703.

Christodoulou M (2012) Neurological nurse specialists: a vital resource under threat. *Lancet Neurology*, **11**: 210–11.

Cleary RA, Thompson PJ, Thom M, *et al* (2013) Postictal psychosis in temporal lobe epilepsy: risk factors and postsurgical outcome. *Epilepsy Research*, **106**: 264–72.

Cuccaro ML, Tuchman RF, Hamilton KL, *et al* (2012) Exploring the relationship between autism spectrum disorder and epilepsy using latent class cluster analysis. *Journal of Autism and Developmental Disorders*, **42**: 1630–41.

De Simone R, Puig XS, Gelisse P, *et al* (2010) Senile myoclonic epilepsy: delineation of a common condition associated with Alzheimer's disease and Down syndrome. *Seizure*, **19**: 383–9.

Department of Health (2001) *Valuing People: A New Strategy for Learning Disability for the 21st Century*. Department of Health.

Emerson E (2001) *Challenging Behaviour: Analysis and Intervention in People with Severe Intellectual Disabilities*. Cambridge University Press.

Farooq S, Sherin A (2008) Interventions for psychotic symptoms concomitant with epilepsy. *Cochrane Database of Systematic Reviews*, CD006118.

Filipek P (2005) Medical aspects of autism. In *Handbook of Autism and Pervasive Developmental Disorders* (eds F Volkmar, A Klin, R Paul, *et al*), pp 534–78. Wiley.

Finegan J-A (1998) Study of behavioral phenotypes: goals and methodological considerations. *American Journal of Medical Genetics*, **81**: 148–55.

Fisher RS, van Emde Boas W, Blume W, *et al* (2005) Epileptic seizures and epilepsy: definitions proposed by the International League Against Epilepsy (ILAE) and the International Bureau for Epilepsy (IBE). *Epilepsia*, **46**: 470–2.

Fombonne E (1999) The epidemiology of autism: a review. *Psychological Medicine*, **29**: 769–86.

Glauser T, Sachdeo R, Ritter F, *et al* (1999) A double-blind, randomized trial of topiramate in Lennox–Gastaut syndrome. *Neurology*, **52**: 1882–7.

Gleissner U, Johanson K, Helmstaedter C, *et al* (1999) Surgical outcome in a group of low-IQ patients with focal epilepsy. *Epilepsia*, **40**: 553–9.

Hannah JA, Brodie MJ (1998) Epilepsy and learning disabilities – a challenge for the next millennium? *Seizure*, **7**: 3–13.

Helbig I, Mefford HC, Sharp AJ, *et al* (2009) 15q13: 3 microdeletions increase risk of idiopathic generalized epilepsy. *Nature Genetics*, **41**: 160–2.

Hoppe C, Elger CE (2011) Depression in epilepsy: a critical review from a clinical perspective. *Nature Reviews: Neurology*, **7**: 462–72.

Kanemoto K, Kawasaki J, Kawai I (1996) Postictal psychosis: a comparison with acute interictal and chronic psychoses. *Epilepsia*, **37**: 551–6.

Kerr MP, Baker GA, Brodie MJ (2005) A randomized, double-blind, placebo-controlled trial of topiramate in adults with epilepsy and intellectual disability: impact on seizures, severity, and quality of life. *Epilepsy and Behavior*, **7**: 472–80.

Kerr MP, Gil-Nagel A, Glynn M, *et al* (2013) Treatment of behavioral problems in intellectually disabled adult patients with epilepsy. *Epilepsia*, **54** (suppl 1): 34–40.

King MA, Newton MR, Jackson GD, *et al* (1998) Epileptology of the first-seizure presentation: a clinical, EEG and MRI study of 300 consecutive patients. *Lancet*, **352**: 1007–11.

Krishnamoorthy E, Trimble M, Sander J, *et al* (2002) Forced normalization at the interface between epilepsy and psychiatry. *Epilepsy and Behavior*, **3**: 303–8.

Langosch JM, Trimble MR (2002) Epilepsy, psychosis and clozapine. *Human Psychopharmacology*, **17**: 115–19.

Lhatoo SD, Sander JW (2001) The epidemiology of epilepsy and learning disability. *Epilepsia*, **42** (suppl 1): 6–9; discussion 19–20.

Lodhi S, Agrawal N (2012) Neurocognitive problems in epilepsy. *Advances in Psychiatric Treatment*, **18**: 232–40.

Malmgren K, Olsson I, Engman E, *et al* (2008) Seizure outcome after resective epilepsy surgery in patients with low IQ. *Brain*, **131**: 535–42.

McGrother CW, Bhaumik S, Thorp CF, *et al* (2006) Epilepsy in adults with intellectual disabilities: prevalence, associations and service implications. *Seizure*, **15**: 376–86.

McKnight K, Jiang Y, Hart Y, *et al* (2005) Serum antibodies in epilepsy and seizure-associated disorders. *Neurology*, **65**: 1730–6.

Mula M, Monaco F (2011) Ictal and peri-ictal psychopathology. *Behavioural Neurology*, **24**: 21–5.

Mula M, Schmitz B (2009) Depression in epilepsy: mechanisms and therapeutic approach. *Therapeutic Advances in Neurological Disorders*, **2**: 337–44.

Pal DK, Evgrafov OV, Tabares P, *et al* (2003) BRD2 (RING3) is a probable major susceptibility gene for common juvenile myoclonic epilepsy. *American Journal of Human Genetics*, **73**: 261–70.

Pandolfo M (2011) Genetics of epilepsy. *Seminars in Neurology*, **31**: 506–18.

Patsalos PN (2013) Drug interactions with the newer antiepileptic drugs (AEDs) – part 1: pharmacokinetic and pharmacodynamic interactions between AEDs. *Clinical Pharmacokinetics*, **52**: 927–66.

Pellock JM, Faught E, Leppik IE, *et al* (2006) Felbamate: consensus of current clinical experience. *Epilepsy Research*, **71**: 89–101.

Pittau F, Grouiller F, Spinelli L, *et al* (2014) The role of functional neuroimaging in pre-surgical epilepsy evaluation. *Frontal Neurology*, **5**: 31.

Qin P, Xu H, Laursen TM, *et al* (2005) Risk for schizophrenia and schizophrenia-like psychosis among patients with epilepsy: population based cohort study. *BMJ*, **331**: 23.

Ring H, Zia A, Bateman N, *et al* (2009) How is epilepsy treated in people with a learning disability? A retrospective observational study of 183 individuals. *Seizure*, **18**: 264–8.

Schoeler NE, Cross JH, Sander JW, *et al* (2013) Can we predict a favourable response to ketogenic diet therapies for drug-resistant epilepsy? *Epilepsy Research*, **106**: 1–16.

Singhi P, Jagirdar S, Khandelwal N, *et al* (2003) Epilepsy in children with cerebral palsy. *Journla of Child Neurology*, **18**: 174–9.

Smith S (2005) EEG in the diagnosis, classification, and management of patients with epilepsy. *Journal of Neurology, Neurosurgery and Psychiatry*, **76**: ii2–ii7.

Spence SJ, Schneider MT (2009) The role of epilepsy and epileptiform EEGs in autism spectrum disorders. *Pediatric Research*, **65**: 599–606.

Striano P, Coppola A, Paravidino R, *et al* (2012) Clinical significance of rare copy number variations in epilepsy: a case-control survey using microarray-based comparative genomic hybridization. *Archives of Neurology*, **69**: 322–30.

Toone B (2000) The psychoses of epilepsy. *Journal of Neurology, Neurosurgery and Psychiatry*, **69**: 1–3.

Tuchman R, Rapin I (2002) Epilepsy in autism. *Lancet Neurology*, **1**: 352–8.

Turk J, Bax M, Williams C, *et al* (2009) Autism spectrum disorder in children with and without epilepsy: impact on social functioning and communication. *Acta Paediatrica*, **98**: 675–81.

Wandinger K-P, Saschenbrecker S, Stoecker W, *et al* (2011) Anti-NMDA-receptor encephalitis: a severe, multistage, treatable disorder presenting with psychosis. *Journal of Neuroimmunology*, **231**: 86–91.

CHAPTER 7

The use of psychotropic medications to manage problem behaviours in adults

Shoumitro Deb

A high proportion of people with disorders of intellectual development (DID) receive medication for both physical and mental health conditions (Deb & Fraser, 1994). Psychotropic medications are commonly used to manage problem behaviours when no diagnosis of a psychiatric disorder can be confirmed. The accurate diagnosis of psychiatric disorders can be particularly difficult in people with DID (Deb *et al*, 2001; Hemmings *et al*, 2013). Problem behaviour in this context is defined as 'socially unacceptable behaviour that causes distress, harm or disadvantage to the person themselves or to other people or damage to property, and usually requires some intervention' (Deb *et al*, 2009: p. 182). Other terms have also been used to describe problem behaviours, such as challenging behaviour, behaviour disorder and behaviour difficulty. Examples of problem behaviours include aggression to other people (physical or verbal aggression), property destruction and self-injurious behaviour (for a more detailed description of problem behaviours see Chapter 5).

There is concern about the use of psychotropic medication in people with DID for the management of problem behaviours in the absence of a diagnosed psychiatric disorder. Some of the reasons for this are:

- perceived excessive use of medication – multiple medications are often used at a high dose for a long period of time without any review, and sometimes exceeding the *British National Formulary* (BNF) (http://www.bnf.org) recommended maximum dose
- adverse events, such as weight gain and somnolence from risperidone, and the difficulty of assessing these in people with DID, including the carrying out of necessary investigations such as serum lithium level and other blood tests
- lack of evidence of effectiveness
- out-of-licence use, as, by and large, these medications are licensed for the treatment of psychiatric disorders, not of problem behaviours
- use of medication without explicit patient consent, as is often the case in relation to people with DID.

Because of this wide public concern, a national guide on the use of medication for the management of problem behaviours in people with DID was developed in the UK on behalf of the Royal College of Psychiatrists (Unwin & Deb, 2010), and subsequently an adapted version of the UK guide was published as an international guide (Deb *et al*, 2009) on behalf of the World Psychiatric Association (WPA). The guide provides advice to people who are considering prescribing medication to manage problem behaviours for adults with DID. It was produced following the guideline development criteria set out by the National Institute for Health and Care Excellence (NICE; http://www.nice.org.uk) and it has been assessed using the internationally accepted Appraisal of Guidelines for Research and Evaluation (AGREE Collaboration, 2001). The guide represents the view of the multidisciplinary Guideline Development Group (GDG). The GDG considered the evidence available and consulted widely before reaching a consensus. The recommendations reflect the principles laid down in *Valuing People Now* (Department of Health, 2010). Health professionals are expected to take it into account fully when exercising their clinical judgement. The guide does not, however, override the individual responsibility of health professionals to make decisions appropriate to the circumstances of the particular situation. Such decisions must be taken after careful consideration of all the possible benefits and potential risks involved with the intervention (as per the NICE criteria). The guide does not consider in any detail the indications for choosing specific medication to manage specific problem behaviours among adults with DID. Rather, it provides recommendations for clinical practice surrounding the use of medication to manage problem behaviours among people aged 18 years and over with DID.

The main recommendations in the national and international guidelines are presented in this chapter, along with some case studies to highlight the issues mentioned in the guideline.

General principles

The primary aim should be not to treat the problem behaviours *per se* but to identify their underlying cause and manage that. (See Appendix 1, which sets out a schema for the assessment of problem behaviours in people with DID.) However, it is not always possible to find a cause for the problem behaviours. When this is the case, the management strategy should be to minimise the impact of the behaviour on the individual, the environment and other people. The ultimate aim should be not only symptom reduction but to improve the quality of life for the person with DID. A thorough assessment of the causes of the behaviour and its consequences, along with a formulation, is an absolute prerequisite in managing any problem behaviours. A proper assessment and formulation will often need input from several disciplines and from families and carers. It is vital that the person with DID is given every opportunity to incorporate her or his views in the decision-making process (see Hall & Deb, 2008). A multi-axial/multilayered diagnostic formulation, such as the one proposed in the *Diagnostic Manual – Intellectual Disability* (DM-ID) (Fletcher *et al*, 2007) may be useful in this context. The assessment should include the behaviour and medical, psychological/psychiatric and social factors (the BMPS model – see Appendix 1). A formulation should be made even in the absence of a medical or psychiatric diagnosis.

Useful sources on assessment are available from the British Psychological Society (2004) and the Royal College of Psychiatrists (Banks *et al*, 2007), and see also the review by Unwin & Deb (2008*a*) on assessment scales for problem behaviours in DID.

As a general rule, the formulation should consist of the following:

- a list of the target behaviours to be managed
- a clear description of the behaviour, including its frequency and severity
- an assessment of the behaviour and its causes
- a differential diagnosis
- a record of reactions to and outcomes of the behaviour
- an assessment of predisposing, precipitating and perpetuating risk factors
- consideration of all management options and their possible outcome
- the rationale for the proposed management option
- a risk assessment
- possible adverse events associated with the proposed intervention(s)
- if appropriate, consideration of previous effectiveness or lack of it (and associated adverse events) for different interventions
- the likely effect of the proposed intervention(s) on the person's quality of life.

When to consider medication

If there is an obvious physical or psychological cause for the behaviour, this should be managed in an appropriate way. Appendix 2 presents case studies that illustrate some of the causes. If an underlying psychiatric disorder is treated with medication, the relevant NICE guidelines (http://www.nice.org.uk) and other appropriate guidelines should be followed (Deb, 2015).

If no psychiatric disorder can be recognised, then non-pharmacological management should be considered, depending on the formulation (Didden *et al*, 2015). Sometimes, after considering the non-pharmacological management options, medication may be used either on its own or as an adjunct to another intervention. Whether medication or other management strategies should be implemented will depend on individual circumstances, and is therefore not within the remit of this guideline. Instead, a number of case studies have been described in Appendix 2 of this chapter to help clinicians deal with different clinical scenarios that they may face in their day-to-day practice. It may be possible to improve the psychological well-being of individuals by providing counselling and addressing social and environmental factors, or by helping them to find more enjoyable activities, and to use medication simultaneously to make the individual with DID less anxious. This strategy may be seen as an interim formulation, which then needs to be monitored carefully at regular intervals to assess its effectiveness (see Appendix 2 case studies).

Main recommendations

A general schema for prescribing medication to manage problem behaviours in adults with DID is set out in Fig. 7.1.

Before prescribing

- The prescriber needs to ensure that an assessment has been conducted and recorded.
- The prescriber should ensure that an appropriate formulation is reached and a treatment plan drawn up.
- The prescriber needs to ensure that, where possible, appropriate physical examinations and investigations have been carried out.

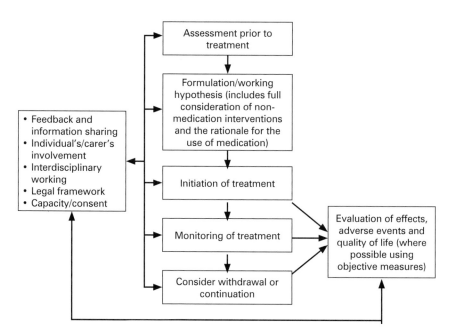

Fig. 7.1 Schema for prescribing: key processes associated with using medication to manage problem behaviours in adults with disorders of intellectual development.

- The prescriber is responsible for assessing the person's capacity to consent to treatment.
- The prescriber should discuss the formulation and treatment plan with the person and family or carers.
- The prescriber should allow the person and family or carers to influence both the decisions that are made and the treatment plan.

When prescribing

- Where possible, and when necessary, the prescriber should discuss the formulation and treatment plan with other relevant professionals, including general practitioners (GPs), as soon as possible. The treatment plan should be part of a broader care plan that takes a person-centred approach.
- The treatment plan must comply with the country's legal framework, including the relevant Mental Health Act and Mental Capacity Act.
- The prescriber should identify a key person who will ensure that medication is administered appropriately and communicate all changes to the relevant parties.
- The prescriber should provide the person and family or carers with a written treatment plan at the time of prescribing. This could be short term (usually covering a period of a few days), medium term (usually covering a period of a few weeks) or long term (usually covering a period of a few months).
- If the prescribing is done over the phone, it should be followed by written confirmation as soon as possible.
- The prescriber should discuss with the person and family, carer, or key person the common and serious adverse events related to the treatment. Where possible, the prescriber should also provide accessible information in writing. Information on commonly used psychotropic medications in accessible format with audio accompaniment is available for downloading free of charge from http://www.ld-medication.bham. ac.uk. The prescriber should advise what action to take if a serious adverse event takes place.
- During the consultation, the prescriber should remember the communication needs of the person with DID, who may need extra time or additional non-verbal communication to be able to understand.

After prescribing

- The method and timing of the assessment of treatment outcome should be set at the beginning of the treatment, along with a follow-up date for review of treatment progress.
- The outcome should be assessed as objectively as possible (ideally, using standardised scales). Some of the rating scales that could be used in this context are: the Modified Overt Aggression Scale (MOAS; Sorgi

et al, 1991), the Aberrant Behavior Checklist (ABC; Aman *et al*, 1985), Positive Goals (Fox & Emerson, 2002) and the Behavior Problems Inventory – Short Form (BPI-S; Rojahn *et al*, 2012) (on assessment scales for problem behaviours in DID, see the review by Unwin & Deb, 2008*a*).

- The route of administration, dosage and its titration over a period should be stated clearly.
- The aim should be to prescribe medication for the minimum period and at the minimum effective dose.
- The prescriber should ensure that follow-up assessments have taken place.
- As far as possible, one medication should be prescribed at a time for each indication.
- As a general rule, the medication should be used within the BNF recommended dose range.
- New medication should begin at a low dose and be gradually increased until there is an improvement in the target behaviour or until any adverse effects are evident.
- As far as possible, the medication should be prescribed to be taken at a time of day that minimises the need for its administration in multiple settings (such as day centres).
- Consideration for withdrawing medication and exploring non-medication management options should be ongoing.
- The prescriber should document all appropriate information and share it with appropriate individuals when necessary.

The evidence base

The management of problem behaviours is discussed in Chapter 5. For a comprehensive review of the evidence base for the effectiveness of psychotropic medication in the management of problem behaviours in DID see Deb (2013, 2015). In summary, there is adequate good-quality evidence based on randomised controlled trials (RCTs) primarily on children with DID with or without autism but also some evidence on adults with DID that risperidone is effective in the management of problem behaviours (with one negative finding out of three RCTs among adults with DID – Tyrer *et al*, 2008) (Deb *et al*, 2007; Deb, 2013, 2015). However, there is concern about adverse events such as somnolence and weight gain (not much evidence is available on other adverse events, such as metabolic and cardiac). Long-term follow-up studies among children are reassuring as regards the adverse events and continued effectiveness (Unwin & Deb, 2011). Two recent RCTs from the pharmaceutical company that produces the drug, written by the same group of authors, with possible overlap of participants included in these studies, show that aripiprazole is effective in improving irritability in children with autism with or without DID (Marcus *et al*, 2009; Owen *et al*, 2009; Deb *et al*, 2014).

There is equivocal evidence, primarily based on prospective and retrospective case studies but not RCTs, on the effectiveness of antidepressants in the treatment of problem behaviours in DID (Sohanpal *et al*, 2007). On average, less than half of the cohort showed improvement in behaviour and the rest either did not improve or deteriorated. The most pronounced effect was found in the presence of anxiety or obsessive–compulsive symptoms. However, there is concern regarding adverse events (sometimes making behaviour worse) (see review by Deb, 2013, 2015).

Among mood stabilisers, there are a few old RCTs based on small sample sizes and which often used non-validated outcome measures, which showed some effectiveness of lithium in the treatment of problem behaviours in hospitalised adults with DID (Deb *et al*, 2008). However, there is concern regarding the use of lithium among those who are not able to give consent and where investigations like blood tests are difficult (Deb, 2013). There is evidence, primarily from small case studies (prospective and retrospective) but not RCTs, to support the use of sodium valproate for the management of problem behaviours in DID (Deb *et al*, 2008). There is currently no evidence available in support of the use of anti-anxiety medications. However, it is worth remembering that absence of evidence is not evidence of absence of effectiveness.

There is currently some equivocal evidence, based primarily on non-randomised trials, for the effectiveness of opioid antagonist medications for the management of problem behaviours in DID (Roy *et al*, 2015a, 2015b). Some showed better results on a lower dose but others showed a better result on a higher dose (see reviews by Deb, 2013, 2015).

Evidence for the choice of medication

No study has directly compared the use of different medications to manage specific problem behaviours such as physical aggression and self-injurious behaviour. Therefore, it is not possible to recommend any specific medication for any specific problem behaviours. However, Unwin & Deb (2008b) carried out a consensus survey among consultant psychiatrists practising in the field of DID in the UK, the results of which are presented below. These findings have to be interpreted with caution because the response rate was slightly below 40% and the clinicians were given forced choices. In real-life situations, they would decide on the type of medication depending on individual clinical circumstances. Also, the current preferences may change when more information becomes available about the efficacy and adverse events of individual medications, and also as new medications become available. However, a recent study has found similar results (Deb *et al*, 2015).

- Most clinicians (96%) preferred non-pharmacological management as the first choice and medication was the second choice for managing problem behaviours in adults with DID.

- Clinicians preferred antipsychotic medication as their first choice, followed by either antidepressants or mood stabilisers, depending on whether they were treating aggression or self-injurious behaviour.
- Clinicians preferred new-generation antipsychotics to older ones.
- Among antidepressants, clinicians preferred newer generations, such as the selective serotonin reuptake inhibitors (SSRIs) rather than older medication, such as the tricyclics.
- Among new-generation antipsychotics, risperidone was the first choice, followed by olanzapine and quetiapine.
- Among antidepressants, citalopram, fluoxetine and sertraline were the preferred choices.
- Among mood stabilisers, carbamazepine and sodium valproate were the preferred choices.
- Clinicians preferred to prescribe antipsychotics, particularly risperidone, in lower doses than is recommended in the BNF for the treatment of schizophrenia.
- Below are some of the situations under which the clinicians stated that they would consider using medications:
  - failure of non-pharmacological interventions
  - risk or evidence of harm or distress to self
  - risk or evidence of harm or distress to others or property
  - high frequency or severity of problem behaviours
  - to treat an underlying mental/psychiatric disorder or anxiety
  - to calm the person to enable implementation of non-pharmacological interventions
  - risk of breakdown to the person's placement
  - lack of adequate or available non-pharmacological interventions
  - good previous response to medication
  - person or carer choice.

Discontinuation of treatment

- Once a medication is prescribed, the prescriber should continue to evaluate the risk–benefit profile regularly, with particular emphasis on the individual's and family's or carers' quality of life.
- Consideration of a reduction in the dose or withdrawing the medication and exploring non-pharmacological options should be ongoing.
- The prescriber should consider withdrawing medication if the problem behaviours do not improve or after a reasonable period of time even if problem behaviours improve. However, the decision about when to withdraw as well as the rate and timing of withdrawal should be based on individual circumstances and the purpose of the medication. For longer-term treatments, withdrawal should be considered within 6–12 months.

- The rate of withdrawal will depend on the type of medication used, the severity of the behaviour, the availability of non-pharmacological options, and previous response to withdrawal.
- The decision to withdraw medication should be made only after discussion with the patient and family or carers, and when necessary with other relevant professionals.
- In the case of a difference of opinion, a multidisciplinary meeting should be organised, at which the best interests of the patient should be borne in mind.
- The withdrawal of medication should be undertaken in a planned and systematic manner, and a contingency plan (relapse plan) should be in place to intervene should a crisis arise (see flow chart in Fig. 7.2).

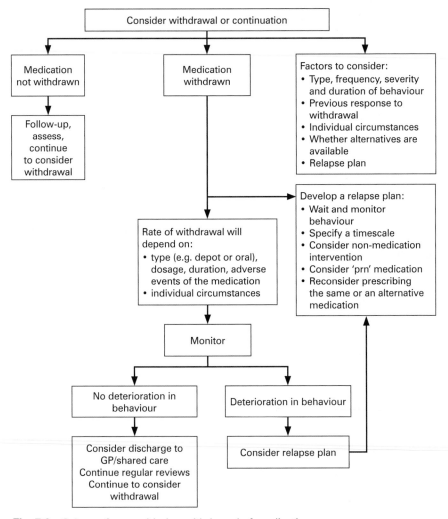

Fig. 7.2 Schema for considering withdrawal of medication.

Conclusion

Proper implementation of the recommendations made in the guideline will depend on timely action on the part of those organisations that are involved in caring for adults with DID for whom medication is either prescribed or considered to manage problem behaviours. These organisations should train and encourage prescribers and other relevant people to use appropriate assessment and review methods for the management of problem behaviours. Documentation of clinical practice in an appropriate manner at the right time and in the right place should be encouraged. Organisations should have mechanisms and resources in place for effective regular communication regarding the management of problem behaviours among the professionals involved as well as the persons with DID and their carers.

Organisations should develop policies to implement the recommendations made here and elsewhere and create mechanisms to regularly monitor and audit the implementation of these recommendations. If necessary, they should take remedial action on time. Organisations should have mechanisms for sharing information among the relevant people on a regular basis. Such information should include evidence of the effectiveness of different interventions for managing problem behaviours in adults with DID. Where necessary, the organisations should provide training for the relevant personnel to enable them to access timely information about the evidence. Organisations should disseminate information about the relevant guidelines to all appropriate people and organisations, including local groups of carers and people with DID (see Deb *et al*, 2006).

Appendix 1 Schema for the assessment of problem behaviours in DID

This list is not a comprehensive, but a broad scheme. Not all assessments will be required in all cases.

The BMPS model

An assessment should address:

- the behaviour (**B**) and the person
- medical and organic factors (**M**)
- psychological and psychiatric factors (**P**)
- social and environmental factors (**S**).

Assessment of the actual behaviour (B)

The type and nature of the behaviour(s)

- history of problem behaviour
- baseline behaviour prior to the onset of problem behaviour
- the pattern of onset of the behaviour

- the frequency, severity and duration of the behaviour
- associated behaviours
- the impact of the problem behaviour on the individual's life, others' lives and the environment
- reactions to the behaviour by the individual, others and services
- the function of the behaviour.

Risk assessment
- the type and the nature of risks:
  - risk to others
  - risk to the individual
  - risk to the environment
  - other risks, including offending history
- methods of risk assessment
- previous risk assessment
- review of risks
- record of reviewing reduction of risks.

Assessment of the person (British Psychological Society, 2004)
- strengths – abilities, opportunities, resources
- needs – impact of disability, service and resource gaps in their lives, mental and physical health needs
- likes, dislikes and preferences and how they express these
- history – social, developmental, psychological and history of use of services
- difficulties in developing fulfilling relationships.

In this context, it is helpful to have a description of the individual's current and past weekly routine.

Medical (M) and organic factors
- chronic physical conditions
- medical conditions
- epilepsy
- other neurological conditions
- genetic conditions
- sensory impairment
- communication problems
- physical disabilities
- use of illicit drugs and alcohol
- use of prescribed drugs
- relevant developmental and medical history.

Psychological/psychiatric (P) factors
- psychiatric disorders
- relevant history of psychological development

- psychological/emotional issues, such as bereavement, relationship, abuse
- new, ongoing or recurrent stress
- difficulty in developing fulfilling relationships
- developmental disorders such as autism spectrum disorder (ASD) and attention-deficit hyperactivity disorder (ADHD), including impulsivity
- impact of neuropsychological factors such as impaired intelligence, memory, attention, communication skills or executive function (including impaired frontal lobe functions such as lack of initiative and apathy) and lower stress tolerance.

Social and environmental (S) factors

- description and assessment of the environment and daily activities
- factors relating to other people around the person, including staff and carers
- change in the environment
- influence of life events
- relationship with peer group, friends, family members and care staff (including any changes)
- effect of daily activities (including any changes)
- effect of (or lack of) leisure and day activities (including any changes)
- the organisational setting – systems and procedures
- absence of appropriate or adequate support for the person and family or carers
- under- or overstimulating environment
- lack of (or opportunity for) appropriate social exposures
- issues relating to integration within the wider society, stigmatisation and discrimination
- carer issues, including levels of stress and lack of support for carers.

Appendix 2 Case examples

- A 56-year-old woman with severe DID suffered from a stroke that led to paralysis of the right side of her body. She started screaming and shouting regularly and the care staff asked for psychotropic medication to manage the behaviour. However, close examination revealed that the woman had developed spasticity in her right hand and she was constantly getting frustrated by not being able to stretch the fingers of her right hand, which led to her screaming. Instead of psychotropic medication, baclofen was prescribed as a muscle relaxant and the behaviour improved.
- A 75-year-old man with moderate DID developed symptoms of dementia. He started screaming and head banging. His sister, who was his primary carer, asked for psychotropic medication but the clinician prescribed a regular dose of paracetamol on the assumption that the

behaviour had been precipitated by headaches. This produced good results: the man stopped screaming and head banging.

- A 19-year-old man with moderate DID and ASD became aggressive towards his parents, who asked for psychotropic medication. He was prescribed a 0.25 mg daily oral dose of risperidone, which was increased to 0.25 mg twice daily, with good effect on the behaviour. However, further assessment revealed this young man's obsession with water and fear of noise. After a few months of behaviour modification his behaviour improved when his risperidone was gradually withdrawn.

- A 26-year-old man with severe DID who had no speech became disturbed when his risperidone, which he had received for many years, was gradually withdrawn. The care staff became very anxious and there was pressure on the clinician through his GP to reinstate the risperidone. However, the clinician explained to the care staff that sometimes, after years of use, drug withdrawal may produce rebound problem behaviours, sometimes caused by withdrawal dyskinesia. The man was treated with p.r.n. medication over the next 3 months and his behaviour gradually settled without the need for any regular medication.

- Care staff asked for psychotropic medication to control problem behaviours in a 36-year-old woman with moderate DID who had no speech. Further assessment by a speech therapist revealed that the care staff usually asked the woman what she wanted for her dinner and gave her two or three choices. She always opted for the last option but sometimes when the food was served she refused to eat it and became disturbed. The speech therapist suggested that instead of giving her choice verbally, the care staff should show pictures of different meals and also involve her in the preparation of her meals. This strategy worked and her behaviour improved without any psychotropic medication.

References

AGREE Collaboration (2001) *Appraisal of Guidelines for Research and Evaluation (AGREE) Instrument*. AGREE Collaboration.

Aman MG, Singh NN, Stewart AW, *et al* (1985) The Aberrant Behavior Checklist: a behavior rating scale for the assessment of treatment effects. *American Journal of Mental Deficiency*, **89**: 485–91.

Banks R, Bush A, Baker P, *et al* (eds) (2007) *Challenging Behaviour: A Unified Approach (Clinical and Service Guidelines for Supporting People with Learning Disabilities Who Are at Risk of Receiving Abusive or Restrictive Practices)* (College Report CR144). Royal College of Psychiatrists.

British Psychological Society (2004) *Psychological Interventions for Severely Challenging Behaviours Shown by People with Learning Disabilities: Clinical Practice Guidelines*. British Psychological Society.

Deb S (2013) Psychopharmacology. In *Handbook of Psychopathology in Intellectual Disability: Research, Practice, and Policy* (eds E Tsakanikos, J McCarthy), pp. 307–24. Springer.

Deb S. (2015) Psychopharmacology. In *Clinical Handbook of Evidence-Based Practices for Individuals with Intellectual and Developmental Disabilities* (ed NN Singh) (Evidence-Based Practice in Behavioral Health Series). Springer (in press).

Deb S, Fraser WI (1994) The use of psychotropic medication in people with learning disability: towards rational prescribing. *Human Psychopharmacology*, **9**: 259–72.

Deb S, Matthews T, Holt G, *et al* (eds) (2001) *Practice Guidelines for the Assessment and Diagnosis of Mental Health Problems in Adults with Intellectual Disability*. Pavilion (now available at http://www.eamhid.org).

Deb S, Clarke D, Unwin G (2006) *Using Medication to Manage Behaviour Problems Among Adults with a Learning Disability: Quick Reference Guide (QRG)*. University of Birmingham (available at http://ld-medication.bham.ac.uk).

Deb S, Sohanpal SK, Soni R, *et al* (2007) The effectiveness of antipsychotic medication in the management of behaviour problems in adults with intellectual disabilities. *Journal of Intellectual Disability Research*, **51**: 766–77.

Deb S, Chaplin R, Sohanpal S, *et al* (2008) The effectiveness of mood stabilisers and antiepileptic medication for the management of behaviour problems in adults with intellectual disability: a systematic review. *Journal of Intellectual Disability Research*, **52**: 107–13.

Deb S, Kwok H, Bertelli M, *et al* (2009) International guide to prescribing psychotropic medication for the management of problem behaviours in adults with intellectual disabilities. *World Psychiatry*, **8**: 181–6.

Deb S, Farmah BK, Arshad E, *et al* (2014) The effectiveness of aripiprazole in the management of problem behaviour in people with intellectual disabilities, developmental disabilities and/or autistic spectrum disorder: a systematic review. *Research in Developmental Disabilities*, **35**: 711–25.

Deb S, Unwin G, Deb T (2015) Characteristics and the trajectory of psychotropic medication use in general and antipsychotics in particular among adults with an intellectual disability who exhibit aggressive behaviour. *Journal of Intellectual Disability Research*, **59**: 11–25.

Department of Health (2010) *Valuing People Now. The Delivery Plan 2010–2011: 'Making it Happen for Everyone*. Central Office of Information.

Didden R, Lindsay W, Lang R, *et al* (2015) Aggression. In *Clinical Handbook of Evidence-Based Practices for Individuals with Intellectual and Developmental Disabilities* (ed NN Singh) ('Evidence-Based Practice in Behavioral Health' Series). Springer (in press).

Fletcher R, Loschen E, Stavrakaki C, *et al* (2007) *Diagnostic Manual – Intellectual Disability: A Clinical Guide for Diagnosis of Mental Disorders in Persons with Intellectual Disability (DM-ID)*. NADD Press.

Fox P, Emerson E (eds) (2002) *Positive Goals; Interventions for People with Learning Disabilities Whose Behaviour Challenges*. Pavilion.

Hall S, Deb S (2008) A qualitative study on the knowledge and views that people with learning disabilities and their carers have of psychotropic medication prescribed for behaviour problems. *Advances in Mental Health and Learning Disabilities*, **2**: 29–37.

Hemmings C, Deb S, Chaplin E, *et al* (2013) Research for people with intellectual disabilities and mental health problems: a view from the UK. *Journal of Mental Health Research in Intellectual Disability*, **6**: 127–58.

Marcus RN, Owen R, Kamen L, *et al* (2009) A placebo-controlled, fixed-dose study of aripiprazole in children and adolescents with irritability associated with autistic disorder. *Journal of American Academy of Child and Adolescent Psychiatry*, **48**: 1110–19.

Owen R, Sikich L, Marcus RN, *et al* (2009) Aripiprazole in the treatment of irritability in children and adolescents with autistic disorder. *Pediatrics*, **124**: 1533–40.

Rojahn J, Rowe EW, Sharber AC, *et al* (2012) The Behavior Problems Inventory – Short Form (BPI-S) for individuals with intellectual disabilities. Part I: Development and provisional clinical reference data. *Journal of Intellectual Disability Research*, **56**: 527–45.

Roy A, Roy M, Deb S, *et al* (2015*a*) Are opioid antagonists effective in attenuating the core symptoms of autism spectrum conditions in children? A systematic review. *Journal of Intellectual Disability Research*, **59**: 293–306.

Roy A, Roy M, Deb S, *et al* (2015*b*) Are opioid antagonists effective in adults with intellectual disability? A systematic review. *Journal of Intellectual Disability Research*, **59**: 55–67.

Sohanpal SK, Deb S, Thomas C, *et al* (2007) The effectiveness of antidepressant medication in the management of behaviour problems in adults with intellectual disabilities: a systematic review. *Journal of Intellectual Disability Research*, **51**: 750–65.

Sorgi P, Ratey J, Knoedler DW, *et al* (1991) Rating aggression in the clinical setting: a retrospective adaptation of the Overt Aggression Scale. Preliminary results. *Journal of Neuropsychiatry*, **3**: 552–6.

Tyrer P, Oliver-Africano PC, Ahmed Z, *et al* (2008) Risperidone, haloperidol, and placebo in the treatment of aggressive challenging behaviour in patients with intellectual disability: a randomised controlled trail. *Lancet*, **371**: 57–63.

Unwin G, Deb S (2008*a*) Psychiatric and behavioural assessment scales for adults with learning disabilities. *Advances in Mental Health in Learning Disability*, **2**(4): 37–45.

Unwin G, Deb S (2008*b*) Use of medication for the management of behaviour problems among adults with intellectual disabilities: a clinicians' consensus survey. *American Journal on Mental Retardation*, **113**: 19–31.

Unwin GL, Deb S (2010) The use of medication to manage problem behaviours in adults with a learning disability: a national guideline. *Advances in Mental Health and Intellectual Disabilities*, **4**(3): 4–11.

Unwin GL, Deb S (2011) Efficacy of atypical antipsychotic medication in the management of behaviour problems in children with intellectual disabilities and borderline intelligence: a systematic review. *Research in Developmental Disabilities*, **32**: 2121–33.

Part 3
Autism spectrum disorder

CHAPTER 8

Overview of autism spectrum disorder

Stelios Georgiades, Terry Bennett and Peter Szatmari

In a classic paper published in 1943, Dr Leo Kanner introduced autism as a distinct disorder by noting

> 'there have come to our attention a number of children whose condition differs so markedly and uniquely from anything reported so far, that each case merits – and I hope will eventually receive – a detailed consideration of its fascinating peculiarities.' (See Kanner, 1968: p. 217)

Around the same time, in an independent report, Dr Hans Asperger published a paper in German describing a form of autism that later became known as Asperger syndrome (Asperger, 1944). Those two landmark papers represent, to this date, the foundation for the clinical presentation of autism spectrum disorder (ASD). ASD is a neurodevelopmental disorder with marked impairments in social communication and a pattern of restricted/repetitive behaviours.

Although age of ASD diagnosis differs across localities and services, nowadays most cases are identified during early childhood. Based on both scientific and empirical evidence, there is now a consensus that ASD is a rather complex, heterogeneous disorder with a clinical presentation that appears to change with development over the life span. Although, in general, individuals with ASD exhibit similar symptoms and behaviours, there is substantial variability in terms of symptom onset, severity, manifestation and configuration.

This chapter provides a brief overview of the prevalence and aetiology of ASD, as well as issues related to the diagnosis and classification of the disorder within the context of the newly published version of the *Diagnostic and Statistical Manual of Mental Disorders*, DSM-5 (American Psychiatric Association, 2013). The chapter also highlights the potential benefits of moving towards a more balanced nosology of ASD that addresses the need for both clinical and research utility.

Prevalence rates

Despite the fact that an experienced clinician can (in most cases) reliably assign an ASD diagnosis to a child as young as 2 years of age, the majority of children do not receive a final, formal diagnosis until 3–4 years of age (Lord *et al*, 2006).

ASD is reported to occur in all ethnic and socioeconomic groups (Baio, 2012) and recent epidemiological studies suggest a dramatic increase in its prevalence (i.e. the number of cases in a defined group of children at a specific point in time). Recently reported rates of ASD range from 1 in every 88 children in a US sample (Baio, 2012) to 1 in every 160 children worldwide (Elsabbagh *et al*, 2012), making ASD a more common neurodevelopmental disorder than previously thought. Some explanations for the increase in prevalence include (but are not limited to) broadening of diagnostic concepts and criteria, growing awareness, improved detection of the disorder, and possibly a true increase in prevalence. Epidemiological studies also suggest that ASD is more common in boys than girls, by a ratio of roughly 4 to 1 (Fombonne *et al*, 2009).

Because ASD appears to be familial (as discussed in the next section) researchers have been investigating the recurrence of the disorder in high-risk younger siblings of children with a confirmed diagnosis. A large multi-site study recently found that the ASD recurrence rate is close to 20% in younger siblings of children with autism (Ozonoff *et al*, 2011). This rate was considerably higher than previously thought and almost 20 times higher than the general population rate. It is important to note that this increased rate may reflect in part a broader conception of the term 'ASD', since most early studies of this type counted only the more narrowly defined 'autism' (as defined by earlier versions of the DSM).

Aetiology and risk factors

Having established that the disorder is familial, researchers went on to try to understand the mechanism of that familiality (genetic and/or environmental). Twin studies have consistently reported that the concordance of ASD is greater in monozygous (MZ) than dyzygous (DZ) twins, which suggests there is an important genetic component (Ronald & Hoekstra, 2011). The MZ concordance rate has never reached 100%, suggesting that there are important factors that prevent complete penetrance and/or that environmental factors play a role in aetiology. The DZ concordance rate in the initial studies was very low, probably as a result of small sample sizes. A recent twin study reports a DZ concordance rate similar to that found in the studies of younger siblings (around 20%), indicating that there may be important shared environmental factors at play in the aetiology of the disorder (Hallmayer *et al*, 2011).

Several different research designs have been used to identify the specific genes that might be involved in the disorder. It is well known that ASD sometimes occurs in the context of a single-gene disorder such as tuberous sclerosis or fragile-X syndrome; these probably account for upwards of 10% of cases of ASD (Abrahams & Geschwind, 2008). Chromosomal abnormalities such as translocations and dislocations can also occur and have been seen all across the genome. These might account for another 5–10% of cases (Devlin & Scherer, 2012). The aetiology of the remaining roughly 80% of cases has been more difficult to determine but recent years have seen important advances in knowledge.

Linkage analysis of genetic markers within specific chromosomal regions that are shared by affected individuals within a family has reported some consistency in results but no autism genetic variants under the linkage peaks have been discovered (Li *et al*, 2012). Genome-wide association studies have tried to identify common genetic variants carried by individuals with ASD more frequently than non-ASD controls but, again, no replicable results reached significance (Sullivan *et al*, 2012).

The real progress in this area has been the result of genome-wide searches for rare copy number variants (CNVs) that affect brain expressed genes (Malhotra & Sebat, 2012). CNVs are structural abnormalities in chromosome sequences greater than 1 kb. These chromosomal abnormalities are not seen by microscopy but by chromosomal micro-arrays or other means. The first rare CNV found in a child with ASD but not seen in controls was in the neurexin gene, which plays an important role in synaptic plasticity and development (Pescosolido *et al*, 2013). Since that time, hundreds of potentially important CNVs have been described in individuals with ASD but are seen rarely, if at all, in non-ASD controls (Betancur, 2011). These CNVs often cross the exons of genes and so potentially lead to abnormalities in gene function. Even though many different CNVs affecting many different genes have been identified, they all seem to belong to several common pathways involved in synaptic plasticity, neuronal development and chromatin remodelling. Most of these CNVs appear to arise *de novo* during meiosis and are not inherited from either parent, thus accounting for upwards of 10% of sporadic cases of ASD. Rare 'inherited' CNVs have also been reported but much less frequently (Pescosolido *et al*, 2013).

The next generation of sequencing studies is likely to add to our understanding of the aetiology of ASD. In these studies, the entire genome (or all the exomes or protein-coding parts of the genes) is sequenced and point mutations can be identified. Several such studies have already been published (Jiang *et al*, 2013; Krumm *et al*, 2013) and the results are promising but the bio-informatics requirements are such that the meaning of these variants remains unclear. However, the field is moving very rapidly.

Nonetheless, environmental risk factors are also important in the aetiology of ASD (Szatmari, 2011). The less than perfect concordance rate in MZ twins and the high concordance rate in DZ twins suggest that some environmental risk factors – either acting alone or in interaction with genetic variants – are important. For instance, it does appear that maternal ingestion of certain anticonvulsants is an important risk factor (Dufour-Rainfray *et al*, 2011). Advanced maternal and paternal age also appear to be important risk factors, possibly associated with an increased risk of chromosomal abnormalities or rare *de novo* CNVs (Hultman *et al*, 2010; Sandin *et al*, 2012). Many other risk factors have been investigated, such as obstetric complications and environmental pollutants, but no consistent picture emerges (Kolevzon *et al*, 2007; Guinchat *et al*, 2012).

Diagnosis and classification

Although age of ASD diagnosis differs across localities and services (Brugha *et al*, 2011), nowadays most cases are identified during early childhood. Children who end up receiving a diagnosis of ASD exhibit deficits related to social communication as well as patterns of restricted/ repetitive behaviours. In most cases, the diagnosis of ASD is associated with additional developmental comorbidities such as lower than average language and IQ scores (Lord & Jones, 2012).

A 'gold standard' diagnosis of ASD involves a comprehensive assessment of behaviours, symptoms, skills and abilities; this information is collected through direct observation of the child by qualified personnel as well as through standardised parent report measures (Falkmer *et al*, 2013).

The two most common systems for diagnosing ASD are ICD-10 (World Health Organization, 1992) and DSM-5. Although there is variability (across localities and service systems) in the way clinicians use these diagnostic systems, certain guidelines exist on best practice related to the recognition, referral and diagnosis of children and young people with ASD (NICE, 2011).

Although the previous version of the *Diagnostic and Statistical Manual* (DSM-IV; American Psychiatric Association, 1994) distinguished between three subtypes of ASD (autistic disorder, Asperger's disorder and pervasive developmental disorder not otherwise specified), the current version does not. In DSM-5, ASD is conceptualised as one 'umbrella' spectrum disorder characterised by two core symptom domains: (1) persistent deficits in social communication and social interaction across multiple contexts; and (2) restricted, repetitive patterns of behaviour, interests or activities. According to DSM-5, these symptoms must be present in the early developmental period, must cause clinically significant impairment in social, occupational, or other important areas of current functioning and must not be better explained by intellectual disability, intellectual developmental disorder or global developmental delay (American Psychiatric Association, 2013).

One noteworthy revision in the DSM-5 criteria is related to the age at onset. Specifically, symptoms can be recognised at any time but must be traced back to early childhood. This change takes into account the notion that sometimes, during the early years, symptoms can go 'unnoticed' until social demands exceed limited capacities.

The revised DSM-5 criteria for ASD also introduce the concept of *clinical specifiers* and *symptom severity*. Recognising that individuals with ASD are usually faced with other challenges, DSM-5 asks clinicians to use clinical specifiers while assigning a diagnosis – that is, to specify whether the disorder presents with or without accompanying intellectual impairment or language impairment, and/or is associated with a known medical or genetic condition or environmental factor. Moreover, to better classify individuals within the autism spectrum, DSM-5 provides a table describing three levels of severity: 'requiring very substantial support' or 'requiring substantial support' or 'requiring support'.

The DSM-5 approach to 'collapse' all autism-related diagnostic subtypes into one umbrella 'ASD' category is viewed by some as 'paradoxical' at a time when clinicians, researchers and parents all seem to accept the notion that ASD is a heterogeneous disorder (Zwaigenbaum, 2012). Furthermore, there is mounting empirical evidence that the 'core' symptoms of ASD (i.e. impaired social communication and restricted/repetitive behaviours) may be more 'fractionable' with respect to genetic and cognitive underpinnings than previously thought (Happe & Ronald, 2008). Therefore, it is likely that categories and subgroups will continue to be used for autism, regardless of how the DSM changes its definition (Mandell, 2011; Rutter, 2012). The development of useful measurement models that have the ability to classify individuals with ASD reliably into more meaningful homogeneous subgroups can serve as a good starting point in our quest for understanding the remarkable heterogeneity seen in this disorder.

Novel statistical methods and recent data from well-designed large studies have changed the nature of the debate on 'categorical versus dimensional' approaches by allowing researchers to explore the notion that 'dimensions can be made into categories by defining thresholds' (Lord & Jones, 2012: p. 492). For example, in an empirical study Georgiades *et al* (2013*a*) examined the underlying structure of the DSM-5 core symptom domains – social communication deficits (SOCOM) and fixated interests and repetitive behaviours (FIRB). By analysing data on 391 newly diagnosed children, this study concluded that the ASD phenotype can be best described using three classes (class 1, 34% of the sample; class 2, 10%; class 3, 56%) based on differential severity gradients on the SOCOM and FIRB symptom dimensions. Children from these classes were diagnosed at different ages and were functioning at different adaptive, language and cognitive levels. This study suggests that the two DSM-5 symptom dimensions of SOCOM and FIRB can be used to stratify children with ASD empirically into three classes/subgroups that are more homogeneous relative to a single class or spectrum (Georgiades *et al*, 2013*a*).

Dimensions, thresholds and categories of ASD may have real-world implications for children and the services they receive. For example, in DSM-5, the diagnosis of social communication disorder (SCD) entails impairment in the social use of language (pragmatic language) as well as deficits in non-verbal communication, without the presence of restricted or repetitive behaviours associated with ASD. SCD falls under the classification of communication disorders, rather than ASD. SCD and ASD are mutually exclusive DSM-5 diagnoses: clinicians must rule out ASD (i.e. a history of restricted or repetitive behaviours) in order to diagnose SCD. Yet SCD is considered by certain experts as an intermediate phenotype, with some overlap with both structural language impairment and ASD (Norbury, 2014). Furthermore, rates of impairment in social communication or pragmatic language may be higher among relatives of individuals with ASD than among low-risk controls (American Psychiatric Association, 2013; Miller *et al*, 2014). More research is needed to test whether the boundaries of SCD are clinically meaningful with respect to specificity of the diagnosis, and whether long-term outcomes will relate the diagnosis more clearly to the spectrum of ASD. In the meantime, naturalistic studies are also required to study whether such shifts in thresholds and diagnostic categories may result in exclusion of children with SCD from important school and healthcare interventions.

The ASD phenotype is multivariate, comprising several developmental domains, including at least one that reflects autistic symptoms and another that reflects adaptive functioning. Factor analytic studies have pointed out the independence of symptoms and functioning, but the true underlying phenotypic structure of ASD is not well understood from a longitudinal perspective. In a recent study, Szatmari *et al* (2015) examined the developmental trajectories of autistic symptom severity and adaptive functioning in a large inception cohort of pre-school children with ASD. Study findings confirmed the heterogeneous nature of developmental trajectories in ASD. Change in adaptive functioning suggests the possibility of notable improvement over the first 12 months after diagnosis in roughly 20% of the sample. Autistic symptom severity appears to be more stable, but here, again, roughly 10% of the children in the sample showed a decline in severity over the first 12 months after diagnosis. Moreover, there appears to be only a moderate amount of 'yoking' of developmental trajectories in autistic symptom severity and adaptive functioning. In other words, progress in one developmental domain does not necessarily correspond to progress in another domain. In general, children with ASD appear to start their course with important baseline differences (i.e. at diagnosis). Therefore, an important time to improve trajectories may be before the diagnosis is officially given, when children present with behavioural or functional concerns during an 'at risk' or 'prodromal' phase.

Future studies must examine the ways in which core symptom domains interact with clinical correlates or specifiers to shape the developmental pathways of individuals with ASD. A recent study investigated patterns of 'cascade effects' between different developmental pathways in children with ASD – the extent to which advantages or impairment in one developmental domain may spread across other domains over time. Such dynamic interactions may explain how so many symptoms and developmental abilities are affected in children with ASD (e.g. social communication, cognition, language, attention, anxiety), as differences, delays or impairments in one domain 'spill over' to others over time. A study of 365 children aged 2–4 who were recently diagnosed with ASD showed evidence of developmental cascades, in which advantages in social competence were strongly associated with improved growth in language ability over 12 months, during which time the two pathways became more specialised and less interrelated (Bennett et al, 2014). Advantages in language did not have the same effect on developing social skills. This supports earlier research which found that emerging social competence is pivotal in influencing other developmental pathways, and suggests that stronger cross-domain interactions may occur in development before the time of diagnosis. Future research will be important to investigate whether other ASD symptoms (e.g. repetitive behaviours) and developmental pathways (e.g. emotion regulation, cognitive abilities) influence each other over longer time periods. Understanding developmental cascades and identifying important 'upstream' skills that influence multiple other symptoms and developmental domains will shed important light on optimal targets for early intervention.

Complexity of the ASD phenotype

Broader autism phenotype

Several studies propose that traits in social communication related to ASD are widely distributed in the general population and in families of affected individuals and that the precise boundaries of the autism diagnosis from these subthreshold traits are currently unclear (Skuse et al, 2005; Constantino, 2011). Moreover, numerous family studies have provided evidence for the existence of what is known as the 'broader autism phenotype' (BAP), a milder (subthreshold) manifestation of autistic-like traits and characteristics in some relatives of individuals with ASD but without serious impairment (Bolton et al, 1994; Bailey et al, 1995; Piven et al, 1997; Szatmari et al, 2008).

Most studies of the BAP focus on parents of children with ASD, although there is a growing literature examining traits related to the BAP in siblings of children with ASD (Constantino et al, 2006; Stone et al, 2007). Georgiades et al (2013b) report that even in younger siblings who do not go on to receive an ASD diagnosis by age 3 there is a risk of more subtle, autism-like traits very early in life. Specifically, approximately 20% of these siblings exhibit delays or difficulties in social communication, cognitive skills and/or anxiety.

Overlap and comorbidities with other disorders

There is a substantial overlap between ASD and other neurodevelopmental and mental disorders, such as attention-deficit hyperactivity disorder

(ADHD), oppositional defiant disorder (ODD), anxiety and mood disorders, developmental coordination disorder and tics/tic disorders (Gadow *et al*, 2004; Brereton *et al*, 2006; Bauminger *et al*, 2010; Lundstrom *et al*, 2014). For example, it is believed that anywhere from 20 to 50% of children with ADHD also meet diagnostic criteria for ASD and 30–80% of children with ASD also meet criteria for ADHD (Lichtenstein *et al*, 2010; Rommelse *et al*, 2010; Rutter, 2012). Moreover, recent genetic findings demonstrate that these neurodevelopmental disorders sometimes also share specific genetic variants, lending support to the idea of common, cross-disorder causal factors and mechanisms (Lichtenstein *et al*, 2010; Lionel *et al*, 2011; Cross-Disorder Group of the Psychiatric Genomics Consortium, 2013).

Georgiades *et al* (2011) examined the phenotypic overlap between core diagnostic features and emotional/behavioural problems in a sample of 335 newly diagnosed pre-school children with ASD. Results demonstrated substantial phenotypic overlap between conventional diagnostic symptoms and problem behaviours in children with ASD, suggesting that ASD might in fact 'share' phenotypes with other childhood-onset neurodevelopmental disorders such as ADHD and OCD. This exploratory study contributes to our understanding of the complexity of the ASD phenotype and supports the inclusion of additional 'clinical specifiers' (e.g. emotional and behavioural problems) as part of the diagnostic characterisation of children with ASD (American Psychiatric Association, 2013). In a way, these findings challenge the current definition of ASD, which is based only on 'core symptoms' (i.e. SCD and FIRB), and call for a systematic investigation that will evaluate the utility of an expanded set of indicators. Emotional and behavioural problems, IQ, language and related cognitive constructs such as theory of mind and executive function are all related to ASD and, again, demonstrate a spectrum of heterogeneity. Although they are not 'core' symptoms of ASD, the ability to self-regulate, to problem solve, to understand and predict others' behaviour, and to plan for the short- and longer-term future are clearly essential to developmental health and well-being. As such, comorbid conditions, skills and deficits should be included as part of a more comprehensive measurement and classification framework for ASD. Future research on this topic should provide evidence on whether these additional indicators often seen in children with ASD are fundamental features of the disorder or whether they should be kept as 'external', associated features of ASD.

Several recent studies have also highlighted the co-occurrence of medical problems in addition to comorbid psychopathology. These might include sleep problems, epilepsy and gastrointestinal symptoms, which are found more commonly in individuals with ASD (Mannion *et al*, 2013; Matson & Goldin, 2013) than in the general population. Taken together, these findings highlight the importance of studying ASD within the larger context of medical and psychiatric nosology in an attempt to better understand how these 'comorbidities' interact with the core autism symptoms to affect both response to treatment and prognosis.

Clinical and research utility of ASD nosology

ASD nosology is constantly updated by new research findings. However, the research utility of new knowledge cannot be directly translated into clinical utility. Owing to the 'Valley of Death' (Szatmari *et al*, 2012) – i.e. our failure to translate scientific knowledge into clinical practice – bridging the gap between researchers and clinicians remains a big challenge. But it is something we need to work on if we are to enhance our understanding of ASD (and other mental and neurodevelopmental disorders).

One possible way of bridging research and clinical practice is to rethink how we evaluate whether a diagnostic category is valid. Currently, this evaluation is based on whether the diagnostic category corresponds to a specific aetiology. That is a naïve bias, based on an outdated 'one cause, one disorder' conception of the aetiology of psychiatric disorders. We now know that both the genetic and the phenotypic architecture of psychiatric disorders (including ASD) is more complex than ever imagined. We also know that many of these disorders show substantial phenotypic and genotypic overlap. So one idea is to try to link cross-disorder information generated from genetic and biological studies to clinical findings and see if they can predict response to treatment and/or developmental outcome. An important example of this different way of studying mental disorders can be found in the Research Domain Criteria (RDoC) project launched by the US National Institute of Mental Health (NIMH) to 'develop, for research purposes, new ways of classifying mental disorders based on behavioral dimensions and neurobiological measures'. The RDoC project aims to integrate data from genetics, neuroscience and behavioural science to study the problems of mental illness, independently from the classification systems by which patients are currently grouped (see http://www.nimh.nih.gov/research-priorities/rdoc/index.shtml).

Acknowledgement

The authors would like to thank all children and families who have participated in their research studies over the years. The authors would also like to thank Kyle Vader, Mike Chalupka and Alessia Greco for their help during the preparation of this chapter.

References

Abrahams BS, Geschwind DH (2008) Advances in autism genetics: on the threshold of a new neurobiology. *Nature Reviews: Genetics*, **9**: 341–55.

American Psychiatric Association (1994) *Diagnostic and Statistical Manual of Mental Disorders* (4th edn) (DSM-IV). APA.

American Psychiatric Association (2013) *Diagnostic and Statistical Manual of Mental Disorders* (5th edn) (DSM-5). APA.

Asperger H (1944) Die 'Autistischen Psychopathen' im Kindesalter [Autistic psychopaths in childhood]. *Archiv für Psychiatrie und Nervenkrankheiten*, **117**: 76–136. doi:10.1007/BF01837709.

Bailey A, Le Couteur A, Gottesman I, *et al* (1995) Autism as a strongly genetic disorder: evidence from a British twin study. *Psychological Medicine*, **25**: 63–77.

Baio J (2012) Prevalence of autism spectrum disorders – autism and developmental disabilities monitoring network, 14 sites, United States, 2008. *Centers for Disease Control and Prevention Surveillance Summaries*, **61**: 1–19.

Bauminger N, Solomon M, Rogers SJ (2010) Externalizing and internalizing behaviors in ASD. *Autism Research: Official Journal of the International Society for Autism Research*, **3**: 101–12. doi: 10.1002/aur.131; 10.1002/aur.131.

Bennett TA, Szatmari P, Georgiades K, *et al* (2014) Do reciprocal associations exist between social and language pathways in preschoolers with autism spectrum disorders? *Journal of Child Psychology and Psychiatry*. doi: 10.1111/jcpp.12356.

Betancur C (2011) Etiological heterogeneity in autism spectrum disorders: more than 100 genetic and genomic disorders and still counting. *Brain Research*, **1380**: 42–77.

Bolton P, Macdonald H, Pickles A, *et al* (1994) A case-control family history study of autism. *Journal of Child Psychology and Psychiatry and Allied Disciplines*, **35**: 877–900.

Brereton AV, Tonge BJ, Einfeld SL (2006) Psychopathology in children and adolescents with autism compared to young people with intellectual disability. *Journal of Autism and Developmental Disorders*, **36**: 863–70. doi: 10.1007/s10803-006-0125-y.

Brugha TS, McManus S, Bankart J, *et al* (2011) Epidemiology of autism spectrum disorders in adults in the community in England. *Archives of General Psychiatry*, **68**: 459–65.

Constantino J, Lajonchere C, Lutz M, *et al* (2006) Autistic social impairment in the siblings of children with pervasive developmental disorders. *American Journal of Psychiatry*, **163**: 294–6.

Constantino JN (2011) The quantitative nature of autistic social impairment. *Pediatric Research*, **69**: 55R–62R.

Cross-Disorder Group of the Psychiatric Genomics Consortium (2013) Genetic relationship between five psychiatric disorders estimated from genome-wide SNPs. *Nature Genetics*, **45**: 984–94.

Devlin B, Scherer SW (2012) Genetic architecture in autism spectrum disorder. *Current Opinion in Genetics and Development*, **22**: 229–37.

Dufour-Rainfray D, Vourc'h P, Tourlet S, *et al* (2011) Fetal exposure to teratogens: evidence of genes involved in autism. *Neuroscience and Biobehavioral Reviews*, **35**: 1254–65.

Elsabbagh M, Divan G, Koh YJ, *et al* (2012) Global prevalence of autism and other pervasive developmental disorders. *Autism Research: Official Journal of the International Society for Autism Research*, **5**: 160–79. doi: 10.1002/aur.239; 10.1002/aur.239.

Falkmer T, Anderson K, Falkmer M, *et al* (2013) Diagnostic procedures in autism spectrum disorders: a systematic literature review. *European Child and Adolescent Psychiatry*, **22**: 329–40. doi: 10.1007/s00787-013-0375-0.

Fombonne E, Quirke S, Hagen A (2009) Prevalence and interpretation of recent trends in rates of pervasive developmental disorders. *McGill Journal of Medicine: MJM: An International Forum for the Advancement of Medical Sciences by Students*, **12**: 73.

Gadow KD, DeVincent CJ, Pomeroy J, *et al* (2004) Psychiatric symptoms in preschool children with PDD and clinic and comparison samples. *Journal of Autism and Developmental Disorders*, **34**: 379–93.

Georgiades S, Szatmari P, Duku E, *et al* (2011) Phenotypic overlap between core diagnostic features and emotional/behavioral problems in preschool children with autism spectrum disorder. *Journal of Autism and Developmental Disorders*, **41**: 1321–9. doi: 10.1007/s10803-010-1158-9.

Georgiades S, Szatmari P, Boyle M, et al (2013a) Investigating phenotypic heterogeneity in children with autism spectrum disorder: a factor mixture modeling approach. *Journal of Child Psychology and Psychiatry and Allied Disciplines*, **54**: 206–15. doi: 10.1111/j.1469-7610.2012.02588.x.

Georgiades S, Szatmari P, Zwaigenbaum L, *et al* (2013*b*) A prospective study of autistic-like traits in unaffected siblings of probands with autism spectrum disorder. *JAMA Psychiatry*, **70**(1): 42–8. doi: 10.1001/2013.jamapsychiatry.1; 10.1001/2013.jamapsychiatry.1.

Guinchat V, Thorsen P, Laurent C, *et al* (2012) Pre-, peri-, and neonatal risk factors for autism. *Acta Obstetricia et Gynecologica Scandinavica*, **91**: 287–300.

Hallmayer J, Cleveland S, Torres A, *et al* (2011) Genetic heritability and shared environmental factors among twin pairs with autism. *Archives of General Psychiatry*, **68**: 1095–102. doi: 10.1001/archgenpsychiatry.2011.76; 10.1001/archgenpsychiatry.2011.76.

Happe F, Ronald A (2008) The 'fractionable autism triad': a review of evidence from behavioural, genetic, cognitive and neural research. *Neuropsychology Review*, **18**: 287–304.

Hultman CM, Sandin S, Levine SZ, *et al* (2010) Advancing paternal age and risk of autism: new evidence from a population-based study and a meta-analysis of epidemiological studies. *Molecular Psychiatry*, **16**: 1203–12.

Jiang YH, Yuen RK, Jin X, *et al* (2013) Detection of clinically relevant genetic variants in autism spectrum disorder by whole-genome sequencing. *American Journal of Human Genetics*, **93**: 249–63.

Kanner L (1968) Autistic disturbances of affective contact. *Acta Paedopsychiatrica*, **35**: 100–36. (Reprint of the original 1943 article in *Nervous Child*, **2**: 217–50.)

Kolevzon A, Gross R, Reichenberg A (2007) Prenatal and perinatal risk factors for autism: a review and integration of findings. *Archives of Pediatric and Adolescent Medicine*, **161**: 326–33.

Krumm N, O'Roak BJ, Shendure J, *et al* (2013) A de novo convergence of autism genetics and molecular neuroscience. *Trends in Neurosciences*, **37**: 95–105.

Li X, Zou H, Brown WT (2012) Genes associated with autism spectrum disorder. *Brain Research Bulletin*, **88**: 543–52.

Lichtenstein P, Carlstrom E, Rastam M, *et al* (2010) The genetics of autism spectrum disorders and related neuropsychiatric disorders in childhood. *American Journal of Psychiatry*, **167**: 1357–63. doi: 10.1176/appi.ajp.2010.10020223; 10.1176/appi.ajp.2010.10020223.

Lionel AC, Crosbie J, Barbosa N, *et al* (2011) Rare copy number variation discovery and cross-disorder comparisons identify risk genes for ADHD. *Science Translational Medicine*, **3**(95): 95ra75.

Lord C, Jones RM (2012) Annual research review: re-thinking the classification of autism spectrum disorders. *Journal of Child Psychology and Psychiatry and Allied Disciplines*, **53**: 490–509. doi: 10.1111/j.1469-7610.2012.02547.x; 10.1111/j.1469-7610.2012.02547.x.

Lord C, Risi S, DiLavore PS, *et al* (2006) Autism from 2 to 9 years of age. *Archives of General Psychiatry*, **63**: 694–701. doi: 10.1001/archpsyc.63.6.694.

Lundstrom S, Reichenberg A, Melke J, *et al* (2014) Autism spectrum disorders and coexisting disorders in a nationwide Swedish twin study. *Journal of Child Psychology and Psychiatry and Allied Disciplines*, doi: 10.1111/jcpp.12329. [Epub ahead of print]

Malhotra D, Sebat J (2012) CNVs: harbingers of a rare variant revolution in psychiatric genetics. *Cell*, **148**: 1223–41.

Mandell D (2011) The heterogeneity in clinical presentation among individuals on the autism spectrum is a remarkably puzzling facet of this set of disorders. *Autism: The International Journal of Research and Practice*, **15**: 259–61.

Mannion A, Leader G, Healy O (2013) An investigation of comorbid psychological disorders, sleep problems, gastrointestinal symptoms and epilepsy in children and adolescents with autism spectrum disorder. *Research in Autism Spectrum Disorders*, **7**: 35–42.

Matson JL, Goldin RL (2013) Comorbidity and autism: trends, topics, and future directions. *Research in Autism Spectrum Disorders*, **7**: 1228–33. doi:10.1016/j.rasd.2013.07.003.

Miller M, Young GS, Hutman T, *et al* (2014) Early pragmatic language difficulties in siblings of children with autism: implications for DSM-5 social communication disorder? *Journal of Child Psychology and Psychiatry and Allied Disciplines.* doi: *10.1111/* jcpp.12342. [Epub ahead of print]

NICE (2011) *Autism Diagnosis in Children and Young People: Recognition, Referral and Diagnosis of Children and Young People on the Autism Spectrum (NICE Clinical Guideline 128).* National Institute for Health and Clinical Excellence.

Norbury CF (2014) Practitioner review: social (pragmatic) communication disorder conceptualization, evidence and clinical implications. *Journal of Child Psychology and Psychiatry and Allied Disciplines,* **55**: 204–16.

Ozonoff S, Young GS, Carter A, *et al* (2011) Recurrence risk for autism spectrum disorders: a Baby Siblings Research Consortium study. *Pediatrics,* **128**: e488–95. doi: 10.1542/peds.2010-2825.

Pescosolido MF, Gamsiz ED, Nagpal S, *et al* (2013) Distribution of disease-associated copy number variants across distinct disorders of cognitive development. *Journal of the American Academy of Child and Adolescent Psychiatry,* **52**: 414–30.

Piven J, Palmer P, Jacobi D, *et al* (1997) Broader autism phenotype: evidence from a family history study of multiple-incidence autism families. *American Journal of Psychiatry,* **154**: 185–90.

Rommelse NN, Franke B, Geurts HM, *et al* (2010) Shared heritability of attention-deficit/ hyperactivity disorder and autism spectrum disorder. *European Child and Adolescent Psychiatry,* **19**: 281–95. doi: 10.1007/s00787-010-0092-x; 10.1007/s00787-010-0092-x.

Ronald A, Hoekstra RA (2011) Autism spectrum disorders and autistic traits: a decade of new twin studies. *American Journal of Medical Genetics Part B: Neuropsychiatric Genetics,* **156**: 255–74.

Rutter M (2012) Changing concepts and findings on autism. *Journal of Autism and Developmental Disorders,* **43**: 1749–57. doi: 10.1007/s10803-012-1713-7.

Sandin S, Hultman CM, Kolevzon A, *et al* (2012) Advancing maternal age is associated with increasing risk for autism: a review and meta-analysis. *Journal of the American Academy of Child and Adolescent Psychiatry,* **51**: 477–86.

Skuse DH, Mandy WP, Scourfield J (2005) Measuring autistic traits: heritability, reliability and validity of the social and communication disorders checklist. *British Journal of Psychiatry,* **187**: 568–72. doi: 10.1192/bjp.187.6.568.

Stone W, McMahon C, Yoder P, *et al* (2007) Early social-communicative and cognitive development of younger siblings of children with autism spectrum disorders. *Archives of Pediatrics and Adolescent Medicine,* **161**: 384–90.

Sullivan PF, Daly MJ, O'Donovan M (2012) Genetic architectures of psychiatric disorders: the emerging picture and its implications. *Nature Reviews: Genetics,* **13**: 537–51.

Szatmari P (2011) Is autism, at least in part, a disorder of fetal programming? *Archives of General Psychiatry,* **68**: 1091–2. doi: 10.1001/archgenpsychiatry.2011.99.

Szatmari P, Georgiades S, Duku E, *et al* (2008) Alexithymia in parents of children with autism spectrum disorder. *Journal of Autism and Developmental Disorders,* **38**: 1859–65. doi: 10.1007/s10803-008-0576-4; 10.1007/s10803-008-0576-4.

Szatmari P, Charman T, Constantino JN (2012) Into, and out of, the 'Valley of Death': research in autism spectrum disorders. *Journal of the American Academy of Child and Adolescent Psychiatry,* **51**: 1108–12.

Szatmari P, Georgiades S, Duku E, *et al* (2015) Developmental trajectories of symptom severity and adaptive functioning in an inception cohort of preschool children with autism spectrum disorder. *JAMA Psychiatry,* **72**: 276–83.

World Health Organization (1992) *International Statistical Classification of Diseases and Related Health Problems* (10th revision) (ICD-10). WHO.

Zwaigenbaum L (2012) What's in a name: changing the terminology of autism diagnosis. *Developmental Medicine and Child Neurology,* **54**: 871–2.

CHAPTER 9

Autism spectrum disorder and Asperger syndrome

Tom Berney

Concepts and labels

Asperger syndrome, a form of autism, is defined solely by its symptoms (Box 9.1). However, our perception of autism together with its terminology and definitions are in flux. The original, florid picture, drawn by Leo Kanner in 1943 (see Chapter 8), still stands – someone who is aloof from or even averse to people, with peculiar speech and markedly rigid, stereotypical and repetitive behaviour. Often with an intellectual disability, sometimes with unusual talents, they represent only one facet of a very varied disorder. The other group, half of those with autism, have neither an intellectual disability nor the obvious anomalies of speech. Some marry or pursue a career, helped as well as hindered by their altered social sensitivity, focused interests, or detached pragmatism, the last being seen as a refreshingly alternative view, a blunt and objective focusing on fact, 'thinking outside the box' or simply eccentricity. It is this picture, initially identified by Hans Asperger as autistic psychopathy in 1944, that emerged as Asperger syndrome (van Krevelen, 1971; Wing, 1981), to become popularised in books, films and plays. Although recently discarded by DSM, the term remains in ICD for the present and continues to have a popular and useful currency, identifying people often overlooked by psychiatry.

The development of the concept, like others in psychiatry, is of clarity alternating with confusion. Bleuler coined the term 'autism' to describe the self-centred social withdrawal of schizophrenia and it was adopted separately by Kanner and Asperger to describe the main thread in their case series.

- Kanner thought autism to be a psychotic process but one separate from schizophrenia: a distinction that was soon lost as it came to be seen simply as the early onset of a unitary psychosis. It was only in 1971, when Kolvin and Rutter showed autism to be substantially different, that it was recognised as a developmental disorder. The defining criteria had passed from Mildred Creak's Nine Points, to Lorna Wing's Triad of Impairment, to those adopted by ICD-9 (World Health Organization, 1978) and DSM-III (American Psychiatric Association, 1980) and now to the latest variant in DSM-5 (American Psychiatric Association, 2013).

Box 9.1 The characteristics of Asperger syndrome in adulthood

- *Difficulties in social interaction.* These may present as social awkwardness, a lack of social responsiveness or failure to take part in a meaningful to-and-fro conversation. Problems in understanding the nuances of social situations may manifest as a proneness to social blunders or as an unthinking lack of concern for others, suggesting a reduced intuitive understanding of how others might think or feel. In the longer term, there may be difficulty in making and maintaining reciprocal friendships (even though the individual may be successful in striking up a series of acquaintances). It is important to review the relationships at work and at home separately, as there is no consistent pattern as to which are the more demanding.

- *Limited non-verbal communication.* This can appear as an unusual use of gaze, facial expression and gesture: elements that may be poorly integrated with each other as well as with what is being said. (This is different to the persistent avoidance of gaze observed in mental disorders such as depression.) Speech may be less vivacious than in most, sounding unusually even in pitch and pace or pedantically correct. This inability to appreciate the non-verbal component of speech not only leaves the person struggling to comprehend what is being said but may lead to serious misunderstanding. This applies particularly where someone appears fluent, demonstrative and well able to express themselves (as it is assumed automatically that comprehension matches expression).

- *Interests and activities that are unusual in their intensity, content or the amount of time they absorb.* This can result in someone whose expertise in a narrow, specialist field is unusual in comparison with their other abilities), unusually set in their ways, with inflexible routines or repetitive behaviour and a rigid aversion to change. It is different from obsessive–compulsive behaviour in that the person does not feel this behaviour to be alien and has no desire to change (particularly if they are doing something they enjoy).

- *Unusual sensory responses.* People with Asperger syndrome are unusually aware of a variety of stimuli (whether drawn to or repelled by them) as diverse as certain sounds, flickering lights, repetitive movement, clothing or minor anomalies such as cracks in walls, the pattern of a fabric or the hum of a neon tube. The result is that the person can seem to be very distracted, day-dreaming or even hallucinating.

- *An inflexibility that results in a person who is very set in their ways with fixed routines and an aversion to anything new.* Again, this differs from obsessive–compulsive behaviour in that the person does not feel this behaviour to be alien and has little desire to change.

- *Something unusual about a comorbid psychiatric disorder.* A failure to respond to treatment may raise the suspicion of Asperger syndrome, although a normal, neurotypical, premorbid personality would seem to make this unlikely. However, symptoms may remain unnoticed until later childhood and even early adolescence if the person has been in supportive circumstances and the symptoms are mild. (However, the older the person is, the less likely it is that there will be an informant available.)

- Asperger, on the other hand, thought the characteristics of his children to be static: an abnormal personality type. Unfortunately, although Lorna Wing had elaborated the cluster of traits that make up Asperger syndrome, there was disagreement over their operationalisation as diagnostic criteria. While many researchers (Gillberg, Szatmari and Tantam) specified that normal syntactical speech be present at the time of diagnosis, the international criteria set out in DSM-IV (American Psychiatric Association, 1994) and ICD-10 (World Health Organization, 1992) went further, requiring that language development had been normal from childhood.

Both forms are part of a wider group of neurodevelopmental disorders, all the result of a varying interaction of genetic predisposition and environmental factors, a group which, although presenting predominantly as a cluster of cognitive and behavioural traits, has a much more widespread effect. Its components vary in form and intensity to fall on a multifaceted, dimensional spectrum of severity that shades from the full-blown syndrome through to those whose symptoms are so mild as to fade imperceptibly into the normality of the neurotypical population. While a categorical label can give a shorthand explanation in clear-cut cases (e.g. the character Raymond Babbitt in the 1988 film *Rain Man*), its validity is less certain both for those individuals who have only a few, albeit florid, symptoms and for those whose milder symptoms put them near the 'normality' end of the spectrum. In the latter, a superficial normality can mask subtle but disabling psychological deficits such as 'mind blindness' or impaired executive function, auditory comprehension or perception. Categorical diagnostic systems combine with the pressure to label to make it tempting to sweep any eccentric, isolated or simply unusual personality under this diagnosis.

This lumping of all socially impaired patients into the autism spectrum disorders (ASD) is offset by efforts to split off syndromes such as pathological demand avoidance (Newson *et al*, 2003), multiplex developmental disorders (Towbin *et al*, 1993) and semantic pragmatic disorder (Bishop & Norbury, 2002); the last has resurfaced as social communication disorder (SCD) in DSM-5. Complicated by synonyms such as right-hemisphere or non-verbal learning disorders (Fitzgerald, 1999), the result is a confusing group of specific disabilities on which we impose recognisable constellations of clinical disorder (Willemsen-Swinkels & Buitelaar, 2002).

Where should we set the boundary for a dimensional disorder? As with the personality disorders, it might be the point at which it causes distress (either to the patient or to those around) or significant problems in social functioning and performance, or at which it requires treatment. This diagnostic threshold is not an absolute, as it will depend on the setting as well as the individual. For example, while the bullied schoolboy may be helped by a diagnosis of Asperger syndrome, it may be less welcome when he becomes a mathematical star enjoying university. This would make for a functional distinction between permanent innate traits and a disorder that depends as much on the setting as on innate characteristics. It also opens to question where a predisposition is to be thought of as a lifelong disorder, which is an issue in all developmental disorders, including epilepsy, which can affect many areas of life, including employability.

The category of Asperger syndrome was introduced by ICD-10 and DSM-IV to discover whether it had an identity discrete from high-functioning autism (HFA; autism unaccompanied by intellectual disability) or was simply autism in a milder form, less coloured by the presence of other disabilities, or was the effect of a different aetiological path (e.g. social impairment that results from problems with early language). After 30 years of research failed to find satisfactory distinguishing criteria (Kugler, 1998), Asperger syndrome, along with other variants, was not included in DSM-5. Ostensibly this leaves the one, all-embracing diagnosis of ASD, although it is unclear how this will sit with SCD, which, although featuring similar (but not identical) social impairment, lacks the requisite repetitive or focused behaviours/interests or sensory anomalies to qualify as ASD. SCD is grouped under 'Language Impairments', a separation that echoes the earlier, experimental distinction of 'Asperger syndrome'.

It remains to be seen how ICD-11 will define the autisms, but for the present, 'Asperger syndrome' identifies a group of people who have autism with no significant intellectual disability and good syntactical speech, although the last tends to mask the very real but sometimes subtle impairment in non-verbal communication (Tantam & Guirgis, 2009; Woodbury-Smith & Volkmar, 2009). It is a useful category, as it describes a group of people who have a social identity and specific service needs. Freed from the constraints of formal criteria, the greater public awareness, the fashionability of the label and a demand to medicalise everyday difficulty, it seems likely that the net will widen. This can only highlight the problem of how to define the point at which an individual's symptoms are sufficiently marked and/or numerous to achieve 'caseness'. On the other hand, the adoption of the term 'autism spectrum condition' (as against 'disorder') reflects an aversion to being pathologised which is carried forward by the neurodiversity movement's preference for terms such as 'autists' or 'aspies'. This emphasises disability as the consequence of living in an alien (neurotypical) environment such that most distinctions would disappear with the development of an inclusive society – analogous to the implications of, and remedies for, gender discrimination (Jaarsma & Welin, 2012).

Epidemiology

Varied definitions make it difficult to disentangle the epidemiology of Asperger syndrome from that of the wider ASD. Kanner's childhood autism is rare, with a population prevalence of about 0.04% (of whom 70–80% have a significant intellectual disability). ASD has extended to become a broader, dimensional disorder with a population prevalence of at least 1% (of whom only about half have a degree of intellectual disability) (Baird *et al*, 2006). Although, as with many neurodevelopmental disorders, ASD improves with age (Balfe *et al*, 2011; Fein *et al*, 2013), its prevalence in adulthood also runs at over 1% but without the comorbid intellectual disability (although this may be because the absence of academic demands allow a wider, functional definition of 'normality') (Brugha *et al*, 2012). It means that, with the selection pressure of other, comorbid disorders, a mainstream mental health service might expect 3–5% of its patients to have an underlying ASD (Nylander & Gillberg, 2001).

The suggestion that we might be in an 'autism epidemic' can be explained by wider recognition, changing concepts and criteria, and better diagnostic services, without calling on an intrinsic increase (Leonard *et al*, 2010).

Numerous reviews but limited data leave us uncertain about the association, if any, between ASD and offending. What determines 'offender' status will depend on the definition of an offence as well as whether an individual is caught, prosecuted and convicted. Studies often lack a normative comparison group and have been hampered by limited sampling or a poor response rate, while varying in the rigour with which they define ASD. Studies of prevalence among offenders have been limited to specialist clinics and institutions and, in the latter case, factors such as structure and limited social demands may minimise symptoms and camouflage cases. Nevertheless, there is some increase in numbers within special hospitals and mental health secure units, ranging from 1.5% to 10%, but it is notable that most of these are new diagnoses. This suggests that studies that follow up those who already have a clinic diagnosis may be focusing on the more law-abiding or that there may be other factors (such as tolerance and support) that prevent someone getting into the justice system. Studies of specialised groups, notably those who have been referred for forensic examination, have found ASD in up to 15–20%, particularly in those convicted of arson, sexual and violent offences (Mouridsen, 2012).

Although about 20% of people with ASD develop epilepsy, much of the association is with intellectual disability; once this has been allowed for, the lifetime risk reduces to 5–8% (Tuchman, 2013), although even this link has been questioned (Berg & Plioplys, 2012). The time of onset is unusual in that, for about half of cases, it does not occur until adolescence.

The presentation in adulthood

Symptoms vary with development and some may even grow out of their ASD (Seltzer *et al*, 2003, 2004; Balfe *et al*, 2011; Fein *et al*, 2013) as a result of innate maturation, learned compensatory skills and a less demanding environment (the last means that symptoms may re-emerge with later events, such as retirement or divorce). The overall result is a syndrome that is often more subtle and ill-defined than in childhood; it may even become subclinical, only to emerge in a crisis or simply in an adverse environment

(Balfe *et al*, 2011; Fein *et al*, 2013). However, even should people fall below the diagnostic threshold, they may retain a number of disabilities in areas such as perception, cognition, communication and motivation, all the more disabling for being hidden and keeping them dependent on others.

Little is known about what happens in later life (Mukaetova-Ladinska *et al*, 2012). An adult population survey did not find that prevalence changed with age (Brugha *et al*, 2012).

However, there is the stress of growing up with Asperger syndrome that arises from unrecognised disability (e.g. poor executive function and idiosyncratic motivation), limited achievement and a sense of failure, often revealed by an increasing contrast with more autonomous and successful siblings or peers. Distorted relationships with family and peers come from their frustration with the person's apparently self-centred insensitivity, obsessiveness and rigid inflexibility. This leads to frequent bullying; irritability and violence are common responses (Balfe & Tantam, 2010). On top of this may be added other, comorbid neurodevelopmental or psychiatric disorders (see below). All these elements add further layers to the person's intrinsic difficulties, resulting in a degree of disability disproportionate to any intellectual impairment (Howlin, 2004: pp. 19–45; Samson *et al*, 2011).

The development of sexual identity and orientation is an under-researched area (Byers *et al*, 2013). It may be delayed and sometimes derailed by confusion about relationships, with social impairment complicated by poorly understood internal feelings. Such factors may contribute to gender identity disorder, while fetishism may be an expression of a focal interest.

While intellectual ability is important in determining independence, it does not guarantee a favourable outcome. Only 16–50% of children with Asperger syndrome but of normal ability become fully independent as adults, the higher end of that range possibly reflecting a community that is unusually supportive (Engstrom *et al*, 2003; Howlin *et al*, 2004; Farley *et al*, 2009).

Diagnosis and assessment

Diagnosis is the allocation of a series of categorical, descriptive labels that summarise whether an individual meets the diagnostic criteria agreed by consensus and set out in such systems as ICD–10 and DSM-5. It is often not appreciated that, as there is no definitive laboratory test for ASD, the diagnosis is part of a clinical formulation, a judgement that can evolve over time as more information is gathered and circumstances change. It has to strike a balance between being too broad and being too selective, a balance that will depend on whether it is:

- for research – where the criteria will depend on the nature of the study, so that a person with ASD may be excluded where there is limited information or simply doubt and it does not mean necessarily that that individual does not have ASD

- clinical – where it is the basis for determining management
- administrative – the diagnosis giving access to services or resources or a different forensic outcome or disposal.

Although ASD is a cluster of dimensional disabilities, the value of a diagnosis lies in its categorical nature (rather than the indeterminate fudge of 'autistic traits'). For some, the achievement of this may be a gateway to a new life, but for most it is of limited benefit without a wider assessment.

Assessment follows diagnosis. It should be multidisciplinary (NICE, 2012) and, depending on the circumstances, might include:

- cognitive ability – measured by various forms of intelligence test, identifying discrepancies between verbal and performance abilities as well as the variety of specific disabilities that can accompany any neurodevelopmental disorder
- functional ability – acknowledging the extent to which there may be difficulties in a wide variety of areas, including social relationships, communication (receptive and expressive), imagination and occupational executive function, the effect of which can be to reduce the extent to which individuals can look after themselves, function independently, take up education, employment or leisure activities, or cope with other people
- coexisting neurodevelopmental disabilities – notably attention-deficit hyperactivity disorder, tics, sensory anomalies and coordination disorder, as well as epilepsy
- coexisting psychiatric disorder – such as anxiety, depression or psychosis
- mental capacity and associated factors such as the risk of coming to harm or of offending
- physical medical issues – such as atopies, gastrointestinal problems or infections.

It is often easier to identify ASD than to exclude it. Should a diagnostic label, which affects the way people are seen as well as the way they see themselves, come to be more hindrance than help, it may be difficult to remove. From the start, it is therefore essential to understand who it is that actually is seeking the diagnosis and why.

Most diagnoses will be straightforward and may simply confirm a conclusion that has already been reached by the person themselves. ASD brings a wide range of symptoms, varied in both nature and intensity, across a wide range of ability and age, and affected by gender. These will colour comorbid disorder, affecting both its presentation and its management. More pronounced under stress (whether psychological or physical), these symptoms may become so intense and sustained as to be difficult to distinguish from distinct, comorbid psychiatric disorder.

The symptoms also may be mistaken for other forms of disorder. An unwitting unconcern for the effect of an action on others can easily be

Box 9.2   Adapting the psychiatric interview

The psychiatrist has to keep in mind the underlying impairment of autism spectrum disorder (ASD) and possibly adapt the interview by the following means.

- Reducing anxiety as far as possible – for example, by structuring the interview, setting out the purpose of the interview, what will happen during it and how long it will last (being guided by the person in this).
- Using short, straightforward, unambiguous sentences, and checking that the individual has understood (fluency and being able to repeat back what has been said do not indicate comprehension). Statements are likely to be taken at face value. It is important not to overload an individual's auditory processing but allow them time to digest and respond.
- Avoiding a dependence on non-verbal elements, such as gesture, facial expression and tone of voice, which may pass unnoticed.
- Appreciating that the person may find difficulty with hypothetical choice, so they may be helped by being presented with a limited range of choices with clear effects.
- Using diagrams and visual text to help comprehension.
- Summarising the main points of an interview in a confirmatory letter.
- Limiting choice to what the individual can manage and making the implications of each choice clear. Indecisiveness may be the result of too many choices or uncertainty about their significance.
- Encouraging the presence of a friend or advocate in the interview, which can allow an individual to discuss afterwards what was said, getting information that was missed and digesting the content of the interview.

These are only examples and adaptations need to be tailored to the needs of the individual.

confused with the ruthless disregard that characterises the dissocial/psychopathic personality disorder, while, particularly in women, borderline personality disorder may be invoked to explain the combination of difficult social relationships, emotional arousal and alexithymia. It is not easy to identify the point at which rigidity and ritual become obsessive–compulsive disorder, nor when a rigidly held, overvalued idea becomes a delusion. Such complexity can be disentangled only by a careful, systematic approach, in the course of which the clinician adapts the interview to the patient's particular needs (Box 9.2).

Differential diagnoses are listed in Box 9.3 (see also 'Comorbid disorder, below).

Diagnostic instruments

A variety of instruments, ranging from screening questionnaires to interview frameworks to structured interview schedules, help clinicians to collect information systematically and consistently, ensure they have the

---

Box 9.3 Differential diagnoses

Anxiety states
- selective mutism
- social anxiety disorder
- generalised anxiety disorder
- panic disorder

Schizophrenia (particularly treatment-resistant)
- paranoid
- chronic
- catatonic
- simple

Personality disorders
- avoidant
- schizoid
- anankastic
- dissocial
- borderline

Attention-deficit hyperactivity disorder
The person flits too actively to relate socially

Obsessive–compulsive disorder
The person is too preoccupied with their pathology to relate socially

---

appropriate information to match against the agreed criteria, and give them a framework against which they might organise their thoughts. Although criteria continually evolve, they do contribute to consistency, holding clinicians to the threshold of that time. The construct may be refined by an algorithm. While algorithms serve to operationalise diagnostic categories and their dimensions, their mechanical simplicity may be misleading when applied to clinical cases, particularly where there is an overlay of comorbid disorder. In the end, a diagnosis is a conclusion (rather than the result of a test) and the data should be available for subsequent review.

The number of instruments reflects not just the different tasks, clinical and research, but also the problem of assessing something that has such a variegated presentation, complicated by a variety of co-occurring disorders. Although narrowing the focus to Asperger syndrome removes the difficulties of distinguishing the effects of significant intellectual disability and language disorder, the symptomatology can be more subtle and much will depend on the clinician's familiarity with autism as well as the ability to draw on childhood (premorbid) as well as current symptoms.

Instruments differ in their evidential underpinning (see review by Lord & Corsello, 2005), the research standard being set by the Autism Diagnostic Instrument – Revised (ADI-R), which uses information gathered from informants over 2–3 hours in a formal, semi-structured interview. It has been complemented by the Autism Diagnostic Observation Scale (ADOS-2), which is designed to elicit, describe and rate autism's symptoms in the course of an interview with the individual, lasting up to an hour. The Diagnostic Instrument for Social and Communication Disorders (DISCO) is a more clinical instrument; it gathers and synthesises information from a variety of informants, including the individual, to give a wider assessment of their developmental disabilities rather than just those relating to autism.

More specific instruments have been designed but are still acquiring the evidential underpinning necessary for their use in research (Stoesz *et al*, 2011). The Adult Asperger Assessment (AAA) incorporates information from standard questionnaires completed beforehand in a semi-structured interview. These questionnaires, plus the Autism Spectrum Quotient (AQ) and the Empathy Questionnaire (EQ), are available online (as are many others) and are widely used in screening and self-diagnosis.

Briefer screening interviews include the Asperger Syndrome Diagnostic Interview (the ASDI) with informants and the Ritvo Autism Asperger Diagnostic Scale – Revised (RAADS-R), a self-completion questionnaire. The Royal College of Psychiatrists has developed a *Diagnostic Interview Guide* to be used in conjunction with the standard psychiatric interview (Berney *et al*, 2011).

Comorbid disorder

Besides its own characteristics, ASD can come with a variety of comorbid conditions. These include other neurodevelopmental disorders, psychiatric illness and relationship difficulties (including family/marital problems) (Tantam & Guirgis, 2009). These may be arbitrarily grouped into:

- other neurodevelopmental disorders – notably attention-deficit hyperactivity disorder (ADHD), tic/Tourette disorder, developmental coordination disorder (DCD) and epilepsy
- psychiatric disorder – anxiety, depression, bipolar disorder, schizophrenia, catatonia and obsessive–compulsive disorder (OCD).

It is becoming clear, though, that, like ASD, these are dimensional disorders that range from the full-blown through to common, population trait. They co-occur, have common predispositional genetic anomalies (e.g. shared copy number variants, particularly affecting genes encoding interacting synaptic proteins, such as neuroligins and neurexins) and common familial inheritance (Sullivan *et al*, 2012; Faraone, 2013), with the dissolution of the discrete, categorical boundaries of ICD and DSM.

Other neurodevelopmental disorders

This comorbidity means that, like troubles and buses, neurodevelopmental disabilities come in clusters rather than singly, and the more severe a disability, the more likely there are to be others: ASD signifies a neurodevelopmental vulnerability which brings disabilities that traditionally belong to other categories of disorder. Although such specific disabilities are grouped into diagnostic clusters, these constellations are neither clear nor discrete; a particular disability may be neither characteristic of nor exclusive to a disorder. For example, inattentiveness and distractibility may be features of ASD as well as central to ADHD, clumsiness may go with ASD as well as DCD, and compulsive behaviour is part of Tourette syndrome as well as of OCD. Other specific disabilities, such as alexithymia and prosopagnosia, have not been allocated a syndromal home but the identification of one disability should trigger a wider enquiry for others.

Obsessive–compulsive disorder (OCD)

While a natural reaction to the mess of everyday life is to establish order, this can reach a maladaptive intensity in someone with ASD. Routines may make it impossible to carry out everyday activities, saving may result in an uncontainable hoard, collecting may resort to theft and a variety of idiosyncratic rules may limit not just the individual's life but also that of those around.

Compulsive traits, increased by anxiety, run through biological psychiatry, but it is the absence of internal resistance in someone with ASD (i.e. it is not egodystonic) which suggests that this is not true OCD. The distinction is an important one, affecting the motivation to change, but it is by no means clear cut. There is common ground between the two disorders (Chasson *et al*, 2011) and individuals may have a variety of obsessive–compulsive symptoms, some acceptable to them and some not, implying the presence of two conditions, to be managed differently.

Anxiety

Anxiety is frequent in ASD and, given the additional difficulties people with ASD typically encounter while growing up, it is unsurprising that this should be a trait. However, anxiety states are also more frequent and, while their form is less clear, ranging from specific phobia to generalised anxiety, they combine to hinder engagement with the wider world. For example, they may present as situational phobias (e.g. social anxiety disorder, performance anxiety and selective mutism), panic (which may result in either paralysis or violent flight) or the intensified symptoms of other disorders described below. Beside their symptom clusters, the later onset of many of these helps to distinguish them from ASD.

Schizophrenia

Schizophrenia's relationship with ASD is close and complex (Palmen & van Engeland, 2012), especially with the pre-schizophrenic, schizoid personality disorder and the residual state (Waris *et al*, 2013), and there are similarities in presentation (Box 9.4). Although Asperger distinguished his syndrome clearly from schizophrenia, it, along with autism, was engulfed in the concept of a unitary psychosis until a distinction was made between the two disorders in 1971, when autism, associated with intellectual disability, epilepsy and a characteristic developmental trajectory, was recognised as a neurodevelopmental disorder (Kolvin, 1971). Yet, although a number of studies have failed to find any specific association with schizophrenia, there is evidence for a link. Sula Wolff's long-running study of 'loners', children who fitted the definition of schizoid personality disorder (later identified with Asperger syndrome), found 5% subsequently developed schizophrenia (Wolff, 1995). A third of those who develop schizophrenia in childhood (an unusual and severe form of psychosis) have pre-existing ASD (Rapoport *et al*, 2009). There is a less specific association with psychosis (Sullivan *et al*, 2013).

Box 9.4 Why Asperger syndrome may be mistaken for psychosis

- Thoughts expressed simply and concretely by someone who has difficulty in describing internal symptoms sound very like hallucinations.
- A very vivid account of events is held consistently but is plainly false. However, these experiences (including perceptions) do not seem to trouble the individual nor to be associated with any functional change. There is the sense that the individual is living in a 'video world', sometimes becoming comprehensible when the interviewer sees the video.
- High arousal in a developmental disorder can produce an acute and transient psychotic state with hallucinations and thought disorder.
- Incomplete answers can sound like psychotic symptoms. For example, a bald report, without elaboration or context, of everyday teasing can sound like persecutory delusions.
- A pragmatic difficulty in appreciating the extent or limitations of someone else's knowledge of a topic, coupled with a tendency to obsessiveness, can result in overinclusive, irrelevant speech that mimics schizophrenic thought disorder.
- Impassivity and a lack of awareness of the emotional climate can look like inappropriate or blunted affect.
- Catatonic symptoms (e.g. odd mannerisms and postures, freezing or difficulty in initiating movement) occur in a variety of neurological conditions, including schizophrenia and autism spectrum disorder.
- The slow and reluctant response of patients asked to perform a task that has no meaning for them resembles the negative symptoms of schizophrenia.
- The symptoms of autism spectrum disorder can show improvement with any anxiolytic drugs, including antipsychotics.

Schizophrenia itself has come to be seen as a neurodevelopmental disorder and its dimensional nature is recognised in the indistinct boundaries with the attenuated psychosis syndrome, simple schizophrenia (which can have a very similar presentation, other than for its late age at onset) and catatonia (see below).

These hints of a return to the unitary psychosis probably reflect association being mistaken for causation: it seems more likely that similar underlying anomalies may give rise to similar, but not identical, symptoms. In the end, it is important to avoid the twin mistakes of overlooking ASD in, or mistaking it for, schizophrenia, which means taking account of the early, childhood history as well as examining the current symptoms (Box 9.4). Where the two disorders do coexist, treatment and rehabilitation have to be aimed at the ASD as well as at the schizophrenia.

Affective disorder

Depression occurs more frequently than in the neurotypical population, although alexithymia and a lack of facial expression mean it may be missed unless an informant's description of behavioural changes is available. However, bipolar disorder also occurs more frequently, both in the individual and in the family, and, as in schizophrenia, there are shared susceptibility genes, with ASD as well as with ADHD (Carroll & Owen, 2009; Sullivan *et al*, 2012; Faraone, 2013).

Catatonia

This ill-defined disorder, primarily impeding voluntary action although it can include overactivity and impulsive actions, was thought to be symptomatic of schizophrenia. However, it became clear that it can occur with other disorders and that its symptoms run through neuropsychiatry. Catatonic symptoms, such as stereotypies, complex mannerisms, a difficulty in initiating voluntary actions, echolalia, unusual slowness, passivity and freezing, are not unusual in ASD. Particularly striking is ambitendence: the person, unable to complete an intended action, withdraws and tries again, turning a straightforward action into a hesitant stutter. However, while the symptoms are frequent, particularly the more severe the degree of autism or intellectual disability, they do not usually interfere with the person's everyday function unless magnified by anxiety (Wing & Shah, 2006). In some, the symptoms are sufficiently sustained, intense and dominant for the syndrome of catatonia; whether this represents a separate, comorbid disorder is unclear but it should be treated as such.

An ordinary life

All individuals vary greatly in the extent to which they have managed to acquire the wide range skills necessary to eventual autonomy. ASD can introduce its own constraints, interfering with the ability to present oneself effectively, to get work and stay in it, coping with people and in the wider world (Balfe *et al*, 2011). At the same time, it can bring areas of skill and talent, such as attention to detail, a tendency to be methodical, to focus on a task and to develop unusual levels of expertise. It is important that such areas are recognised and the initial assessment should help everyone, including the individual, to recognise these talents and limitations, to build on the former and to remedy the latter. The management of ASD itself is therefore primarily about education, training and social support and care. This can come from a range of resources as well as the individual's family and peers. Some of the more important areas are:

- the provision of support, which can range from mentoring or a part-time personal assistant through to a full-time residential placement
- formal teaching in areas such as:
  - social skills (how to cope with others), which may extend to social and sexual rules
  - emotional management, which covers areas such as emotional literacy (the ability to identify and describe feelings), relaxation training, stress reduction and anger management, and throughout which there may be as much emphasis on averting arousal as on dealing with it
  - independent living skills, which might equip someone to leave home, and which include for example shopping, budgeting, housekeeping, laundry and personal hygiene
  - work skills, such as how to apply for a job, interview skills and how to cope with a job and a work environment (as employers and services become more familiar with, and appreciative of, ASD, so it becomes more feasible to adapt occupations and their environments)
- peer group support, which may come through the internet as well as from voluntary groups.

Legal issues

Mental capacity

While ASD entails communication difficulties (see Boxes 9.2 and 9.5) that can affect decision-making, it can also affect the ability to weigh up information, bringing rigid views as to how the world works (or should work) and a perception of cause and effect that may not reflect reality. It can be difficult for an individual to judge the authority and motivation of informants, and this can emerge, for example, as a strong belief that something on the internet must be true or that anything from someone in authority will be false. There may simply be an overriding aversion to change or choice, but, whatever lies underneath, people with ASD are likely to find decisions difficult (Luke *et al*, 2012).

Reliability as a witness

A report of an event depends not just on what the person actually saw, but also on their interpretation of the scene and on their memory: we have a natural tendency to fill in what we expected to see. Certain characteristics of Asperger syndrome can colour the understanding and recall of a situation (Box 9.5).

Any difficulty in picking up the overall narrative may interfere with the recall of events. For example, the UK police are encouraged to use the cognitive interview, in which, after a detailed narrative account, the person is asked to re-examine the events in a different order and from a different perspective. However, for people with ASD this increases errors in recall (Maras & Bowler, 2010).

Consequently, in deciding on somebody's fitness to act as a witness it is important to assess their ability to give a reliable account. This means enough specific, concrete, verifiable material such as details of the scene (e.g. the design of a ring or the colour and pattern of the wallpaper) as well as of the events preceding and following the episode to be able to identify any temporal confusion. The individual's ability to comprehend and to respond to questions must also be assessed. Allowance must be made for

---

Box 9.5 Characteristics that might affect the reliability of a person with autism spectrum disorder as a witness

- Misinterpretation of the event, whether experienced or observed (e.g. was someone being coerced or helped?).
- Difficulty with the dimension of time. Although the person may recall the sequence of events correctly, their perception of the relative periods of intervening time may be so inaccurate as to make it unclear as to whether they are recounting something that happened the previous day, week or year.
- Difficulties in remembering people, their appearance and their actions.
- Difficulty in distinguishing the person's own actions from those of others, which may extend to a confusion of reality with observed fiction.
- Difficulties with attention and concentration (which may be as much to do with anxiety as innate attention-deficit hyperactivity disorder), made worse by discomfort or sensory distraction.
- Susceptibility to inappropriate interviewing (e.g. the Cognitive Interview), unfamiliar surroundings and circumstances (whether the police station or the witness box) and relationships.
- Distortion by the misinterpretation of rules and relationships, with undue compliance complicated by a rigid tendency to adhere to (and believe in) a story once it is in their head.

communication problems such as using words without understanding their significance, a very literal comprehension, and difficulty in grasping non-verbal components.

Their ability will be influenced by their role, whether accused, observer or victim. There is a risk that an adult may not be recognised as vulnerable,

---

Box 9.6 Characteristics of autism spectrum disorder that may predispose to criminal offending

- A misinterpretation of relationships can leave the individual open to being drawn into illicit relationships, to intimidation, or to exploitation as a stooge. Limited emotional knowledge hinders understanding of adult situations and relationships and can, for example, lead to social attraction or friendship being mistaken for love.
- A misinterpretation of rules, particularly social ones, can lead someone, who does not grasp the point at which 'no' means 'no', to stumble into offences such as 'date rape' and stalking. Their understanding of rules may be undermined by failing to recognise the extent to which television and video scenarios present fictional standards.
- Innate difficulty in reading social signals and cues (e.g. a difficulty in judging the age of others) can lead to, for instance, sexual advances to somebody under age (which is particularly likely where social ineptness has made it more comfortable to associate with a younger peer group).
- An unusual passivity can leave the individual open to being influenced and exploited by others.
- Impulsivity, sometimes violent, may be a component of a comorbid attention-deficit hyperactivity disorder, a state of anxiety turning into panic or a confusing blend of both. The result can be an emotional response (e.g. a tantrum) that is out of proportion to the situation that others then misinterpret as threatening to them.
- A limited awareness of the outcome of their actions, its seriousness or its impact on others can lead the individual to embark on a course of behaviour irrespective of its consequences. For example, what starts as fire setting may result in a building's destruction or what starts as a minor assault might become disproportionately intense and damaging.
- Overriding preoccupations can lead to offences such as stalking or compulsive theft. Here, admonition may increase anxiety and consequently a ruminative thinking of the unthinkable that increases the likelihood of action.
- Misjudging the nature of an interview may encourage an incautious frankness, which can confirm the interviewer's suspicion that the individual is an offender or, at least, a potential offender. Private fantasies may be no more lurid than those of many in the wider population but may be startling in terms of their clinical detachment, their obsessional quality and the lack of insight, leading to socially inappropriate disclosure.
- A failure to appreciate any need to change (or finding change inordinately difficult) can leave the individual stuck in a risky pattern of behaviour – a problem that may be made worse by comorbid dysphoria, anxiety or any other mental state that reduces flexible thinking.

---

particularly where there is an academic awareness of right from wrong. The ability to challenge evidence depends on understanding it and the removal of the right to silence puts even more weight on how someone presents themselves in court and can affect their fitness to stand trial without compensatory arrangements (Gray et al, 2001; Freckelton & List, 2009).

Offending

People with ASD can work out the rules as long as they are not destabilised by emotional arousal (whether anxiety or excitement) or their enthusiasm, either of which can make them overlook the consequences of their actions. These and other factors (Box 9.6) may lead an individual to stumble into offending; such characteristics need to be identified and taken into account in the person's management.

Conclusion

The characteristics of Asperger syndrome can range from a subtle variant of the personality through to a florid disorder. Its importance to the psychiatrist is its contribution to associated comorbid conditions, which themselves can vary from non-specific anxiety and malaise to more definite psychiatric disorder. It is as prevalent and, particularly if unrecognised, as disabling as any other psychiatric disorder. In addition, other disorders may mimic features of the syndrome. All this makes the psychiatrist an essential component of the multidisciplinary team, not just in terms of the diagnosis and management of these individuals, but also in promoting their wider social inclusion.

References

American Psychiatric Association (1980) *Diagnostic and Statistical Manual of Mental Disorders* (3rd edn) (DSM-III). APA.

American Psychiatric Association (1994) *Diagnostic and Statistical Manual of Mental Disorders* (4th edn) (DSM-IV). APA.

American Psychiatric Association (2013) *Diagnostic and Statistical Manual of Mental Disorders* (5th edn) (DSM-5). APA.

Baird G, Simonoff E, Pickles A, *et al* (2006) Prevalence of disorders of the autism spectrum in a population cohort of children in South Thames: the Special Needs and Autism Project (SNAP). *Lancet*, **368**: 210–15.

Balfe M, Tantam D (2010) A descriptive social and health profile of a community sample of adults and adolescents with Asperger syndrome. *BMC Research Notes*, **3**: 300.

Balfe M, Tantam D, Campbell M (2011) Possible evidence for a fall in the prevalence of high-functioning pervasive developmental disorder with age? *Autism Research and Treatment*, article ID 325495 (Epub 19 June 2011).

Berg AT, Plioplys S (2012) Epilepsy and autism: is there a special relationship? *Epilepsy and Behavior*, **23**: 193–8.

Berney T, Brugha T, Carpenter P (2011) *Diagnostic Interview Guide for the Assessment of Adults with Autism Spectrum Disorder (ASD)*. Royal College of Psychiatrists.

Bishop DVM, Norbury CF (2002) Exploring the borderlands of autistic disorder and specific language impairment: a study using standardised diagnostic instruments. *Journal of Child Psychology and Psychiatry and Allied Disciplines,* **43**: 917–29.

Brugha T, Cooper SA, McManus S, *et al* (2012) *Estimating the Prevalence of Autism Spectrum Conditions in Adults: Extending the 2007 Adult Psychiatric Morbidity Survey.* NHS Health and Social Care Information Centre.

Byers ES, Nichols S, Voyer SD, *et al* (2013) Sexual well-being of a community sample of high-functioning adults on the autism spectrum who have been in a romantic relationship. *Autism,* **17**: 418–33.

Carroll LS, Owen MJ (2009) Genetic overlap between autism, schizophrenia and bipolar disorder. *Genome Medicine,* **1**: 102.

Chasson GS, Timpano KR, Greenberg JL, *et al* (2011) Shared social competence impairment: another link between the obsessive–compulsive and autism spectrums? *Clinical Psychology Review,* **31**: 653–62.

Engstrom I, Ekstrom L, Emilsson B (2003) Psychosocial functioning in a group of Swedish adults with Asperger syndrome or high-functioning autism. *Autism,* **7**: 99–110.

Faraone SV (2013) Attention-deficit hyperactivity disorder and the shifting sands of psychiatric nosology. *British Journal of Psychiatry,* **203**: 81–3.

Farley MA, McMahon WM, Fombonne E, *et al* (2009) Twenty-year outcome for individuals with autism and average or near-average cognitive abilities. *Autism Research,* **2**: 109–18.

Fein D, Barton M, Eigsti I-M, *et al* (2013) Optimal outcome in individuals with a history of autism. *Journal of Child Psychology and Psychiatry,* **54**: 195–205.

Fitzgerald M (1999) Differential diagnosis of adolescent and adult pervasive developmental disorders/autism spectrum disorders (PDD/ASD): a not uncommon diagnostic dilemma. *Irish Journal of Psychological Medicine,* **16**: 145–8.

Freckelton I, List D (2009) Asperger's disorder, criminal responsibility and criminal culpability. *Psychiatry, Psychology and Law,* **16**: 16–40.

Gray NS, O'Connor C, Williams T, *et al* (2001) Fitness to plead: implications from case-law arising from the Criminal Justice and Public Order Act 1994. *Journal of Forensic Psychiatry,* **12**: 52–62.

Howlin P (2004) *Autism and Asperger Syndrome: Preparing for Adulthood* (2nd edn). Routledge.

Howlin P, Goode S, Hutton J, *et al* (2004) Adult outcome for children with autism. *Journal of Child Psychology and Psychiatry and Allied Disciplines,* **45**: 212–29.

Jaarsma P, Welin S (2012) Autism as a natural human variation: reflections on the claims of the neurodiversity movement. *Health Care Analysis,* **20**: 20–30.

Kolvin I (1971) Studies in childhood psychoses. I. Diagnostic criteria and classification. *British Journal of Psychiatry,* **118**: 381–4.

Kugler B (1998) The differentiation between autism and Asperger syndrome. *Autism,* **2**: 11–32.

Leonard H, Dixon G, Whitehouse AJO, *et al* (2010) Unpacking the complex nature of the autism epidemic. *Research in Autism Spectrum Disorders,* **4**: 548–54.

Lord C, Corsello C (2005) Diagnostic instruments in autistic spectrum disorders. In *Handbook of Autism and Pervasive Developmental Disorders: Volume 1, Diagnosis, Development, Neurobiology, and Behavior* (eds FR Volkmar, R Paul, A Klin, *et al*): pp 730–71. Wiley.

Luke L, Clare ICH, Ring H, *et al* (2012) Decision-making difficulties experienced by adults with autism spectrum conditions. *Autism,* **16**: 612–21.

Maras KL, Bowler DM (2010) The Cognitive Interview for eyewitnesses with autism spectrum disorder. *Journal of Autism and Developmental Disorders,* **40**: 1350–60.

Mouridsen SE (2012) Current status of research on autism spectrum disorders and offending. *Research in Autism Spectrum Disorders,* **6**: 79–86.

Mukaetova-Ladinska EB, Perry E, Baron M, *et al* (2012) Ageing in people with autistic spectrum disorder. *International Journal of Geriatric Psychiatry,* **27**: 109–18.

Newson E, Le Marechal K, David C (2003) Pathological demand avoidance syndrome: a necessary distinction within the pervasive developmental disorders. *Archives of Disease in Childhood*, **88**: 595–600.

NICE (2012) *Autism: Recognition, Referral, Diagnosis and Management of Adults on the Autism Spectrum* (Clinical Guideline 142). National Institute for Health and Clinical Excellence.

Nylander L, Gillberg C (2001) Screening for autism spectrum disorders in adult psychiatric out-patients: a preliminary report. *Acta Psychiatrica Scandinavica*, **103**: 428–34.

Palmen S, van Engeland H (2012) The relationship between autism and schizophrenia: a reappraisal. In *Brain, Mind, and Developmental Psychopathology in Childhood* (eds ME Garralda, J-P Raynaud): pp 123–44. Jason Aronson.

Rapoport J, Chavez A, Greenstein D, *et al* (2009) Autism spectrum disorders and childhood-onset schizophrenia: clinical and biological contributions to a relation revisited. *Journal of the American Academy of Child and Adolescent Psychiatry*, **48**: 10–18.

Samson A, Huber O, Ruch W (2011) Teasing, ridiculing and the relation to the fear of being laughed at in individuals with Asperger's syndrome. *Journal of Autism and Developmental Disorders*, **41**: 475–83.

Seltzer MM, Krauss MW, Shattuck PT, *et al* (2003) The symptoms of autism spectrum disorders in adolescence and adulthood. *Journal of Autism and Developmental Disorders*, **33**: 565–81.

Seltzer MM, Shattuck P, Abbeduto L, *et al* (2004) Trajectory of development in adolescents and adults with autism. *Mental Retardation and Developmental Disabilities Research Reviews*, **10**: 234–47.

Stoesz BM, Montgomery JM, Smart SL, *et al* (2011) Review of five instruments for the assessment of Asperger's disorder in adults. *Clinical Neuropsychologist*, **25**: 376–401.

Sullivan PF, Magnusson C, Reichenberg A, *et al* (2012) Family history of schizophrenia and bipolar disorder as risk factors for autism family history of psychosis as risk factor for ASD. *Archives of General Psychiatry*, **69**: 1099–103.

Sullivan S, Rai D, Golding J, *et al* (2013) The association between autism spectrum disorder and psychotic experiences in the Avon Longitudinal Study of Parents and Children (ALSPAC) birth cohort. *Journal of the American Academy of Child and Adolescent Psychiatry*, **52**: 806–14.

Tantam D, Guirgis S (2009) Recognition and treatment of Asperger syndrome in the community. *British Medical Bulletin*, **89**: 41–62.

Towbin KE, Dykens EM, Pearson GS, *et al* (1993) Conceptualizing 'borderline syndrome of childhood' and 'childhood schizophrenia' as a developmental disorder. *Journal of the American Academy of Child and Adolescent Psychiatry*, **32**: 775–82.

Tuchman R (2013) Autism and social cognition in epilepsy: implications for comprehensive epilepsy care. *Current Opinion in Neurology*, **26**: 214–18.

van Krevelen DA (1971) Early infantile autism and autistic psychopathy. *Journal of Childhood Autism and Schizophrenia*, **1**: 82–6.

Waris P, Lindberg N, Kettunen K, (2013) The relationship between Asperger's syndrome and schizophrenia in adolescence. *European Child and Adolescent Psychiatry*, **22**: 217–23.

Willemsen-Swinkels SHN, Buitelaar JK (2002) The autistic spectrum: subgroups, boundaries, and treatment. *Psychiatric Clinics of North America*, **25**: 811–36.

Wing L (1981) Asperger's syndrome: a clinical account. *Psychological Medicine*, **11**: 115–29.

Wing L, Shah A (2006) A systematic examination of catatonia-like clinical pictures in autism spectrum disorders. *International Review of Neurobiology*, **72**: 21–39.

Woodbury-Smith M, Volkmar F (2009) Asperger syndrome. *European Child and Adolescent Psychiatry*, **18**: 2–11.

Wolff S (1995) *Loners: The Life Path of Unusual Children*. Psychology Press.

World Health Organization (1978) *International Statistical Classification of Diseases and Related Health Problems* (9th revision) (ICD-9). WHO.

World Health Organization (1992) *International Statistical Classification of Diseases and Related Health Problems* (10th revision) (ICD-10). WHO.

CHAPTER 10

Pharmacological management of core and comorbid symptoms in autism spectrum disorder

Rachel Elvins and Jonathan Green

Autism spectrum disorder (ASD) is one of the leading causes of lifetime developmental disability (Fombonne, 2003). The diagnosis includes childhood autism, atypical autism and Asperger syndrome; these are often alternatively grouped as pervasive developmental disorders. DSM-5 has integrated these separate disorders into a single 'autism spectrum disorder' diagnosis (American Psychiatric Association, 2013). They are recognised as complex neurodevelopmental disorders, often becoming clinically apparent in the second to third year of life. The DSM-5 diagnosis is based on disturbance in two domains: persistent deficits in social communication and social interaction across multiple contexts; and restricted, repetitive patterns of behaviour, interests or activities. Up to two-thirds of affected individuals will present with a degree of global intellectual disability, although some may have a very uneven profile of abilities. Accurate diagnosis, usually made by a combination of direct observation of behaviour and informant history, is complicated by considerable heterogeneity in the manifestation of these core deficits, by variation in ability level and by developmental changes. However, it is clear that ASD persists across the life span, and produces varied and complex needs in adult life (Lord *et al*, 2001). The course of development into old age is, as yet, largely unknown.

Prevalence figures vary widely, depending on the definition of 'caseness' and assessment tools used. UK studies have reported a prevalence of around 1.2% (Baird *et al*, 2006). There are no accurate prevalence figures available for adults but in 2011 it was estimated there were 5.3 million adults with diagnosed ASD across Europe, the USA and Japan (Nightingale, 2012). A male excess of between 3:1 and 4:1 is generally observed (Fombonne, 2003). ASD is associated with an estimated annual UK cost in childhood of £3.1 billion (Buescher *et al*, 2014), greater than asthma, diabetes or other intellectual disability.

Maladaptive behaviours and comorbid psychiatric symptoms are common in individuals with ASD and are strongly associated with carer stress (Lecavalier *et al*, 2006).

Autism spectrum disorder is thus a relatively common, chronic, potentially substantially disabling disorder, with significant costs both to the affected individual and to family members. There are no established definitive treatments for the core social impairment. Both the severity of the disorder and the lack of effective treatments continue to promote keen public interest and to prompt research. Controversies surrounding environmental causes of autism and novel (unproven) treatments serve to keep this set of disorders in the public eye and increase referrals to both paediatric and psychiatric services. Since the publication of guidance from the National Institute of Health and Care Excellence (NICE) on assessment (NICE, 2011) and treatment (NICE, 2013), there has been a further focus on early intervention as well as assessment. More people are now first diagnosed with ASD as adolescents and adults, possibly owing to increased public and professional recognition (Mesibov & Handlan, 1997). For many families, the transition from adolescence to adulthood will be a period of increased need. As a result, more referrals may be seen across adult psychiatry.

Medication management in autism

Alongside burgeoning professional interest, increasingly rigorous clinical trials have attempted to elucidate evidence-based pharmacological strategies for both the core ASD syndrome and comorbidity. In the field of neurodevelopmental disability there has traditionally been a dearth of independent, well-powered randomised controlled trials (RCTs). However, more rigorous psychopharmacology studies have started to be published.

Educational and psychosocial interventions are the mainstay of treatment, with the aim of improving language acquisition and maximising communication and social skills (NICE, 2013). However, medication management, particularly of maladaptive behaviours, is common and possibly increasing (Aman *et al*, 2005). Such behaviours or symptoms of comorbid disorders may interfere with socialisation and educational progress, and severely impair individuals' and families' quality of life. A UK study found that up to 75% of individuals with ASD and disorders of intellectual development (DID) were prescribed at least one psychotropic medication (Tsakanikos *et al*, 2006). Factors associated with increasing medication use include greater age, poorer functioning and higher levels of challenging behaviour (Aman *et al*, 2005).

There are, however, no currently available standard medication regimes. Medications that are commonly used belong to diverse groups and are non-specific to the target symptoms identified. They may affect a wide range of neurological functions, with subsequent unwanted effects. An attempt to elucidate the evidence base for the use of such treatments is therefore helpful for prescribers and case managers alike.

The aim of this chapter is to discuss and summarise clinical pharmaco-therapy for ASD, based upon target domains of behaviour (Table 10.1).

Table 10.1 Selected medication for use in domains of behaviour in autism

Symptom cluster	Medications	Common/important adverse effects	Supporting references
Stereotypical and compulsive/repetitive behaviours	SSRI (fluoxetine, fluvoxamine)	Irritability, activation, insomnia, gastrointestinal upset, potential increase in suicidal ideation	McDougle et al, 1996; Hollander et al, 2005; Posey et al, 2006
	Second-generation antipsychotic (risperidone, aripiprazole)	Appetite increase, weight gain, sedation, glucose dysregulation, extrapyramidal symptoms, QTc prolongation, neuroleptic malignant syndrome	Scahill et al, 2002; McDougle et al, 2005; Ching & Pringsheim, 2012
Irritability, aggression and self-injury	Second-generation antipsychotic (risperidone and aripiprazole)	As above	McDougle et al, 1998; Shea et al, 2004; Ching & Pringsheim 2012
	Opiate antagonist (naltrexone)	Headaches and dizziness	Symons et al, 2004
	Typical antipsychotic (haloperidol)	Extrapyramidal symptoms, akathisia, weight gain, QTc prolongation, neuroleptic malignant syndrome	Remington et al, 2001
Hyperkinesis and inattention	Immediate-release methylphenidate	Appetite suppression, weight loss, insomnia, rebound hyperkinesis, tachycardia, hypertension	RUPP Autism Network, 2005a
	Alpha-2 agonist (clonidine)	Fatigue, hypotension	Jaselskis et al, 1992
	Atomoxetine	Gastrointestinal upset, fatigue, appetite suppression, liver dysfunction, suicidal ideation, hypertension, tachycardia	Arnold et al, 2006; Zeiner et al, 2011
	Antipsychotics (aripiprazole, risperidone)	As above	Aman et al, 2010; Ching & Pringsheim, 2012
Depressive symptoms	SSRI	As above	Posey et al, 2006
Manic symptoms	Anticonvulsant mood stabiliser (valproate/divalproex)	Weight gain, sedation, gastrointestinal upset, platelet suppression, liver dysfunction, pancreatitis, teratogenicity	Hollander et al, 2001
	Second-generation antipsychotics	As above	Joshi et al, 2012
Anxiety symptoms	SSRI	As above	Posey et al, 2006
	Buspirone	Dyskinesia	Buitelaar et al, 1998
Sleep dysfunction	Melatonin	Somnolence	Owens et al, 2005; Gringras et al, 2012
	Antihistamine	Irritability, somnolence	Owens et al, 2005

RUPP, Research Units of Pediatric Psychopharmacology; SSRI, selective serotonin reuptake inhibitor.

Such symptoms, which are difficult to manage, are often the reason why families seek medical treatments. We first evaluate treatments targeted at the underlying core social deficit of ASD and then address certain target clusters of symptoms, such as stereotypical and compulsive/ritualistic behaviours, and serious aggressive and self-injurious behaviour. The distinction between core syndrome phenomena and co-occurring symptoms is important in assessment and treatment planning, even though this distinction is sometimes subtle and takes detailed assessment: improvement in one area may lead to global improvements, and some drugs may play a role in several symptom clusters. However, a systematic approach that makes this distinction will help clinicians organise their thinking when deciding on a particular medication strategy, allowing them to focus on exactly which presenting problem they are trying to treat, and with what. A methodical approach of this kind is also essential to minimise polypharmacy and the development of potentially disastrous management strategies in which further medication has to be used to treat emerging unwanted effects of previous medications.

We will focus on RCTs, where available, as well as the common unwanted effects of particular drugs and shortcomings of the published data. Although the field is not yet at a stage at which treatment protocols or algorithms can usefully be written, the aim is to identify medication regimes which are most likely to be clinically useful for each domain. Medication management of common psychiatric comorbidities in ASD will also be discussed. The NICE (2013) guidance on the management and support of young people on the autistic spectrum is discussed and the recommendations and the evidence base on which these are made are highlighted.

Finally, future directions of pharmacotherapeutic research will be discussed.

Core symptoms

Social deficits

The detailed underlying pathophysiology of social impairments in ASD is still unclear. Their treatment has been subject to many 'false dawns' in the literature, with therapeutic approaches often based on questionable theory. Rigorous trials have reduced interest in some unproven approaches, despite their active promotion by vested interests. Recently, secretin, a gastrointestinal peptide, and fenfluramine, an indirect 5-HT partial agonist, have been widely trialled, with nearly 500 children with ASD being recruited to RCTs for secretin alone. Both drugs were shown in preliminary trials to have prosocial effects in autism. However, placebo-controlled trials have failed to show consistent improvements (McDougle et al, 2006). Neither medication has any evidence base in autism management at this time.

Diet

Vitamins and minerals have been widely trialled, with broadly disappointing results, a recent example being a Cochrane review of RCTs studying the use of vitamin B6 and magnesium (Nye & Brice, 2005). It was concluded that their use cannot be supported in ASD based on the available evidence, and that larger, better-designed studies are needed. There is widespread interest in exclusion diets, but as yet there have been no good-quality RCTs in this area.

Immune function

Infectious and immune mechanisms have been popular candidate aetiological agents in autism (although there is no significant support for this from basic science). A limited number of related treatment studies have been carried out. One trial of vancomycin (Sandler *et al*, 2000) showed that improvements in communication returned to baseline when the drug was stopped. Pentoxifylline (a methylxanthine that has immunological and serotonergic effects) has been shown to improve irritability and social withdrawal in combination with risperidone, an antipsychotic drug (Akhondzadeh *et al*, 2010). RCTs of other drugs having a direct effect upon immune function in autism have not so far been conducted.

There is, at present, no place for immunotherapy in the management of autism in standard clinical practice. There is also no reliable evidence that anti-fungal treatments are effective in the treatment of ASD.

Vaccinations, particularly the combined measles, mumps and rubella (MMR) vaccine, have long been the subject of controversy with regard to aetiological mechanisms and ASD. Several large studies have refuted a causal link between MMR and ASD (Honda *et al*, 2005).

Antidepressants and antipsychotics

Clinical studies (mostly open label) of selective serotonin reuptake inhibitors (SSRIs) and second-generation antipsychotics such as risperidone have suggested that some individuals with ASD show improvement in aspects of social relatedness following treatment (McDougle *et al*, 2006). Risperidone does have a proven effect on arousal states and behaviour (see below) and any effect on prosocial behaviour is likely to be secondary to this. Aripiprazole, a partial D2 agonist, has demonstrated improvements in measures of social withdrawal and inappropriate speech in recent trials (Marcus *et al*, 2009; Owen *et al*, 2009). However, NICE guidance specifically recommends against the use of antipsychotics or antidepressants for the core features of autism at this time owing to the adverse balance of risks and benefits (see Kendall *et al*, 2013).

Glutamate-active medication

Glutamatergic function has been the focus of recent extensive research in neuropsychiatric disorders. Glutamate is the primary excitatory amino acid in the brain and is thought to be important in regulating neuronal plasticity and higher cognitive functions (Carlsson, 1998). Both ASD and schizophrenia are postulated to be hypoglutamatergic disorders and parallels have been drawn between the negative symptoms of schizophrenia and the social impairment in autism (Nikolov *et al*, 2006).

Further interest has been excited by a large pooled genetic analysis (Autism Genome Project Consortium, 2007) which used linkage and copy number variation analysis respectively to implicate candidate gene loci on chromosome 11p12-p13 and neurexins. Neurexins and neuroligins (independently linked with autism in other analyses) are implicated in glutamatergic synaptogenesis, highlighting glutamate-related genes as promising candidates in ASD. One glutamate-active drug of interest is D-cycloserine, a partial agonist at the N-methyl-D-aspartate (NMDA) receptor complex. It has been used with benefit when added to conventional antipsychotics in schizophrenia and this benefit has been associated with enhanced temporal lobe function (Yurgelun-Todd *et al*, 2005). A small single-blind pilot study of D-cycloserine targeting the core social impairment in children with ASD (Posey *et al*, 2004) showed a dose–response relationship with improvements in social withdrawal. Adverse effects were reported only at higher doses. However, Posey recently reported a larger, double-blind parallel-groups study which showed that D-cycloserine did not improve social relatedness in young children (Posey, 2008). Large neurobiological and pharmaceutical trials involving this drug are under development (Wink *et al*, 2010).

Other drugs currently being trialled include amantadine and memantine, which act as non-competitive antagonists at the NMDA receptor. Open-label and retrospective studies of memantine have had mixed results in the domain of social relatedness (Owley *et al*, 2006; Chez *et al*, 2007) and side-effects have included irritability and excessive sedation. One small controlled trial of amantadine in children (King *et al*, 2001) showed a trend towards greater treatment response based on ratings on the Clinical Global Improvement (CGI) scale. Other studies have had less favourable results; for example, lamotrigine (an anticonvulsant which attenuates cortical glutamate release) was found to be no better than placebo on any outcome measure employed in a small RCT in children (Belsito *et al*, 2001).

The active research interest in this area parallels that in schizophrenia and more work will undoubtedly follow. However, work is still at a preliminary stage and at present the available evidence would not support the clinical use of glutamate-active medications in ASD.

Clinical implications

The core social impairments in ASD remain relatively intractable. In childhood and adolescence, psychosocial and education management strategies should be the first line in management and do have an early evidence base for efficacy. The current small evidence base for a pharmacological approach to long-term disabilities means that at present medication does not have a place in practice for the management of core symptoms. Future advances may change the situation.

Stereotypical and ritualistic/compulsive behaviours

These behaviours are defined as part of the core of ASD. They include verbal and motor rituals, obsessive questioning, rigid adherence to routine, preoccupation with details and obsessive desire for maintenance of sameness. Such symptoms are commonly the most functionally impairing aspect of the syndrome and interfere significantly with an individual's progression in educational and socialisation programmes. They have similarities with the phenomena of obsessive–compulsive disorder (OCD) and thus medications such as tricyclic antidepressants and SSRIs with known efficacy in OCD are obvious candidate drugs.

Antidepressants

Clomipramine is a non-selective tricyclic antidepressant that affects uptake of serotonin, noradrenaline and dopamine. Two cross-over RCTs using children and young adults provide some evidence that clomipramine is superior to placebo on measures such as anger and obsessive symptoms (Gordon et al, 1993; Remington et al, 2001). Remington et al (2001) found no gains in areas such as hyperactivity and global symptom severity. Concerns about adverse effects of clomipramine make this drug less widely used than SSRIs.

Using the SSRI fluvoxamine, a short-term RCT in adults with autism showed improvements in both compulsive and prosocial behaviour (McDougle et al, 1996). Trials with children have had more mixed results. A short-term RCT involving children with ASD showed that fluvoxamine had no advantage over placebo (McDougle et al, 2000). Adverse effects were noted in 78%. More encouragingly, another 12-week RCT cross-over study of 18 children with ASD judged that 10 were treatment responders on the CGI scale. However, a placebo response rate is not recorded, and adverse events occurred in 39%, although this was not considered significant (Sugie et al, 2005).

Improvements in repetitive behaviours have been shown in two very small cross-over RCTs in children and adults using fluoxetine (Buchsbaum et al, 2001). There were no differences in side-effects between drug and placebo in children (Hollander et al, 2005). Unpublished data of a recent large RCT of fluoxetine in children showed that repetitive behaviours were reduced in those taking either placebo or fluoxetine but there were no statistically significant differences in response between the two groups (Autism Speaks, 2009). Large-scale trials of fluoxetine aiming to identify responders and non-responders to SSRIs are in development (Nightingale, 2012).

Evidence regarding other antidepressant use is scant and of less quality. Open-label trials of sertraline, citalopram and escitalopram in children and adults have shown benefits in reducing aggression and repetitive behaviours (e.g. Owley *et al*, 2005). An open-label study using paroxetine in adults showed improvements at 1-month but not at 4-month follow-up (Davanzo *et al*, 1998). There are no studies using paroxetine in children as yet. A larger RCT of citalopram in children with ASD and repetitive behaviours showed no significant differences in response between the citalopram- and placebo-treated groups, although both groups showed improvements. Citalopram was more likely to be associated with adverse events such as increased energy levels and insomnia (King *et al*, 2009). Open-label studies of venlafaxine have suggested efficacy in repetitive behaviours in some children and adults (Hollander *et al*, 2000).

SSRIs may be more effective and give rise to fewer side-effects in adolescents and adults with ASD than in children (Erickson *et al*, 2007).

Antipsychotics

Two large multi-site trials in children (Shea *et al*, 2004; McDougle *et al*, 2005) showed that risperidone was significantly more effective than placebo for reducing interfering behaviours. However, in smaller RCTs with pre-school children with autism, risperidone was not meaningfully superior to placebo (Luby *et al*, 2006). Adverse effects of second-generation antipsychotics include increased appetite and weight gain, dyslipidaemia and insulin resistance, somnolence, extrapyramidal symptoms and prolactin elevation. One study looking at the prescribing of risperidone over the course of 12 months used a pooled database of prolactin levels in 700 children (Dunbar *et al*, 2004). Mean levels were found to increase and peak in the first 1–2 months and then return to near normal by 3–5 months. There was no associated delay in growth or sexual maturation.

Prolongation of the QTc interval with risperidone has been reported, but studies in both adults and children did not find prolongation beyond the threshold accepted as being associated with *torsade de pointes* or other significant changes on the electrocardiogram (ECG) (see e.g. Harrigan *et al*, 2004).

Clinical implications

In this domain of the core symptoms of ASD, the situation is rather the reverse of the social deficits. Psychosocial or cognitive–behavioural interventions can be useful adjuncts but may be less effective in this patient group than they can be, for example, in people with autism and comorbid obsessive–compulsive symptoms. Medication effects do show a great deal of individual variation, and patients and families need to understand that trials of medication may be exploratory and subject to careful monitoring and dosage adjustment. A review (McDougle *et al*, 2006) suggests that, given the side-effect profile of risperidone, low-dose SSRIs should be used as first-line treatment if repetitive behaviour is the main focus of treatment. Even with newer antipsychotics such as aripiprazole, the extent of weight gain and long-term neurological effects is not yet clear. However, the current evidence base for SSRIs consists of small short-term RCTs with heterogeneous populations and varying outcome measures. Ongoing trials of SSRIs should address the limitations of the current published data. At this time, as above, NICE does not recommend use of SSRI or antipsychotic medication for treatment of this domain of core autism symptoms any more than for the social impairment domain (Kendall *et al*, 2013).

Co-occurring or comorbid psychiatric symptoms

There is a high prevalence of both psychiatric and physical comorbidities in ASD (Broadstock *et al*, 2007). These tend to emerge in middle childhood and wax and wane according to circumstances. At a theoretical level, it is not always clear that such symptoms constitute a true psychiatric comorbidity; commonly, symptoms will co-occur with autism because of the interaction between the developmental disorder and concurrent stressors such as increased social demands, inadequately adapted schooling, a sense of rejection or poor self-image, bullying or family conflict. These symptoms are important to understand, since they are often as functionally impairing and yet more tractable than the core disorder, and are often a key target for intervention.

Accurate diagnosis of comorbid psychiatric disorders can be difficult. Modifications of diagnostic criteria may be necessary to account for differing clinical presentations in individuals with developmental disability. 'Diagnostic overshadowing' may prevent the accurate detection of symptoms; even if detected, they may be spuriously attributed to the core disorder (Dykens, 2000). It is also clear, however, that a condition like autism will be associated with additional symptoms which may not rise to the level of 'disorder'. Deciding when and whom to treat may be largely based on functional impairment. Conditions such as depression and anxiety (as opposed to the core syndrome) may be eminently treatable and tackling them may vastly improve patients' and families' quality of life.

A growing body of literature is focused on the evidence base for treating symptoms of hyperkinetic disorder in autism. However, there is a relative dearth of high-quality data considering other psychiatric comorbidities. Most of the available data come from trials designed to assess core and behavioural symptoms associated with autism but which also found improvements in other domains, such as depressive or anxious symptoms. RCTs studying patients with both ASD and adequately defined psychiatric comorbidities are urgently needed, but are difficult to design and carry out. Much of the data on psychiatric comorbidity in adolescents and adults are based on case reports and are difficult to interpret, given the potential for selection, referral or reporting biases.

Maladaptive aggression and self-injury

Self-injurious behaviour and aggression can severely disrupt the management of autism. Many pharmacological treatments have been trialled.

Antipsychotics

Second-generation antipsychotics are the most frequently used psychotropic medication for aggression and serious self-injury in people with ASD (Erickson *et al*, 2007). Moderately sized RCTs of risperidone in both adults and children (Shea *et al*, 2004) have shown beneficial effects. Open-label studies with a double-blind discontinuation component have suggested both longer-term benefits and tolerance (e.g. Research Units on Pediatric Psychopharmacology Autism Network, 2005*b*). In 2006, the US Food and Drug Administration approved risperidone for the symptomatic treatment of irritability (including aggression and self-injury) in children and adolescents. In the UK, a Cochrane review (Jesner *et al*, 2007) concluded that risperidone can be beneficial, but that the lack of a single standardised outcome measure did not allow direct comparison of studies. Aripiprazole has demonstrated improvements in irritability, aggression and self-injury (Stigler *et al*, 2009; McPheeters *et al*, 2011) and a Cochrane review (Ching & Pringsheim, 2012) concluded that it is effective in the short-term treatment of irritability, hyperactivity and repetitive movements in children. However, the long-term safety of aripiprazole needs further investigation.

Evidence of the efficacy of other antipsychotics is very preliminary. One small RCT of olanzapine found it to be effective in about 50% of children (Hollander *et al*, 2006*a*). However, olanzapine is strongly associated with weight gain and other physical morbidity. Open-label trials of quetiapine indicate that the response rate and tolerability are poor (e.g. Martin *et al*, 1999). Clozapine and ziprasidone are rarely used because of the risk of blood dyscrasias and QTc prolongation, respectively.

Several large, well-designed RCTs (e.g. Remington *et al*, 2001) have studied haloperidol and found it efficacious in both children and adults with autism and behaviour problems. Adverse events, including dyskinesia and sedation, are common, however, and it is therefore more often reserved for treatment-refractory symptoms.

Opiate antagonists

Initial findings of open-label studies of naltrexone seemed promising (Panksepp & Lensing, 1991) but subsequent placebo-controlled studies showed no positive effects for the core social deficits. The most consistent finding is a modest reduction in hyperactivity (Feldman *et al*, 1999). A quantitative review of the literature suggests that naltrexone might be beneficial for reducing self-injurious behaviours in individuals with mental retardation, including those with ASD (Symons *et al*, 2004).

Mood stabilisers

Hepatotoxicity, weight gain, sedation and teratogenicity are important side-effects for this group of drugs. Evidence regarding the effects of mood stabilisers on ASD is mixed. A small RCT of valproate (Hellings *et al*, 2005) involving 30 adolescents could not demonstrate a significant difference between the drug and placebo, but a small trial of 13 children treated with divalproex (Hollander *et al*, 2006*b*) demonstrated benefits. A further trial indicated it confers benefits on measures of global irritability (Hollander *et al*, 2010). Published data for carbamazepine are limited to case reports. There are no controlled trials of the use of lithium in ASD. Evidence for alpha-2 agonists such as clonidine and beta-blockers are limited to small RCTs and case reports (Myers, 2007).

Clinical implications

Severe maladaptive aggression and self-injury can be the most disturbing and impairing co-occurring symptoms in ASD, particularly in individuals with intellectual disability. Medication management has a clear role here. Antipsychotics, particularly risperidone and aripiprazole, have a consistent evidence base, are increasingly prescribed and can be very useful. NICE recommends consideration of antipsychotic medication management after assessment has ruled out treatable causes and if psychosocial or other interventions are insufficient or could not be delivered because of the severity of the behaviour (Kendall *et al*, 2013). Medication management should be done carefully and well monitored; doses should be titrated up from a low base to the 'minimum effective dose', using frequent detailed symptom monitoring. In this way the emergence of medication side-effects (so easily confused with the target symptoms themselves) can be identified and the real effect of the drug can be assessed. Another reason for detailed assessment and targeting of symptoms is that families may be unrealistic about the limitations of medication in complex situations; the placebo response in parental report is often strong. Specific medications should not be pursued if there is no evidence of their benefit; but withdrawal should be slow and judicious to avoid withdrawal effects. The limitations of published studies and drug side-effect profiles should be carefully considered; however, judged carefully and used with persistence, medication management can transform children's development and families' lives.

Hyperkinesis and inattention

Symptoms of hyperkinetic disorder (inattention, impulsivity, distractibility and hyperactivity) are very common in autism, particularly in children and adolescents (Lee & Ousley, 2006). Traditionally in UK diagnostic schemes, a diagnosis of hyperkinetic disorder is not made if it occurs exclusively during the course of ASD (the diagnostic hierarchy concept). However, this has the limitation of tending to underplay or even obscure significant and treatable symptom co-occurrence. These symptoms may severely impair an individual's functioning and warrant treatment in their own right. A comorbidity approach is thus increasingly appropriate, as in DSM-5.

Psychostimulants

Randomised controlled trials of methylphenidate have shown its benefits in childhood autism (Quintana *et al*, 1995; Research Units on Pediatric Psychopharmacology Autism Network, 2005*a*). This applies to immediate-release preparations, but it is unclear whether the results can be applied to other stimulants. Trials suggest that the response rate in people with autism is lower than that in people without autism, and that side-effects such as irritability and poor appetite are more common (Erickson *et al*, 2007). One trial suggested that patients with Asperger syndrome may respond more positively than those with other types of autism, but not better than neurotypical individuals (Stigler *et al*, 2004). However, a more recent, large, open-label study found no statistically significant difference in degree of response or adverse events between those with ASD and those without (Santosh *et al*, 2006). Secondary analysis of the trial by the Research Units on Pediatric Psychopharmacology Autism Network (2005*a*) also suggested that psychostimulants may have a positive effect on some aspects of social communication in children with ASD and hyperactivity, such as joint attention initiations (Jahromi *et al*, 2009).

Atomoxetine

Atomoxetine is a selective noradrenaline inhibitor. Recently, open-label studies (e.g. Zeiner *et al*, 2011) and a small pilot RCT (Arnold *et al*, 2006) have suggested its effectiveness for hyperactivity, impulsivity and oppositional behaviour in ASD. Atomoxetine is often well tolerated but common side-effects include nausea, increased heart rate and fatigue.

Alpha-2 adrenergic agonists

Two very small RCTs involving a total of 17 patients (Fankhauser *et al*, 1992) have suggested modest benefits of clonidine, and one small cross-over study suggested similar effects for lofexidine (Niederhofer *et al*, 2002). A small cross-over RCT in children indicated that guanfacine may also be helpful for hyperactivity (Handen *et al*, 2008). Common side-effects include sedation and hypotension.

Cholinergics

Open-label trials and case series of the acetylcholinesterase inhibitors donepezil, galantamine and rivastigmine have indicated improvements in hyperactivity, inattention and irritability (Chez *et al*, 2004).

Amantadine

One RCT of amantadine for children (Ing *et al*, 2001) showed some improvements in hyperactivity and impulsivity on observer measures but not on parent-scored measures. Amantadine may therefore be useful in modulating behaviour in some young patients, but it is not clear whether this is because of its glutamatergic activity or enhancement of dopaminergic neurotransmission.

Antipsychotics

Aripiprazole has produced short-term improvements in measures of hyperactivity in RCTs in children (Ching & Pringsheim, 2012). Open-label trials of risperidone also indicate it may be helpful in this domain, particularly when combined with behavioural therapy (Aman *et al*, 2010) or other drugs, for example mood stabilisers such as topiramate (Rezaei *et al*, 2010).

Clinical implications

In children with any form of developmental disability, hyperkinesis and inattention are more complex to treat than in neurotypical children: the response is more idiosyncratic and unwanted effects are more common. Thus far, immediate-release methylphenidate has the most consistent evidence base with regard to symptoms of motor hyperactivity and inattention in children and adolescents, although there is increasing interest in antipsychotics. Research involving adults with ASD who experience these symptoms, as in the non-autism adult population with such problems, continues to lag far behind. NICE guidance for autism recommends that comorbidities such as ADHD within autism are treated with the appropriate evidence-based treatments from NICE guidance for those disorders. In this case, the relevant NICE guidance (2008) does not specifically mention individuals with ASD who also have significant problems with hyperkinesis. However, it states that drug treatments should be offered as first-line treatment only to patients with severe symptoms or impairment, and always in combination with psychosocial interventions. Methylphenidate, dexamphetamine and atomoxetine are all regarded as options for management.

Mood disorders

Patients with autism have been reported to be at increased risk of depression (prevalence of about 2% among all those with ASD), particularly those who are more cognitively able (Ghaziuddin *et al*, 2002). However, a recent follow-up study suggests that the incidence of mood disorder may be no different from that in the general population (Hutton *et al*, 2008). Nevertheless, depressive symptoms remain an important treatable cause of deterioration in functioning.

Mood disorder in ASD tends to emerge from middle childhood and is often associated clinically with the child's increased self-awareness of difference and the increasing social demands of peers. As in other children with mood disorders, psychosocial management is the first-line approach, and adaptation of the social and educational environment is often a first-line target.

For persistent and/or severe depressive disorder in children and adolescents, open-label trials of SSRIs, including fluoxetine, fluvoxamine, sertraline, citalopram and escitalopram, in children and adults have been associated with improvements in a depressive phenotype, including such symptoms as social withdrawal, irritability, sadness or crying, decreased energy and weight loss. Systematic reviews have confirmed that SSRIs should be considered for the treatment of depressive symptoms in autism (Posey *et al*, 2006).

Anticonvulsants such as divalproex have been posited to be useful in mood lability (Myers, 2007). Several case reports describe patients with autism and atypical bipolar disorder who responded well to open-label treatment with lithium (e.g. Kerbeshian *et al*, 1987). Open-label trials of second-generation antipsychotics suggest no difference in response to treatment between those with autism and a concurrent diagnosis of bipolar disorder and those without autism (Joshi *et al*, 2012).

Anxiety disorders

Individuals with ASD are at increased risk of anxiety disorders (Kim *et al*, 2000). It is often particularly intense and sometimes atypical, and sometimes interacts with core symptoms to such an extent that it mimics thought disorder. One double-blind trial showed evidence of fluvoxamine's efficacy (McDougle *et al*, 1996), and case reports of other SSRIs indicate improvements in anxiety symptoms with their use (Posey *et al*, 2006).

An open-label study as well as case reports suggest that buspirone (a 5-HT agonist) may also be effective for anxiety (Buitelaar *et al*, 1998). Beta-blockers may be appropriate where panic is a component.

Clinical implications

Anxiety in ASD has particular qualities and is often underrecognised. It can significantly increase presenting social symptoms and social anxiety, or specific phobias can contribute to social avoidance and functional social impairment. Anxiety management strategies and desensitisation for behavioural avoidance can usefully be combined with medication.

Tic disorders and OCD

Tourette syndrome has been shown to be comorbid in over 6% of autism cases, more than would be expected by chance (Baron-Cohen *et al*, 1999). There are increasingly recognised overlaps between ASD, OCD and tic disorders. There is no evidence that pharmacological treatment of these disorders should differ from that used in each disorder alone. The use of haloperidol, clonidine and risperidone for tics, and clomipramine or SSRIs for obsessions and compulsions is well described in the literature (Gringras, 2000).

Sleep disorders

There is some evidence of abnormal melatonin regulation in autism (Paavonen *et al*, 2003). Open-label studies suggest melatonin may be effective for improving sleep onset, but controlled trials are lacking (Gringras, 2000). Alpha-2 agonists, antihistamines, ramelteon (a melatonin receptor agonist) and mirtazapine have all been reported to have some effect on sleep in open-label trials and case reports (e.g. Owens *et al*, 2005).

A carefully designed placebo-controlled RCT across neurodevelopmental disorders including autism (Gringras *et al*, 2012) found that immediate-release melatonin did show an effect in improving sleep onset latency, although total sleep time was not increased. The drug was well tolerated and further study on sustained-release preparations is indicated.

Clinical implications

Sleep disorder is common and often underrecognised. It is the cause of long-term debility for families and daytime symptoms in patients. Many parents are focused on medication management for these problems, and it can be effective, but equally important is systematic sleep hygiene and behavioural measures.

Thought disorder

There is a consensus in the clinical literature on the occurrence of atypical quasi-psychotic symptoms in autism. These are often transient but can be recurring or persist in mild form. Such symptoms are important to recognise as they often cause diagnostic confusion and inappropriate treatment response. The nosological status of such states is not agreed: they do not necessarily represent a psychotic prodrome and the prevalence of psychosis is not markedly increased. The acute transient form can often be appropriately classified as a brief reactive psychosis; a useful syndromic account of the relapsing form has been given under the descriptive, if inelegant, term 'multiplex complex developmental disorder' (Buitelaar & van der Gaag, 1998).

These states can often be managed conservatively, without medication, by identification and reduction of relevant environmental stressors. However, the more recurrent forms will often need pharmacological management, and the correct response here is for titrated antipsychotic medication, often with low-dose maintenance treatment to prevent a relapsing course. There are rarer states that also need consideration in a differential diagnosis, such as emerging developmental abnormalities in adolescence associated with microdeletion on 22q11 (the velo-cardio-facial syndrome).

Discussion

Research in many of the areas discussed is still in its early phases, and the ongoing limitations of the evidence and intrinsic difficulties of measurement are important for clinicians to remember when discussing things with often well-informed and frustrated families. Box 10.1 highlights some of the evidential shortcomings of the published literature. There are few RCTs, and trials are often small and underpowered. Long-term studies of unwanted effects are often lacking. The population studied is not homogeneous and many trials use disparate outcome measures, which makes comparisons difficult or simply invalid. Many outcome measures subsume a variety of elements of behaviour, making it hard to be clear about what the data actually show for specific areas (Wisniewski *et al*, 2007).

Moreover, there is the inherent difficulty of studying pharmacological response in developmental disorders themselves. Measuring change in ASD is complex and must take into account day-to-day fluctuations, powerful placebo effects and idiosyncratic responses. The examples of fenfluramine and secretin illustrate these particular difficulties. Reasons for a large placebo response in children with autism include heightening of positive expectancy by media attention, by sensory experiences associated with intravenous injections, and participation effects modifying carers' behaviour. Sandler (2005) discusses these issues in detail.

The underlying developmental trajectory of individual patients is highly variable and may confound apparent positive responses to medication. This issue is more widely recognised now and researchers (e.g. Research Units on Pediatric Psychopharmacology Autism Network, 2005a,2005b; Scahill *et al*, 2006) are attempting to address these concerns; however, the field awaits a critical mass of larger, more robust clinical trials with more specific measurements and sophisticated analyses of clinical effectiveness.

Box 10.1 Shortcomings of published data on the pharmacological management of symptoms in autism spectrum disorder

- Few randomised controlled trials
- Underpowered trials
- Short follow-up periods
- Lack of safety data
- Lack of trials in adult populations
- Heterogeneous populations studied (need for appropriate case definitions)
- Heterogeneous clinical outcome measures used make it difficult to compare trials
- Powerful placebo responses
- Problems in measuring change in people with autism

Clinicians will need to interpret the clinical evidence carefully and make active adjustments in applying it to the specific situation of their patients.

Despite the limitations, however, both the quantity and the quality of medication trials targeting symptom domains in ASD have increased in recent years. There remains a lack of important information on the long-term safety and efficacy of drugs, and the standard of evidence so far does not allow for definitive treatment protocols for various symptom clusters. However, the aggregation of data suggests that SSRIs, risperidone and immediate-release methylphenidate can be of great value within the domains discussed. There are as yet no proven treatments for the underlying social deficit in autism and medication management here is not recommended.

We have emphasised that medication management is only one strand of interventions for people with autism and the mainstay of treatment remains educational and psychosocial. Pharmacological management needs to be undertaken after thorough assessment and accurate diagnosis, and with regular monitoring of target symptom clusters, comorbid diagnoses and response to treatment (Box 10.2).

Looking to the future

There are several exciting new developments within the field of pharmacology research in ASD. Large trials in glutamatergic function are currently ongoing, particularly in the USA. Arbaclofen, a GABA

Box 10.2 Important considerations when prescribing for autism

To make informed decisions about a potential role for medication, the prescriber must:

- clarify the characteristics of the challenging behaviours, including frequency, intensity, duration and degree of interference with functioning
- be clear about the target symptoms to be treated (differentiate core from comorbid symptoms)
- identify exacerbating and ameliorating factors, including response to psycho-therapeutic interventions
- assess existing and available health, educational and social supports, and the strengths of the family (e.g. the family's ability to support the individual)
- assess comorbid physical problems by thorough history and examination, and consider their impact on presentation and treatment of the challenging behaviours
- consider potential adverse events and drug interactions
- avoid polypharmacy
- use a 'start low and go slow' treatment strategy

receptor agonist, is currently undergoing trial development for the core symptoms of ASD. Most studies to date have focused on the use of one drug to target one group of related symptoms. One such study is the phase III development of fluoxetine in a novel strategy aiming to identify and target likely responders (Nightingale, 2012). Memantine is one of the only candidate drugs in development for treating symptoms in both children and adults. Studies using more than one drug to target more than one symptom domain (so-called 'coactive studies') are also being considered further in treatment trials. Researchers are beginning to consider the value of a more formal combination of behavioural and medical interventions in complex treatment trials designed to alter the developmental trajectory of those with autism. Advances in neurophysiology and genetics, such as stem-cell therapy, may also make it possible to delineate subgroups who may be particularly responsive to particular treatments. Such developments may pave the way for a more integrated consensus on an overall approach to the treatment of ASD across the life span.

References

Akhondzadeh S, Falleh J, Mohammadi MR, *et al* (2010) Double blind placebo controlled trial of pentoxifylline added to risperidone: effects on aberrant behaviour in children with autism. *Programme of Neuropsychopharmacological and Biological Psychiatry*, **34**: 32–6.

Aman MG, Lam KSL, Van Bourgondien ME (2005) Medication patterns in patients with autism: temporal, regional, and demographic influences. *Journal of Child and Adolescent Psychopharmacology*, **15**: 116–26.

Aman MG, McDougle CJ, Scahill L, *et al* (2010) Medication and parent training in children with pervasive developmental disorders and serious behavior problems: results from a randomized clinical trial. *Journal of the American Academy of Child and Adolescent Psychiatry*, **48**: 1143–54.

American Psychiatric Association (2013) *Diagnostic and Statistical Manual of Mental Disorders* (5th edn) (DSM-5). APA.

Arnold LE, Aman MG, Cook AM, *et al* (2006) Atomoxetine for hyperactivity in autism spectrum disorders: placebo-controlled crossover pilot trial. *Journal of the American Academy of Child and Adolescent Psychiatry*, **45**: 1196–205.

Autism Genome Project Consortium (2007) Mapping autism risk loci using genetic linkage and chromosomal rearrangements. *Nature Genetics*, **39**: 319–28.

Autism Speaks (2009) *Autism Speaks Announces Results Reported for the Study of Fluoxetine in Autism (SOFIA)*. Autism Speaks.

Baird G, Simonoff E, Pickles A, *et al* (2006) Prevalence of disorders of the autism spectrum in a population cohort of children in South Thames: the Special Needs and Autism Project (SNAP). *Lancet*, **368**: 210–15.

Baron-Cohen S, Mortimore C, Moriarty J, *et al* (1999) The prevalence of Gilles de la Tourette's syndrome in children and adolescents with autism. *Journal of Child Psychology and Psychiatry*, **40**: 213–18.

Belsito KM, Law PA, Kirk KS, *et al* (2001) Lamotrigine therapy for autistic disorder: a randomized, double-blind, placebo-controlled trial. *Journal of Autism and Developmental Disorders*, **31**: 175–81.

Broadstock M, Doughty C, Eggleston M (2007) Systematic review of the effectiveness of pharmacological treatments for adolescents and adults with autism spectrum disorder. *Autism*, **11**: 335–48.

Buchsbaum MS, Hollander E, Haznedar MM, *et al* (2001) Effect of fluoxetine on regional cerebral metabolism in autistic spectrum disorders: a pilot study. *International Journal of Neuropsychopharmacology*, **4**: 119–25.

Buescher AV, Cidav Z, Knapp M, *et al* (2014) Costs of autism spectrum disorders in the United Kingdom and the United States. *JAMA Pediatrics*, **168**: 721–8.

Buitelaar J, van der Gaag R (1998) Diagnostic rules for children with PDDNoS and multiple complex developmental disorder. *Journal of Child Psychology and Psychiatry*, **39**: 911–19.

Buitelaar JK, van der Gaag RJ, van der Hoeven J (1998) Buspirone in the management of anxiety and irritability in children with pervasive developmental disorders: results of an open-label study. *Journal of Clinical Psychiatry*, **59**: 56–9.

Carlsson ML (1998) Hypothesis: is infantile autism a hypoglutamatergic disorder? Relevance of glutamate–serotonin interactions for pharmacotherapy. *Journal of Neural Transmission*, **105**: 525–35.

Chez MG, Aimonovitch M, Buchanan T, *et al* (2004) Treating autistic spectrum disorders in children: utility of the cholinesterase inhibitor rivastigmine tartrate. *Journal of Child Neurology*, **19**: 165–9.

Chez MG, Burton Q, Dowling T, *et al* (2007) Memantine as adjunctive therapy in children diagnosed with autistic spectrum disorders: an observation of initial clinical response and maintenance tolerability. *Journal of Child Neurology*, **22**: 574–9.

Ching H, Pringsheim T (2012) Aripiprazole for autistic spectrum disorders. *Cochrane Database of Systematic Reviews*, **5**: CD009043.

Davanzo PA, Belin TR, Widawski MH, *et al* (1998) Paroxetine treatment of aggression and self-injury in persons with mental retardation. *American Journal on Mental Retardation*, **102**: 427–37.

Dunbar F, Kusumakar V, Daneman D, *et al* (2004) Growth and sexual maturation during long-term treatment with risperidone. *American Journal of Psychiatry*, **161**: 918–20.

Dykens EM (2000) Annotation: psychopathology in children with intellectual disability. *Journal of Child Psychology and Psychiatry and Allied Disciplines*, **41**: 407–17.

Erickson CA, Posey DJ, Stigler KA, *et al* (2007) Pharmacologic treatment of autism and related disorders. *Pediatric Annals*, **36**: 575–85.

Fankhauser MP, Karumanchi VC, German ML, *et al* (1992) A double-blind, placebo-controlled study of the efficacy of transdermal clonidine in autism. *Journal of Clinical Psychiatry*, **53**: 77–82.

Feldman HM, Kolmen BK, Gonzaga AM (1999) Naltrexone and communication skills in young children with autism. *Journal of the American Academy of Child and Adolescent Psychiatry*, **38**: 587–93.

Fombonne E (2003) The prevalence of autism. *JAMA*, **289**: 87–9.

Ghaziuddin M, Ghaziuddin N, Greden J (2002) Depression in persons with autism: implications for research and clinical care. *Journal of Autism and Developmental Disorders*, **32**: 299–306.

Gordon CT, State RC, Nelson JF, *et al* (1993) A double-blind comparison of clomipramine, deipramine, and placebo in the treatment of autistic disorder. *Archives of General Psychiatry*, **50**: 441–7.

Gringras P (2000) Practical paediatric psychopharmacological prescribing in autism: the potential and the pitfalls. *Autism*, **4**: 229–47.

Gringras P, Gamble C, Jones AP, *et al* (2012) Melatonin for sleep problems in children with neurodevelopmental disorders: randomised double masked placebo controlled trial. *BMJ*, **345**: e6664.

Handen BL, Sahl R, Hardan AY (2008) Guanfacine in children with autism and/or intellectual disabilities. *Journal of Developmental and Behavioral Pediatrics*, **29**: 303–8.

Harrigan EP, Miceli JJ, Anziano R, *et al* (2004) A randomized evaluation of the effects of six antipsychotic agents on QTc, in the absence and presence of metabolic inhibition. *Journal of Clinical Psychopharmacology*, **24**: 62–9.

Hellings JA, Weckbaugh M, Nickel EJ, et al (2005) A double-blind, placebo-controlled study of valproate for aggression in youth with pervasive developmental disorders. *Journal of Child and Adolescent Psychopharmacology*, **15**: 682–92.

Hollander E, Kaplan A, Cartwright C, et al (2000) Venlafaxine in children, adolescents, and young adults with autism spectrum disorders: an open retrospective clinical report. *Journal of Child Neurology*, **15**: 132–5.

Hollander E, Dolgoff Caspar R, Cartwright C, et al (2001) An open trial of divalproex sodium in autism spectrum disorders. *Journal of Clinical Psychiatry*, **62**: 530–4.

Hollander E, Phillips A, Chaplin W, et al (2005) A placebo controlled crossover trial of liquid fluoxetine on repetitive behaviors in childhood and adolescent autism. *Neuropsychopharmacology*, **30**: 582–9.

Hollander E, Wasserman S, Swanson EN, et al (2006a) A double-blind placebo-controlled pilot study of olanzapine in childhood/adolescent pervasive developmental disorder. *Journal of Child and Adolescent Psychopharmacology*, **16**: 541–8.

Hollander E, Soorya L, Wasserman S, et al (2006b) Divalproex sodium vs. placebo in the treatment of repetitive behaviours in autism spectrum disorder. *International Journal of Neuropsychopharmacology*, **9**: 209–13.

Hollander E, Chaplin W, Soorya L, et al (2010) Divalproex sodium vs. placebo for the treatment of irritability in children and adolescents with autism spectrum disorders. *Neuropsychopharmacology*, **35**: 990–8.

Honda H, Shimizu Y, Rutter M (2005) No effect of MMR withdrawal on the incidence of autism: a total population study. *Journal of Child Psychology and Psychiatry*, **46**: 572–9.

Hutton J, Goode S, Murphy M, et al (2008) New-onset psychiatric disorders in individuals with autism. *Autism*, **12**: 373–90.

Ing BH, Wright DM, Handen BL, et al (2001) Double blind, placebo controlled study of amantadine hydrochloride in the treatment of children with autistic disorder. *Journal of the American Academy of Child and Adolescent Psychiatry*, **40**: 658–65.

Jahromi LB, Kasari CL, McCracken JT, et al (2009) Positive effects of methylphenidate on social communication and self-regulation in children with pervasive developmental disorders and hyperactivity. *Journal of Autism and Developmental Disorders*, **39**: 395–404.

Jaselskis CA, Cook EH, Fletcher KE, et al (1992) Clonidine treatment of hyperactive and impulsive children with autistic disorder. *Journal of Clinical Psychopharmacology*, **12**: 322–7.

Jesner OS, Aref-Adib M, Coren E (2007) Risperidone for autism spectrum disorder. *Cochrane Database of Systematic Reviews*, **1**: CD005040.

Joshi G, Beiderman J, Wozniack J, et al (2012) Response to second generation antipsychotics in youth with comorbid bipolar disorder and autism spectrum disorder. *CNS Neuroscience and Therapeutics*, **18**: 28–33.

Kendall T, Megnin-Viggars O, Gould N, et al (2013) Management of autism in children and young people: summary of NICE and SCIE guidance. *BMJ*, **347**: f4865.

Kerbeshian J, Burd L, Fisher W (1987) Lithium carbonate in the treatment of two patients with infantile autism and atypical bipolar symptomatology. *Journal of Clinical Psychopharmacology*, **7**: 401–5.

Kim JA, Szatmari P, Bryson SE, et al (2000) The prevalence of anxiety and mood problems among children with autism and Asperger syndrome. *Autism*, **4**: 117–32.

King BH, Wright DM, Handen BL, et al (2001) Double-blind, placebo-controlled study of amantadine hydrochloride in the treatment of children with autistic disorder. *Journal of the American Academy of Child and Adolescent Psychiatry*, **40**: 658–65.

King BH, Hollander E, Sikich L, et al (2009) Lack of efficacy of citalopram in children with autism spectrum disorders and high levels of repetitive behavior: citalopram ineffective in children with autism. *Archives of General Psychiatry*, **66**: 583–90.

Lecavalier L, Leone S, Wiltz J (2006) The impact of behaviour problems on caregiver stress in young people with autism spectrum disorders. *Journal of Intellectual Disability Research*, **50**: 172–83.

Lee DO, Ousley OY (2006) Attention-deficit hyperactivity disorder symptoms in a clinic sample of children and adolescents with pervasive developmental disorders. *Journal of Child and Adolescent Psychopharmacology*, **16**: 737–46.

Lord C, Leventhal BL, Cook EH (2001) Quantifying the phenotype in autism spectrum disorders. *American Journal of Medical Genetics Part B: Neuropsychiatric Genetics*, **105**: 36–8.

Luby J, Mrakotsky C, Stalets MM, *et al* (2006) Risperidone in preschool children with autistic spectrum disorders: an investigation of safety and efficacy. *Journal of Child and Adolescent Psychopharmacology*, **16**: 575–87.

Marcus RN, Owen R, Kamen L, *et al* (2009) A placebo controlled, fixed dose study of aripiprazole in children and adolescents with irritability associated with autistic disorder. *Journal of the American Academy of Child and Adolescent Psychiatry*, **48**: 1110–9.

Martin A, Koenig K, Scahill L, *et al* (1999) Open-label quetiapine in the treatment of children and adolescents with autistic disorder. *Journal of Child and Adolescent Psychopharmacology*, **9**: 99–107.

McDougle CJ, Naylor ST, Cohen DJ, *et al* (1996) A double-blind, placebo-controlled study of fluvoxamine in adults with autistic disorder. *Archives of General Psychiatry*, **53**: 1001–8.

McDougle CJ, Holmes JP, Carlson DC, *et al* (1998) A double blind placebo controlled study of risperidone in adults with autistic disorder and other pervasive developmental disorders. *Archives of General Psychiatry*, **55**: 633–41.

McDougle CJ, Kresch LE, Posey DJ (2000) Repetitive thoughts and behavior in pervasive developmental disorders: treatment with serotonin reuptake inhibitors. *Journal of Autism and Developmental Disorders*, **30**: 427–35.

McDougle CJ, Scahill L, Aman MG, *et al* (2005) Risperidone for the core symptom domains of autism: results from the study by the Autism Network of the Research Units on Pediatric Psychopharmacology. *American Journal of Psychiatry*, **162**: 1142–8.

McDougle CJ, Stigler KA, Erickson CA, *et al* (2006) Pharmacology of autism. *Clinical Neuroscience Research*, **6**: 179–88.

McPheeters ML, Warren Z, Sathe N, *et al* (2011) A systematic review of medical treatments for children with autism spectrum disorders. *Pediatrics*, **127**: e1312–21.

Mesibov GB, Handlan S (1997) Adolescents and adults with autism. In *Handbook of Autism and Pervasive Developmental Disorders* (eds DJ Cohen, FR Volkman): pp. 309–22. Wiley.

Myers SM (2007) The status of pharmacotherapy for autism spectrum disorders. *Expert Opinion in Pharmacotherapy*, **8**: 1579–603.

NICE (2008) *Attention Deficit Hyperactivity Disorder: Diagnosis and Management of ADHD in Children, Young People and Adults* (CG72). National Institute for Health and Clinical Excellence.

NICE (2011) *Autism Diagnosis in Children and Young People: Recognition, Referral and Diagnosis of Children and Young People on the Autism Spectrum* (CG128). National Institute for Health and Clinical Excellence.

NICE (2013) *Autism: The Management and Support of Children and Young People on the Autism Spectrum* (CG170). National Institute for Health and Care Excellence.

Niederhofer H, Staffer W, Mair A (2002) Lofexidine in hyperactive and impulsive children with autistic disorder. *Journal of the American Academy of Child and Adolescent Psychiatry*, **41**: 1396–7.

Nightingale S (2012) Autism spectrum disorders. *Nature Reviews: Drug Discovery*, **11**: 745–6.

Nikolov R, Jonker J, Scahill L (2006) Autistic disorder: current psychopharmacological treatments and areas of interest for future developments [Portuguese, English]. *Revista Brasileira de Psiquiatria*, **28** (suppl 1): S39–46.

Nye C, Brice A (2005) Combined vitamin B6–magnesium treatment in autism spectrum disorder. *Cochrane Database of Systematic Reviews*, **4**: CD003497.

Owen R, Sikich L, Marcus RN, *et al* (2009) Aripiprazole in the treatment of irritability in children and adolescents with autistic disorder. *Pediatrics*, **124**: 1533–40.

Owens JA, Babcock D, Blumer J, et al (2005) The use of pharmacotherapy in the treatment of pediatric insomnia in primary care: rational approaches. A consensus meeting summary. *Journal of Clinical Sleep Medicine*, 1: 49–59.

Owley T, Walton L, Salt J, et al (2005) An open-label trial of escitalopram in pervasive developmental disorders. *Journal of the American Academy of Child and Adolescent Psychiatry*, 44: 343–8.

Owley T, Salt J, Guter S, et al (2006) A prospective open label trial of memantine in the treatment of cognitive, behavioral and memory dysfunction in pervasive developmental disorders. *Journal of Child and Adolescent Psychopharmacology*, 16: 517–24.

Paavonen EJ, Nieminen-von Wendt T, Vanhala R, et al (2003) Effectiveness of melatonin in the treatment of sleep disturbances in children with Asperger disorder. *Journal of Child and Adolescent Psychopharmacology*, 13: 83–95.

Panksepp J, Lensing P (1991) A synopsis of an open-trial of naltrexone treatment of autism with four children. *Journal of Autism and Developmental Disorders*, 21: 243–9.

Posey DJ (2008) A double-blind placebo-controlled study of D-cycloserine in children with autistic disorder. In *Proceedings of the 55th Annual Meeting of the American Academy of Child and Adolescent Psychiatry*: abstract 3.53. AACAP.

Posey DJ, Kem DL, Swiezy NB, et al (2004) A pilot study of D-cycloserine in subjects with autistic disorder. *American Journal of Psychiatry*, 161: 2115–7.

Posey DJ, Erickson CA, Stigler KA, et al (2006) The use of selective serotonin reuptake inhibitors in autism and related disorders. *Journal of Child and Adolescent Psychopharmacology*, 16: 181–6.

Quintana H, Birmaher B, Stedge D, et al (1995) Use of methylphenidate in the treatment of children with autistic disorder. *Journal of Autism and Developmental Disorders*, 25: 283–94.

Remington G, Sloman L, Konstantareas M, et al (2001) Clomipramine versus haloperidol in the treatment of autistic disorder: a double-blind, placebo-controlled, crossover study. *Journal of Clinical Psychopharmacology*, 21: 440–4.

Research Units on Pediatric Psychopharmacology Autism Network (2005a) Randomised, controlled, crossover trial of methylphenidate in pervasive developmental disorders with hyperactivity. *Archives of General Psychiatry*, 62: 1266–74.

Research Units on Pediatric Psychopharmacology Autism Network (2005b) Risperidone treatment of autistic disorder: longer term benefits and blinded discontinuation after 6 months. *American Journal of Psychiatry*, 162: 1361–9.

Rezaei V, Mohammadi MR, Ghanizadeh A, et al (2010) Double blind, placebo controlled trial of risperidone plus topiramate in children with autistic disorder. *Programme of Neuropsychopharmacological and Biological Psychiatry*, 34: 1269–72.

Sandler A (2005) Placebo effects in developmental disabilities: implications for research and practice. *Mental Retardation and Developmental Disabilities Research Reviews*, 11: 164–70.

Sandler RH, Finegold SM, Bolte ER, et al (2000) Short-term benefit from oral vancomycin treatment of regressive-onset autism. *Journal of Child Neurology*, 15: 429–35.

Santosh PJ, Baird G, Pityaratstian N, et al (2006) Impact of comorbid autism spectrum disorders on stimulant response in children with attention deficit hyperactivity disorder: a retrospective and prospective effectiveness study. *Child: Care, Health and Development*, 32: 575–83.

Scahill L, McCracken JT, McGough J, et al (2002) Risperidone in children with autism and serious behavioral problems. *New England Journal of Medicine*, 347: 314–21.

Scahill L, Aman MC, McDougle CJ, et al (2006) A prospective open trial of guanfacine in children with pervasive developmental disorders. *Journal of Child and Adolescent Psychopharmacology*, 16: 589–98.

Shea S, Turgay A, Carroll A, et al (2004) Risperidone in the treatment of disruptive behavioral symptoms in children with autistic and other pervasive developmental disorders. *Pediatrics*, 114: e634–41.

Stigler KA, Desmond LA, Posey DJ, *et al* (2004) A naturalistic retrospective analysis of psychostimulants in pervasive developmental disorders. *Journal of Child and Adolescent Psychopharmacology*, **14**: 49–56.

Stigler KA, Diener JT, Kohn AE, *et al* (2009) Aripiprazole in pervasive developmental disorder not otherwise specified and Asperger's disorder: a 14-week, prospective, open-label study. *Journal of Child and Adolescent Psychopharmacology*, **19**: 265–74.

Sugie Y, Sugie H, Fukuda T, *et al* (2005) Clinical efficacy of fluvoxamine and functional polymorphism in a serotonin transporter gene on childhood autism. *Journal of Autism and Developmental Disorders*, **35**: 377–85.

Symons FJ, Thompson A, Rodriguez MC (2004) Self injurious behaviour and the efficacy of naltrexone treatment: a quantitative synthesis. *Mental Retardation and Developmental Disability Research Review*, **10**: 193–200.

Tsakanikos E, Costello H, Holt G, *et al* (2006) Psychopathology in adults with autism and intellectual disability. *Journal of Autism and Developmental Disorders*, **36**: 1123–9.

Wink LK, Plawecki M, Erickson C, *et al* (2010) Emerging drugs for the treatment of symptoms associated with autism spectrum disorders. *Expert Opinion on Emerging Drugs*, **15**: 481–94.

Wisniewski, T, Brimacombe MB, Ming X (2007) Pharmaceutical treatment studies in autism and ADHD: a design based review of study quality. *Journal of Pediatric Neurology*, **5**: 189–97.

Yurgelun-Todd DA, Coyle JT, Gruber SA, *et al* (2005) Functional magnetic resonance imaging studies of schizophrenic patients during word production: effects of D-cycloserine. *Psychiatry Research*, **138**: 23–31.

Zeiner P, Gjevik E, Weidle B (2011) Response to atomoxetine in boys with high functioning autism spectrum disorders and attention deficit/hyperactivity disorder. *Acta Paediatrica Scandinavica*, **100**: 1258–61.

CHAPTER 11

Psychological treatment of autism spectrum disorder

Jo-Ann Reitzel, Jane Summers and Irene Drmic

In the past 60 years there has been significant progress in the identification, treatment and understanding of autism spectrum disorder (ASD) as a severe neurodevelopmental disorder (Rutter, 2005). The prevalence rates have increased dramatically over time and are currently 1 in 68 according to the US Centers for Disease Control and Prevention (Developmental Disabilities Monitoring Network Surveillance Year 2010 Principal Investigators, 2014). In DSM-IV-TR (American Psychiatric Association, 2000), ASD diagnoses consisted of four separate disorders that fell under the broad umbrella term 'pervasive developmental disorder'. In DSM-5 (American Psychiatric Association, 2013), ASD is one disorder of varying degrees of defined severity that may coexist with other disorders, such as attention-deficit hyperactivity disorder and intellectual disability.

The core symptoms of ASD include social-communication deficits, such as difficulties in reciprocal social interactions, and restrictive and repetitive interests. The severity of social-communication difficulties and restrictive and repetitive interests may fluctuate from day to day, and may vary with age. There can also be a range of associated complex issues that may or may not fluctuate over the course of the life span. These include intellectual and learning difficulties, as well as social, emotional, behavioural and mental health problems such as depression and anxiety. Furthermore, ASD often affects the family, school and community.

There is no known cure or medication that modifies the core symptoms of ASD; however, with careful treatment planning and monitoring, problems arising from the core features of ASD and related difficulties can be managed and improved. Evidence-based behavioural and psychological therapies can modify and improve symptoms of ASD and problems associated with ASD (Maglione *et al*, 2012; Anagnostou *et al*, 2014). Psycho-social supports, psycho-education and training can be incorporated into treatment plans, depending on the strengths and needs of the family, as well as their levels stress, and their values and culture. In addition to intervention and psycho-social supports, some persons with ASD require assistance and supervision to help them and their family and carers address problems. The amount of support needed may vary. Even though there has been a steady increase in the awareness of the need for assistance, services and treatments, no one service or treatment package has been found to suit all. There is a proliferation of treatments in the field of ASD in response to the desperate need for assistance, but caution is needed when recommending therapies and treatment centres and selecting therapists.

Understandably, parents and families can be overwhelmed when their child is diagnosed with ASD and many seek information and search for treatments or a cure for ASD. Parents and carers may be vulnerable and there is an unfortunate propensity for fad ASD treatments that often have misleading or little evidence to support their pseudo-scientific claims. Standards of care for children and adults with ASD are required, as well as effective psychological treatments.

In the UK, the National Institute for Health and Care Excellence (NICE, 2014) has developed a quality standard of care for ASD. The intention of this quality standard is to direct and measure quality improvements in the social care and health of persons with ASD. The standard was informed by research findings and other NICE guidelines for ASD that address the assessment and diagnosis and clinical care of children and adults with ASD (NICE, 2011, 2012) and the management of and supports for children and youths (NICE, 2013). Implementation steps address improvement in access to health and social services, knowledge and competence of health and social work professionals, as well as improvement in adjustments to social and physical environments, in psychological and pharmacological interventions for behaviour problems, in care for families and carers, and in the transition to adult services.

Evidence-based treatment standards have also been set in the USA. The National ASD Center (NAC) has developed standards for non-medical ASD treatments (NAC, 2009). The NAC convened internationally renowned ASD experts to systematically review the research literature on interventions for ASD and determine the strength of the evidence. The National ASD Standards, also referred to as NAS (NAC, 2009), were then developed to inform families and clinicians about empirically validated and effective ASD treatments for persons up to age 22 and to assist in making treatment decisions. Evidence-based psychological interventions for children and youths with ASD, recommended by the NAS, are primarily from the field of applied behaviour analysis (ABA). Other recommended interventions that are not directly behaviour analytic incorporate aspects of ABA. More traditional talk-based therapies have not been found to be effective to date, probably because of the social-communication difficulties inherent in ASD. However, there is some emerging evidence supporting the use of cognitive–behavioural therapy (CBT) to address mental health problems in children and youths with ASD; however, there is little study of the effectiveness of other psychological interventions for adults.

This chapter focuses on ABA interventions and the emerging evidence for CBT for children and youths with ASD. The ABA section will provide an overview of the science of ABA, review the evidence for more focused ABA interventions aimed at improving the core symptoms of ASD through the acquisition of skills and by reducing problem behaviour, as well as review the evidence for comprehensive early intensive behaviour intervention (IBI) aimed at changing the child's ASD symptoms and developmental trajectories in relation to cognitive, language and adaptive behaviour. The CBT section will review the emerging evidence for the use of CBT as a mental health intervention.

Although parent, carer, family and community social supports play important roles in ASD treatment plans, reducing stress and improving the quality of life for the person with ASD and the family, such support programmes will not be addressed in this chapter.

Applied behaviour analysis and ASD

Applied behaviour analysis (ABA), which is the science of behaviour change to address problems of social importance (Baer *et al*, 1968), has served as a foundation for improving the quality of life for children and adults with ASD for several decades. Owing largely to the pioneering efforts of O. Ivar Lovaas in the 1960s and 1970s , evidence began to emerge regarding the effectiveness of ABA-based procedures for teaching a variety of skills to children with ASD (Smith & Eikeseth, 2011). Until that point, many children were considered to be untreatable. In the years since Lovaas's landmark research, thousands of studies and numerous research reviews attesting to the effectiveness of ABA interventions have been published (Matson *et al*, 2012*a*, 2012*b*). Presently, evidence-based ABA strategies are used in comprehensive early intensive behaviour interventions that have generated the strongest evidence base for improving cognitive, language, social and adaptive outcomes for many young children with ASD (Smith *et al*, 2000; Howard *et al*, 2005; Sallows & Graupner, 2005; Eldevik *et al*, 2009; Makrygianni & Reed, 2010). In addition, ABA interventions have been found to be effective for enhancing the skill development of individuals with ASD and reducing disruptive and harmful behaviours that interfere with their ability to learn and to function in society.

While ABA is most often associated with addressing the needs of individuals with ASD and developmental disabilities (Axelrod *et al*, 2012), it can be applied to a wide range of populations and problems (Dillenburger & Keenan, 2009). ABA as a discipline provides the scientific framework and technology: (1) to assess a broad range of social and environmental factors that influence behaviour; (2) to manipulate these variables to bring about changes in behaviour; (3) to demonstrate that the interventions used are responsible for improvements in behaviour; and (4) to optimise opportunities for behavioural improvements to occur and be sustained under 'real life' conditions. Here, after a brief overview of the key elements of ABA, a review is provided of the evidence in support of using ABA approaches for teaching specific skills to individuals with ASD in the areas of communication, social skills and daily living, as well as for the management of problem behaviour. Each of these areas has been studied extensively; however, for the purpose of brevity, only key findings will be presented.

Key elements of ABA for core and associated features of ASD

The starting point for intervention is the selection of a behavioural target that will result in a functionally important outcome for the individual with ASD, such as a skill to be increased or a problem behaviour to be decreased. A key element of ABA approaches is the emphasis on defining target behaviour in objective, observable terms that allow for accurate and consistent measurement. Behaviour can be measured across different dimensions, including frequency, duration and intensity. Measurement of a behaviour prior to the initiation of an intervention as well as following its termination yields evidence regarding the effectiveness of the treatment.

Another important element of ABA approaches is the analysis of environmental variables that can affect behaviour. These variables include people, activities and events that are present before the behaviour occurs ('antecedents') and events that follow the behaviour ('consequences') which increase or decrease the likelihood it will occur again in the future. These variables can be manipulated to prevent or minimise the occurrence of problem behaviour and promote the acquisition of new skills or improve existing skills. Different experimental designs can be used to demonstrate functional control of variables, either for a single person or across a group of individuals, such as multiple baseline, multi-element and reversal designs.

A third element of ABA approaches is the application of scientifically validated teaching and behaviour-reduction procedures. This process is guided by consideration of the individual's characteristics and the specific environmental/contextual factors that affect their learning and behaviour. Precise and detailed information is necessary to facilitate the implementation and replication of behavioural procedures, another important element of ABA approaches.

Finally, ABA should be effective (Ringdahl *et al*, 2009), producing changes in behaviour that occur across time, people and settings, and that generalise to behaviour that has not been the focus of training (Stokes & Baer, 1977).

Communication

Perhaps the area that has received the greatest attention in the ABA literature is in relation to improving communication outcomes in individuals with ASD, since communication impairments are central to the diagnosis. These outcomes can range from training a non-verbal individual to make requests using an exchange-based communication system to teaching a verbal individual to understand the subtleties of humour. Teaching approaches share a number of commonalities, including the use of models/demonstrations, shaping, prompting and prompt fading and differential reinforcement. These various components are active ingredients in comprehensive treatment packages that will be reviewed later in this chapter.

The most widely studied approach is known as discrete trial training (DTT). DTT is a highly structured, tightly controlled and fast-paced instructional approach in which an individual is presented with multiple brief learning opportunities in the form of 'trials'. During DTT, skills are broken down into small steps and teaching occurs in a carefully prescribed manner (Smith, 2001). Goldstein (2002) reviewed empirical evidence that had been gathered over 20 years regarding the effectiveness of DTT approaches for teaching receptive and expressive language skills to children with ASD. A total of 12 small studies were identified that were methodologically sound and had been subject to peer review. DTT approaches were shown to have been successful in expanding children's comprehension and verbal responses and often resulted in generalisation of newly acquired language skills outside of the treatment setting. One of the potential benefits of DTT approaches is that they may result in faster acquisition of skills owing to rapid and repeated learning trials, particularly with regard to basic learning skills such as attending, cooperation, imitation and following instructions (Ghezzi, 2007), which are prerequisites for more advanced skills. Owing to their systematic and stepwise nature, they may be easier for less experienced staff to implement (Kodak & Grow, 2011). However, some of the criticisms of the 'first-generation behaviour protocols' (Delprato, 2001) were that they were too far removed from real-life conditions and did not promote spontaneous communication or generalise well to less structured environments.

Over time, more naturalistic or 'normalised' interventions have gained popularity for teaching language skills to children with ASD and have become a required step for them to master a skill that can be fully used in the real world. The term 'natural environment training' (NET) is used to refer to several different approaches, including pivotal response training, incidental teaching and milieu teaching (Vismara & Rogers, 2010). These approaches have a number of key features in common. Language instruction occurs within the context of naturally occurring events, promotes child self-initiations and makes use of reinforcers that have a functional relationship to the language skills being taught. Some of the benefits of using NET approaches are that they provide a means to maximise the child's motivation to communicate, reduce dependence on adult prompting, can be implemented at home, at school and in the community, and pay particular attention to generalisation of language skills (Charlop-Christy et al, 1999). However, NET approaches may be difficult to implement where the child's behaviour is not under instructional control and may result in slower gains due to fewer learning opportunities.

Goldstein (2002), in his review of 12 treatment studies that reported the outcome of naturalistic teaching approaches, concluded there was no clear evidence that they are more effective than DTT approaches. Rather than trying to oversimplify a complex clinical issue by adopting a narrow 'DTT versus NET' focus, it may be more advantageous to draw from a broad range of empirically validated intervention procedures that use the principles of ABA to address the communication needs of specific individuals with ASD.

For individuals with little or no expressive speech, augmentative and alternative communication (AAC) approaches are used to enhance their communicative competence by supplementing or replacing their natural speech (e.g. Schlosser & Wendt, 2008). The Picture Exchange Communication System (PECS; Bondy & Frost, 1994, 2001) is a popular intervention that was developed to teach children with ASD who have little or no functional speech to initiate communicative interactions within a social context. PECS draws on ABA principles such as prompting and reinforcement to teach a variety of communicative functions, including requesting, labelling and commenting. Initially, the child (or adult) is taught to pick up a picture of a desired item that is in full view, reach towards a communicative partner and place the picture in his or her open hand; the picture is then 'exchanged' for the item itself. In later phases of PECS training, the child is taught: (1) to seek out a communicative partner who may be 'busy' or is not in the immediate vicinity; (2) to request specific items by including descriptive information about particular features (e.g. size, colour, shape); and (3) to respond to questions by using sentence starters such as 'I want' or 'I see'. Throughout PECS training, a strong emphasis is placed on spontaneous, functional communication and generalisation of communication skills to different people, situations and reinforcing items. Preston & Carter (2009) conducted a comprehensive review of 27 studies that reported the outcomes of PECS interventions for children and adults (the majority of whom had a diagnosis of ASD) who were non-verbal or had minimal or no functional speech. Variables of interest consisted of independent exchanges, speech and vocalisations, social-communicative behaviours and problem behaviours. The majority of studies used single-participant designs, and only three randomised controlled trials were available for review. The review yielded promising results, in that most individuals were able to master some phases of PECS and many were able to generalise their skills to different people, settings and stimuli. However, many questions still remain unanswered about PECS, such as whether it produces improvements in comprehension and speech production and which components of the programme contribute most to positive outcomes.

Social skills

Impairments in social and emotional responsiveness are among the earliest concerns that are identified by parents of infants and very young children who eventually receive a diagnosis of ASD (Zwaigenbaum *et al*, 2013). Along with communication deficits, abnormalities in social development and function are a defining feature of ASD and are present in varying degrees among individuals of all ages and ability levels (Howlin *et al*, 2004). The basis for social impairments is complex and can be linked in part to underlying problems with social cognition, attention and motivation (Baron-Cohen & Belmonte, 2005; Stavropoulos & Carver, 2013). Social skills deficits can run the gamut from lack of eye contact and avoidance of social interactions at one extreme to 'reading' more subtle social and emotional cues such as facial expressions and body language at the other extreme. Impairments in social functioning are associated with reduced opportunities for inclusion, independence and employment, increased risks of bullying and victimisation, and high rates of mental health and behaviour problems. The goal of social skills intervention programmes is to improve the social competence of individuals with ASD, since social impairments are arguably the most disabling feature and have greatest impact on functioning. However, total remediation of social skills deficits has not been demonstrated (Reichow *et al*, 2012).

Social skills can be subdivided into positive or prosocial behaviours that promote and sustain social interactions, and negative or challenging behaviours that interfere with socialisation (Walton & Ingersoll, 2013). The selection of which specific social skills to target for intervention is often based on a consideration of the individual's age and characteristics, along with the demands of their particular social environment. For young children, this may involve teaching sharing and turn-taking skills. For adolescents, recognition and regulation of emotional responses may be important targets, whereas for adults, making friends, interacting with co-workers and participating in social events may have the greatest relevance.

Social skills interventions may be implemented on an individual basis or within a group format, take place in contrived or naturally occurring situations and environments, and involve more socially competent peers in the process. Key elements of social skills training programmes that are drawn from ABA principles include direct skills-based instruction, along with *in vivo* or video modelling, rehearsal and role-plays, task analysis, prompting, performance feedback and differential reinforcement (DeMatteo *et al*, 2012). Other procedures that have been used to teach social skills include social stories, social scripts and visual schedules. Interventions can be adult- or peer-mediated and can also involve teaching the individual with ASD to self-manage their own behaviour in social situations (Weiss & Harris, 2001). Group-based interventions, which are becoming increasingly popular, often utilise a curriculum and manualised treatment approach (Kaat & Lecavalier, 2014). Matson *et al* (2007) evaluated trends in social skills treatments for children with ASD by conducting a selective review of 79 studies that had been published over a 25-year period. The number of publications and variety of social skills interventions being reported increased sixfold over this period. The majority of interventions took place in school settings and involved small groups of children; the most widely used behavioural intervention procedures were modelling, feedback and reinforcement.

With the growing recognition of the importance of increasing the social competency of individuals with ASD, it is somewhat surprising to find relatively few well designed behavioural skills training studies. Moreover, much of the evidence regarding positive outcomes has been gathered from studies using single-case methodology, rather than larger investigations that can use statistical methods to help answer broader questions about the relative effectiveness of different interventions (Thomson *et al*, 2011). Two recent meta-analyses may shed some light on this issue. Wang *et al* (2013) conducted a meta-analysis of social skills interventions for studies that used single-case methodology. Using hierarchical linear modelling (HLM), the investigators found that social skills interventions were generally effective and that outcomes were related to the design of the study itself (in particular, multiple baseline and reversal designs) rather than specific characteristics of the participants or quality indicators for treatment. Reichow *et al* (2012) evaluated social skills groups for children and youths with ASD with average cognitive ability. Their meta-analysis synthesised results from five randomised controlled trials and yielded some emerging evidence for improved social competence and quality of friendships among the individuals in the treatment groups. At the present time, social skills training packages are classified as emerging treatments for children and adolescents with ASD (NAC, 2009), with more high-quality studies being needed to firmly establish effectiveness.

Daily living

Functional life skills are important at any age, but take on greater importance as individuals enter adolescence and adulthood, when expectations for independence increase. In general, lower levels of daily living skills are correlated with higher support needs, greater carer strain and reduced opportunities for self-sufficiency and community integration. Interest in teaching functional life skills to individuals with ASD has traditionally lagged behind efforts to improve their cognitive and language outcomes. However, there is increasing awareness of the importance of treating adaptive skill deficits of individuals with ASD (Minshawi *et al*, 2009) and a growing literature related to the use of ABA-based approaches for teaching functional life skills (Matson *et al*, 2012a).

Activities of daily living include personal, domestic and community skills, academic skills, and work and leisure skills. Interventions for teaching such skills to individuals with ASD have largely relied on a variety of behavioural techniques, such as task analysis, prompting and prompt fading, error correction, modelling and demonstrations, chaining, shaping and differential reinforcement (Minshawi *et al*, 2009). Verbal and visual supports (written, pictorial, *in vivo* or video modelling and prompting) form an important part of treatment packages that have been successfully used to teach individuals with ASD to carry out sequences of steps (Matson *et al*, 2012*a*), such as those involved in performing hygiene tasks (Mays & Heflin, 2011; Reitzel *et al*, 2013), following cooking recipes (Mechling *et al*, 2013), washing dishes (Canella-Malone *et al*, 2011), setting the table (Shipley-Benamou *et al*, 2002), folding laundry (Van Laarhoven *et al*, 2010), making purchases (Haring *et al*, 1987), performing clerical tasks (Bennett *et al*, 2013) and following directions to seek assistance when lost (Hoch *et al*, 2009). There is emerging evidence that mobile hand-held devices (such as the iPod® and iPad®) that have multimedia capabilities and employ touch-screen technology can play a valuable role in intervention programmes for teaching daily living skills to individuals with ASD or other developmental disabilities (Kagohara *et al*, 2013).

In summary, impairments in adaptive and self-help skills can have a detrimental impact on the lives of individuals with ASD. Fortunately, there is a growing body of literature that attests to the effectiveness of ABA-based interventions for teaching daily living skills to children, adolescents and adults with ASD. Real-life application of teaching programmes, by embedding instructional opportunities within natural contexts and regularly occurring routines, may go a long way to remediating skill deficits in individuals with ASD and, in doing so, improving their quality of life.

Problem behaviour

Given that deficits in communication and social skills are core features of ASD, it is not surprising that approximately 50% of individuals with ASD and other developmental disabilities display challenging or problematic behaviour. Aggression, self-injury, tantrums, elopement, property destruction, non-compliance and disruptive behaviour have all been reported (Doehring *et al*, 2014). Challenging behaviour can place individuals with ASD and those around them at risk of injury, increase carer stress and result in more restrictive placements and reduced opportunities for community and social integration.

Applied behaviour analytic research has advanced our understanding of variables that underlie the development and maintenance of problem behaviour such as aggression and self-injury, and ABA has provided a technology for demonstrating causal relations between environmental events and the occurrence/non-occurrence of the problem behaviour. A key issue is the identification of reinforcers that maintain a problem behaviour. Carr (1977) proposed that seemingly senseless or bizarre behaviour such as self-injury can be linked to 'extrinsic reinforcement' (e.g. positive social and negative social reinforcement that is controlled by other people) and 'intrinsic reinforcement' (e.g. when occurrence of the behaviour generates sensory stimulation or brings about relief from pain or discomfort). In his view, it was necessary to correctly identify the underlying motivation(s) for an individual's self-injurious behaviour in order to design effective treatment approaches. Iwata *et al* (1982) outlined a methodology for identifying functional relationships between problem behaviour and specific environmental events. They systematically and repeatedly manipulated elements of the social and physical environment and measured rates of self-injurious behaviour under these different conditions in a group of children with developmental disabilities. Possible reinforcers for self-injurious behaviour could be identified for a number of children in the study, based on the finding of consistently higher rates of self-injurious behaviour under specific physical and/or social conditions.

Function-based behavioural interventions are now standard for individuals with ASD (Ward-Horner *et al*, 2011). Along with level of intellectual disability and severity of autism symptoms, communication deficits are a known risk factor for problem behaviour in individuals with ASD. Functional communication training (FCT) involves teaching a socially acceptable communicative response that is functionally equivalent to the problem behaviour (Carr & Durand, 1985). The literature on FCT has grown considerably over the years, and FCT been classified as a well-established treatment for a range of problem behaviours in children with ASD (Kurtz *et al*, 2011).

Distinguishing between ABA interventions and intensive behavioural interventions

The terms 'intensive behavioural intervention' (IBI) and 'applied behaviour analysis' can be confusing. To make the situation even more confusing, in the research and clinical literature IBI is at times referred to as early intensive behavioural intervention (EIBI), as well as intensive ABA, but to reduce confusion only the term IBI will be used in this chapter. ABA interventions and IBI both use the principles and evidence-based techniques of applied behaviour analysis. However, there are important differences, as outlined in Table 11.1.

The use of IBI to improve cognitive, language and adaptive behaviour outcomes

IBI is often recommended clinically for pre-school children at the time of diagnosis with ASD (Johnson & Myers, 2007; Anagnostou *et al*, 2014). The earlier the intervention starts, the better the potential for improvements in the child's development as well as in the support for parents and in the training for parents, other carers and teachers (National Research Council, 2001; NICE, 2013). Intensive early intervention means that intervention is provided for many hours a week, and 25 hours or more per week have been consistently recommended for young children with ASD for well over a decade (National Research Council, 2001; NAC, 2009).

There is well-established research evidence supporting the effectiveness of IBI programmes from numerous meta-analyses (e.g. Eldevik *et al*, 2009; Makrygianni & Reed, 2010); however, there is also some evidence for other approaches to early intervention for young children with ASD. Pivotal response training (Koegel *et al*, 1999) is an early intervention that focuses on the development of pivotal learning skills such as motivation, responding to multiple cues and self-regulation; it is designed to have positive and widespread effects on other behaviours in other settings, rather than focusing on teaching specific skills. There is also promising emerging evidence for the Early Start Denver Model (ESDM; Dawson *et al*, 2009), which incorporates a developmental and relationship-based approach with behavioural strategies for toddlers and pre-schoolers. To date, no study has compared the outcomes from these approaches and curricula to the

Table 11.1 Similarities and differences between intensive behavioural intervention (IBI) and applied behaviour analysis (ABA)

Variables	IBI	ABA
Age	Effective for some children up to age 8	Early childhood to adulthood
Aim	Improve developmental trajectories, master skills, reduce problem behaviour	Master skills, reduce problem behaviour
Intensity	20–40 hours per week; at least 25 hours per week recommended	Typically a few hours per week of direct or consultation intervention
Duration	1–3 years, depending upon child's response	Typically short term, up to 6 months
Direct intervention	Comprehensive programme across all early developmental domains	Focused programme in one area of skill development at a time
Strategies	Written programmes and data collection, evidenced-based ABA procedures	Written programme and data collection, evidence-based ABA procedures
Staff:child ratios	1:1, <1:1, small groups, dyads	1:1, <1:1, small groups, dyads
Primary ratio	1:1	Less than 1:1
Supervision	Trained staff supervised by behavioural psychologists and behaviour analysts	Trained staff supervised by behavioural psychologists and behaviour analysts
Settings	Clinic, home, community	Clinic, home, community
Parent involvement	Training, coaching, workshops	Training, coaching, workshops
School and other professionals	Workshops, hands-on demonstrations, case consultation	Workshops, hands-on demonstrations, case consultation

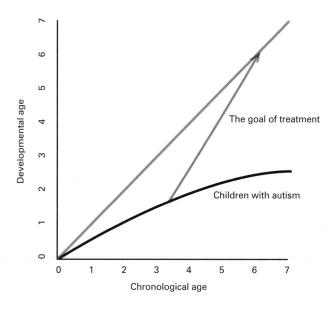

Fig. 11.1 The goal of intensive behavioural intervention (IBI): closing the gap between developmental and chronological age (reproduced by kind permission, McMaster Children's Hosptial, Autism, Developmental Pediatrics and Rehabilitation Services).

outcomes from IBI, although one is currently being conducted comparing the ESDM and IBI.

Given the large amount of converging evidence supporting the effectiveness of IBI for young children with ASD from studies run from universities and from community-based studies, and the common clinical recommendations for IBI, the remainder of this section will focus on IBI.

The aim of IBI is to improve or accelerate the rate of cognitive, language and adaptive behaviour development by providing a young child with ASD with an intensive and comprehensive behavioural programme across all developmental domains (Rogers & Vismara, 2008; Reichow & Wolery, 2009) to achieve functioning within the normal range. When children with ASD achieve best outcomes from IBI, their development catches up with their chronological age by closing the learning gaps between their developmental trajectories and those of their neurotypical peers. This is illustrated in Fig. 11.1.

Unfortunately, studies consistently show that only some children achieve best outcomes: the proportion of children reported to have achieved best outcomes from IBI ranges from 47–48% (Lovaas, 1987; Sallows & Graupner, 2005) to 11% in a community-based programme that served children at the severe end of the spectrum (Perry *et al*, 2008). Most IBI outcome studies have not found that IBI has had the same magnitude of effect as was found for the children in the original Lovaas (1987) study. However, IBI outcome studies have also consistently found that another portion of children make substantial, clinically significant improvements in cognitive and adaptive behaviour functioning, while not actually achieving 'best outcome' status', while the remainder make little or no change.

Key clinical features of IBI

The amount of IBI – intensity and duration – are key ingredients. Clinically, IBI is provided at an intensity of 20–40 hours per week for approximately 1–3 years, depending on whether the child is responding. Studies of 10–12 hours per week have not reported the same developmental changes (Smith *et al*, 1997; Eldevik *et al*, 2006) and there is no research to date comparing outcomes for children who received different dosages of IBI within the range 20–40 hours per week. In addition, research studies have typically shown that IBI is a relatively short-term intervention, with a duration from 1 to 3 years, with only one study of children who were in IBI for up to 4 years (Sallows & Graupner, 2005).

Assessment is another key feature of IBI. IBI begins with a baseline assessment. The baseline assessment is actually a comprehensive child assessment protocol with information gathered from multiple methods, sources and perspectives, including parents. Both standardised norm-referenced cognitive, language and adaptive behaviour measures and criterion-referenced curriculum and behavioural assessments are included.

The baseline assessment and curriculum results inform the child's individualised IBI treatment or programme plan for setting goals, designing programmes and determining the settings and intensity, as well as parent and carer involvement. Fig. 11.2 depicts these features of the IBI treatment model used at McMaster Children's Hospital in the Hamilton-Niagara Regional Autism Intervention Program (H-NRAIP), in Ontario, Canada. It shows the progression from an early learning level of programming to teach consistent attending, requesting and responding to simple instructions, to an intermediate learning level of activity-embedded communication and cognitive skills generalised across settings and people and materials, to advanced learning and self-regulation with typical peers in natural learning situations.

The individualised goals and programmes in the child's treatment plan are delivered by highly trained staff who are supervised on a regular basis by qualified psychologists and behaviour analysts. The child's programming is reviewed weekly and revised in accordance with the data collected. The assessment protocol is repeated to measure the child's progress at least every 6 months. The updated assessment data are helpful in making the difficult clinical decisions about whether the child is benefiting from IBI and whether IBI should be continued or discontinued and whether the child's treatment should be transitioned from IBI to another treatment

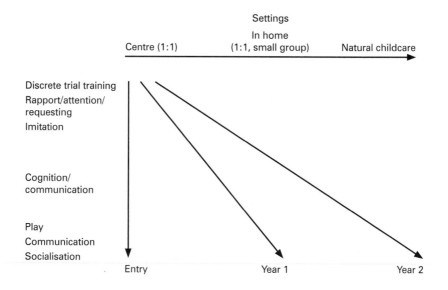

Fig. 11.2 McMaster Children's Hospital H-NRAIP 2-spectra IBI treatment model (reproduced by kind permission, McMaster Children's Hosptial, Autism, Developmental Pediatrics and Rehabilitation Services)

approach that would be more appropriate to the child's needs. Consistent and transparent IBI continuation decision criteria have been developed by the Regional Autism Providers of Ontario (RAPON, 2012) to guide IBI treatment decision-making (available from the first author on request).

The essential ingredients of IBI are summarised in Table 11.2.

Evidence for the effectiveness of IBI

Studies of IBI have accumulated internationally over decades. It has been well established as an effective intervention for young children with ASD in many meta-analyses (Eldevik *et al*, 2009; Reichow & Wolery, 2009; Makrygianni & Reed, 2010) and systematic reviews (Warren *et al*, 2011) as well as in rigorous research studies, including randomised controlled trials (Smith *et al*, 2000; Sallows & Graupner, 2005). IBI has also been found to be more effective in many controlled comparison studies comparing IBI with eclectic treatments (Eikeseth *et al*, 2007), community-based programmes (Howard *et al*, 2005), clinic-directed treatment (Remington *et al*, 2007), parent training (Smith *et al*, 2000) and school (Sheinkopf & Seigel, 1998; Cohen *et al*, 2006). Perry *et al* (2008) evaluated the effectiveness of the Ontario community-based IBI programme. Similar results were obtained with another sample of children who received IBI through the H-NRAIP

Table 11.2 Essential ingredients of intensive behavioural intervention (IBI)

Essential feature of IBI	Description
Staff training and evaluation of IBI implementation	Standardised curriculum of initial staff training on applied behaviour analysis (ABA) and autism spectrum disorder (ASD) and hands-on skills and evaluation
Direct supervision	Supervised programming a minimum of 10% of each child's IBI hours by qualified and registered child psychologist and behaviour analyst with extensive experience supervising IBI for children with ASD
Amount of IBI	Intensity: at least 20 hours per week Duration: minimum trial of 6 months; up to 1–3 years
Baseline and discharge assessment protocol	Standard assessment protocol at IBI entry and exit to measure effectiveness of treatment
Manualised curriculum	Criterion-referenced curriculum assessment to identify skills and skills deficits, to guide programming and measure skills growth: Assessment of Behaviour Language and Learning Skills – Revised (ABLLS-R; Partington, 2006); Verbal Behavior Milestones Assessment and Placement Program (VB-Mapp; Sundberg, 2008). Supplementary programming may include PECS (Frost & Bondy, 2002); social skills (Maurice *et al*, 2001); functional skills (Partington & Mueller, 2012) and early learning skills (Teaford, 2010)
Individualised treatment plan goals, programming and settings	Individualised goal-setting based on needs of child identified in current assessment with parent/carer input ABA-based teaching strategies in written programmes with data collection systems for learning and behaviour. Settings can be clinic, home and natural learning community locations Written proactive positive behaviour strategies (Dunlap & Fox, 1999)
Functional approach to problem behaviours	Functional assessment approach to problem behaviours and written behaviour reduction plans with data collection and parent input (O'Neil *et al*, 1990)
Systematic process of assessment and treatment	Standard update protocol of curriculum, programming and standardised assessments to measure progress in IBI and determine next steps in treatment planning for child at least every 6 months
Consistent and transparent decision-making criteria	To determine ongoing effectiveness of IBI for each individual child
Parent and family involvement	Parent, carer and family involvement in assessment and treatment planning, as well as training, workshops, generalisation of skills
Transition planning	Planning transition to the child's next learning environment

Adapted from Dawson & Osterling (1997).

IBI programme at McMaster Children's Hospital (details available from the first author on request).

As noted above, IBI child outcome studies have consistently shown that IBI is effective for only a portion of children who receive the treatment. Studies are searching for child characteristics that predict successful response to IBI, including age, level of functioning, rate of learning and severity of symptoms. There is some variability in the conclusions for age as a predictor. The age range of the children in IBI studies is somewhat restricted to pre-school and young school-age children, and some studies indicate that age as a predictor is confounded by length of treatment (i.e. younger children received longer durations of IBI). Results from some studies indicated that the earlier children started IBI (preferably before age 4), the better the outcomes (Luiselli et al, 2000; Perry et al, 2011) but this was not concluded from some other studies (Sallows & Graupner, 2005; Magiati et al, 2007; Hayward et al, 2009). Intellectual functioning at entry to IBI has also been studied as a predictor, and results generally support the conclusion that children with higher IQ scores at the time of entry to IBI have better outcomes (Eikeseth et al, 2007; Magiati et al, 2007; Remington et al, 2007; Hayward et al, 2009; Perry et al, 2011); however, higher IQ did not predict better outcomes in the randomised controlled trial by Smith et al (2000). Interestingly, at the lower end of cognitive functioning, Sallows & Graupner (2005) found that limited progress in IBI was predicted by IQ scores below 44 and no words at 36 months of age. Rapid acquisition of early learning skills at the beginning of IBI has also been studied and results indicate that the children who learn skills quickly have better outcomes (Weiss, 1999; Sallows & Graupner, 2005; Summers et al, 2012).

Current interventions for children with ASD often incorporate parent skills training, and parent involvement may play a role in children's outcome (Osborne et al, 2008). Strauss (2011) discussed the beneficial implications of parent inclusion for their child's progress with IBI. The implementation of parent training within the treatment group led to less challenging behaviours, increased commitment to treatment and an overall direct change in behaviour. Relatively little is known about the family factors that may influence a child's response to IBI; however, there are some preliminary results indicating that parental stress may affect parent involvement in IBI and child outcomes (Strauss et al, 2012).

In summary, research has consistently concluded that IBI is effective in improving cognitive, language and adaptive behaviour, all of which may reach the normal range of functioning for some young children with ASD. Research also broadly supports the need for IBI to start as soon as possible, because children who start IBI at under 4 years and who are higher functioning at the time of entry to IBI are among those who achieve better outcomes. It is also known that, unfortunately, not all children with ASD respond to IBI and they need other ABA approaches. However, this is a challenge, as alternative ABA interventions are underdeveloped, making it difficult to match a child's needs to the right treatment at the right time. More research is needed to better tailor treatment plans and set appropriate goals for the child. Additional research is needed on parent involvement and the other family factors that may have an impact on child outcomes.

Currently, there is some variability in the research evidence on the child characteristics that predict best outcomes from IBI or no change. This is complicated by the fact that there is a great deal of heterogeneity in medical conditions and developmental and behavioural characteristics among young children with ASD (Georgiades *et al*, 2013). Taken together, it is difficult to recommend other ABA treatments for a young child with ASD prior to a trial of IBI to assess the child's response to the treatment. A trial of IBI would inform the next steps for treatment planning, education and care for young children with ASD.

Mental health in ASD

Individuals with ASD experience high levels of emotional and behavioural problems. There is a growing body of literature showing that, in addition to struggles related to the core ASD symptoms, psychiatric concerns are common, with 28–84% meeting criteria for one psychiatric disorder and 27–50% for two or more (e.g. Farley *et al*, 2009; for reviews see Leyfer *et al*, 2006; Simonoff *et al*, 2008; Mattila *et al*, 2010; Memari *et al*, 2012; Drmic & Szatmari, 2014). These findings, though variable, highlight the potential impact of mental health symptoms on the lives of individuals with ASD and their families. People with ASD experience more severe psychiatric symptoms than typically developing peers (Gadow *et al*, 2004; Farrugia & Hudson, 2006; Turek *et al*, 2014) and similar or higher rates than other clinical groups (e.g. Green *et al*, 2000; Evans *et al*, 2005; Totsika *et al*, 2011a, 2011b; Tureck *et al*, 2014). Evidence is beginning to demonstrate that psychiatric problems in ASD are present at a young age, and persist from childhood to adolescence and into adulthood (Gadow *et al*, 2004; Billstedt *et al*, 2005; Eaves & Ho, 2008; Farley *et al*, 2009; Davis *et al*, 2010; Gray *et al*, 2012; Simonoff *et al*, 2013); however, a better understanding is needed of how symptoms change throughout the life course. Furthermore, many individuals do not quite meet full criteria for a psychiatric disorder and are 'sub-syndromal', implying that many individuals are experiencing concerning mental health symptoms and would likely benefit from additional support and treatment (Leyfer *et al*, 2006). Recognising comorbid symptoms early and providing treatments that target mental health concerns are important for a good quality of life, as well as better prognosis and long-term outcomes (White *et al*, 2009).

Assessment of comorbidity

Mental health problems in individuals with ASD are often underdiagnosed despite growing evidence that they are common. There are challenges with assessment and differential diagnosis that may help explain why these concerns are largely unrecognised. Individuals with ASD may have difficulty with introspection, that is, recognising and describing their internal states, symptoms and physiological experiences; the clinician therefore needs to gather clinical information from a variety of sources and using a variety of techniques. There is also a tendency for clinicians to falsely attribute psychiatric symptoms to the ASD or intellectual disability, thereby overlooking the psychiatric diagnosis (termed diagnostic overshadowing). Indeed, determining whether the psychiatric symptoms in ASD are part of the same dimension (part of the autism spectrum) or a different dimension (part of comorbid psychiatric disorder) is challenging owing to symptom overlap between psychiatric symptoms and core ASD symptoms (e.g. social withdrawal may be characteristic of ASD or depression), atypical presentation of psychiatric concerns and masking of psychiatric problems by ASD symptoms (Skokauskas & Gallagher, 2010). Furthermore, few tools (i.e. questionnaires, interviews) have been specifically developed, modified or validated in individuals with ASD or other intellectual disabilities, making it difficult validly and efficiently to identify and diagnose psychiatric disorders, although progress is being made in this area (Leyfer *et al*, 2006; Hermans *et al*, 2011). Recommendations to assist with differential diagnosis include determining: whether the impairment is over and above the impairment caused by the primary diagnosis (ASD); whether the behaviour is seen in all situations (due to ASD) or only certain situations (when anxious); whether there has been a change in the behaviour over time; whether there has been a deterioration in adaptive functioning (Kim *et al*, 2000; Tantum, 2000; MacNeil *et al*, 2009; Szatmari & McConnell, 2011). Lastly, Werner & Stawski (2012) conducted a review examining the knowledge, attitudes and training of mental health professionals regarding service provision to individuals with developmental disabilities, and found a need to improve the knowledge, competence and attitudes of practitioners through training and practice opportunities.

Cognitive–behavioural therapy and ASD: treatment of mental health concerns

Given the increasing recognition of the presence of mental health problems in individuals with ASD, research has started to examine interventions that target these problems. Being able to recognise that a problem is related to a mental health concern, as opposed to a symptom related to ASD or a problem behaviour, will allow for appropriate treatment decisions that target the specific problem (Leyfer *et al*, 2006). There is an extensive literature about the use of ABA techniques to target various problem behaviours, social skills deficits and poor adaptive skills (see previous section). Significantly less work has been done specifically targeting mental health concerns. There is a fast-growing literature examining the use of cognitive–behavioural therapy (CBT) to address comorbid anxiety in individuals with ASD (Lang *et al*, 2010), and a few studies are emerging that use cognitive and behavioural strategies to target other areas, such as emotion regulation (Scarpa & Reyes, 2011), increasing understanding and expression of affectionate behaviour (Sofronoff *et al*, 2011; Attwood, 2013), as well as social skills (Bauminger-Zviely, 2013). Data on the treatment of other psychiatric disorders is limited, although some work is beginning to emerge to address depression (Spek *et al*, 2013), anger and aggression (Sofronoff *et al*, 2007; Frazier *et al*, 2010; Singh *et al*, 2011), self-management and emotional regulation (Scarpa & Reyes, 2011; Singh *et al*, 2011) and attention (Safren, 2006) in individuals with ASD and other neurodevelopmental disorders. Furthermore, the utility and effectiveness of other intervention approaches are being explored, including mindfulness-based strategies (Singh *et al*, 2011; Spek *et al*, 2013) and narrative methods such as the use of externalising metaphors (McGuinty *et al*, 2011) or perhaps addressing factors that are common across emotional and behavioural problems, using a trans-diagnostic approach (Norton, 2012; Norton & Barrera, 2012; Weiss, 2014). Since the majority of the evidence relates to the treatment of anxiety disorders in ASD using CBT, this will be the primary focus of the remainder of this chapter.

What is CBT?

CBT is one of the most commonly used and researched treatment approaches, and has garnered evidence as being effective for a range of psychological problems in children and adolescents (e.g. James *et al*, 2013; Munoz-Solomando *et al*, 2008; Reynolds *et al*, 2012), as well as adults (Hofmann & Smits, 2008). CBT is a structured and brief therapy that focuses on current problems and can be delivered in various formats – individual, group, parents or family. In CBT, the therapist's roles include diagnostician, consultant and educator (Kendall & Panichelli-Mindel, 1995). CBT targets many areas of potential vulnerability, including thoughts, feelings and behaviours, which are thought to be causally related. The goal of CBT is to identify, challenge and change dysfunctional beliefs, catastrophic cognitions and problematic behaviours and create new cognitive and behavioural coping techniques that result in better outcomes (Kendall, 2000). CBT consists of a number of components, including psycho-education, the development of coping skills (e.g. somatic management), modifying self-talk (i.e. cognitive restructuring), problem solving, and self-reflection, as well as practising these skills while in the feared or stressful situation in a gradual but incremental fashion (in the exposure phase) (Kendall & Gosch, 1994; Kendall & Panichelli-Mindel, 1995; Benjamin *et al*, 2011; Scarpa & Lorenzi, 2013). The variety of strategies used reflects its rich history and the integration of behavioural, cognitive and other theories of human development and psychopathology (Benjamin *et al*, 2011).

CBT to treat anxiety disorders in ASD

There is mounting evidence that CBT is an effective approach for treating mental health symptoms in individuals with ASD, with the majority of studies being conducted in the treatment of comorbid anxiety. CBT was considered an 'emerging' treatment according to the 2009 National Autism Center's *National Standards* report, and since that time evidence continues to emerge supporting claims that CBT is effective in this population. Indeed, support for the effectiveness of CBT in reducing anxiety has been demonstrated in various studies, including case studies, small-group studies and randomised clinical trials (Lang *et al*, 2010). The majority of studies have been conducted with children and adolescents and only a few with adults (e.g. Sofronoff *et al*, 2005; Sze & Wood, 2007; Reaven *et al*, 2012b; Binnie & Blainey, 2013). Both individually based (e.g. Storch *et al*, 2013; Wood *et al*, 2009) and group-based (e.g. Sofronoff *et al*, 2005; Reaven *et al*, 2012a, 2012b) treatment formats have been shown to be effective, although a direct comparison of the two formats has not been conducted in this population. Furthermore, the CBT programmes that have been utilised have either been developed specifically for children and youths with ASD, or were originally developed for typically developing anxiety-disordered individuals and modified for ASD. It is not clear whether an ASD-specific programme is more beneficial than a general programme that is modified for ASD. It is also noteworthy that evidence on the treatment of anxiety in individuals with an intellectual disability is limited; there is some support for the use of CBT for anger, depression and phobia, although evidence is scant and studies are generally of low quality (Hagopian & Jennett, 2008; Jennett & Hagopian, 2008; Sturmey, 2012). Thus, more research is needed to determine whether cognitive–behavioural strategies would be effective, and if so, the modifications needed to support individuals with intellectual disability and mental health problems.

On the whole, individuals with ASD who struggle with anxiety show improvement following participation in a CBT programme compared with a control group (i.e. treatment as usual or a waiting-list control condition; see Table 11.3). The rate of treatment response, those achieving a clinically meaningful improvement relative to baseline, has ranged from 46 to 77% in individuals who received CBT, compared with 9–14% with treatment as usual (see Table 11.3), which is similar to rates in typically developing anxiety-disordered youths (60–78%) (Walkup *et al*, 2008; Wood *et al*, 2009). Treatment gains were maintained at short-term follow-up (i.e. 3 and 6 months) (Reaven *et al*, 2012a, 2012b; Storch *et al*, 2013), but no studies have examined longer-term outcomes. One study reported that the number needed to treat (NNT) was 1.72 (McNally Keehn *et al*, 2013), which is similar to the typically developing population (NNT = 2.8; Walkup *et al*, 2008). The proportion of individuals who no longer met criteria for an anxiety diagnosis (i.e. remission rate) ranged from 38 to 71% in the ASD group, versus less than 9% in the control groups (Chalfant *et al*, 2007;

Table 11.3 Rates (%) of treatment response and remission from cognitive–behavioural therapy (CBT) for children with autism spectrum disorder

Reference	CBT programme	% treatment response (CGI-I)		% treatment remission (ADIS-P/C/CSR)		
		CBT	TAU	CBT	TAU or (WL)	NNT
Storch et al (2013)	BIACA* 3-month follow-up	75 73	14	38	5	–
McNally Keehn et al (2013)	Coping Cat (modified)* 2-month follow-up	–	–	58 36	(0)	1.72
Reaven et al (2012a)	Facing Fears 3- and 6-month follow-up	50 Gains maintained	8.7	–	–	–
Reaven et al (2012b)	Facing Fears 3-month follow-up	46 Gains maintained	–	–	–	–
Wood et al (2009)	Building Confidence (modified)** 3-month follow-up	76.5	8.7	52.9 80	8.7	–
Chalfant et al (2007)	Cool Kids (modified)*	–	–	71.4	(0)	–

*No longer met criteria for primary anxiety diagnosis (remission rates). ** No longer met criteria for all anxiety diagnoses (remission rates).

ADIS-P/C/CSR, Anxiety Disorder Interview Scale – Parent/Child Clinical Severity Rating; BIACA, Behavioral Interventions for Anxiety in Children with Autism (Wood & Drahota, 2005); CGI-I, Clinical Global Impressions Scale – Improvement; NNT, number needed to treat; TAU, treatment as usual; WL, waiting-list control.

Wood *et al*, 2009; McNally Keehn *et al*, 2013; Storch *et al*, 2013); and in the typical population ranged from 64 to 70% (Kendall, 1994; Barrett *et al*, 1996; Kendall *et al*, 2008). At follow-up (2 or 3 months) remission rates ranged from 36 to 80%. Given the broad range of remission rates reported in the ASD population following treatment and at follow-up, it seems a potentially large proportion of individuals maintain their anxiety diagnosis, regardless of their response to treatment. This may reflect difficulties with generalisation, child characteristics (e.g. cognitive delay, comorbidity) or parent factors (e.g. stress, mental health concerns) (Storch *et al*, 2013). Thus, research is needed to delineate the factors that lead to improved treatment outcomes, such as examining the impact of parental inclusion, length of treatment, inclusion of booster sessions, or modifications that are made to CBT for individuals with ASD.

Studies examining CBT in ASD and comorbid anxiety have typically used a quasi-experimental pre–post study design without a control group, or a randomised controlled trial design using a control group; none has compared CBT with an active control condition, such as another form of supportive psychotherapy or pharmacotherapy. However, Sung *et al* (2011) compared a 16-week CBT programme with a 16-week social recreational programme on anxiety symptoms in children with ASD, and found lower anxiety symptoms at 6-month follow-up for both programmes. The authors suggested that both programmes offer an effective framework (e.g. consistent sessions and therapists, structured setting, social exposure) to help manage anxiety, but more work is needed to determine what components contribute to effectiveness. It is important to note that although anxiety was measured using a child-based questionnaire and clinical impression, no information was provided by parents and no determination was made of the presence of an anxiety disorder. Although it was noted that the pre-treatment total anxiety scores were higher than the normative sample, the level of impairment and interference with daily functioning is not known and the study sample may represent a less psychiatrically impaired group of children. Nonetheless, this study highlights the benefits of structured programming in supporting vulnerable children who struggle with anxiety symptoms (or other emotional or behavioural concerns), and such programmes may be a valuable tool in the prevention of more serious mental health concerns. Most of the research to date has examined treating existing mental health disorders; less has examined prevention, resiliency and the promotion of mental health and well-being (Wilson *et al*, 1997).

Although progress is being made in the recognition and treatment of mental health disorders in this population, numerous areas require further investigation. The treatment studies have not considered the impact of other emotional or behavioural disorders on outcome, nor have they examined changes in other internalising or externalising symptoms following treatment. For example, a study examining outcomes following participation in a structured social skills programme found that children with ASD (and no comorbid psychiatric diagnosis) and children with ASD and comorbid anxiety showed improved social skills, whereas children with ASD and comorbid attention-deficit hyperactivity disorder failed to improve (Antshell *et al*, 2011). Thus, the presence of a psychiatric disorder may affect improvement in other skill areas, and may signal or provide information about the best order of treatment participation. Future studies should compare CBT with another active form of therapy. It is also important to examine outcomes in various domains of functioning (e.g. social, school, daily living) and to utilise better outcome measures that look at functional outcomes of success and translate to better functioning in the individual's daily life. Treatment needs to extend to individuals who are younger and older, and to those individuals with an intellectual disability. A better understanding of moderating and mediating factors may help us to better understand the factors that predict or promote treatment success, thereby allowing treatments to be tailored to an individual's unique needs and learning style.

Modifications to CBT

The basic CBT techniques and structure are similar regardless of whether they are used with children or adults. However, when working with children many considerations and adjustments are recommended. Friedburg & McClure (2002) noted that it is important to consider the child's cognitive and verbal abilities and deliver the therapy at a developmentally appropriate level. It is also valuable to consider the child's interests and preferences, and to keep in mind that children are more action oriented (i.e. learn by doing) and may require more explicit reinforcement than adults. Given that CBT is a treatment package made up of multiple techniques, it is not uncommon to modify or tailor components to accommodate individual needs (Sze & Wood, 2008).

Participation in CBT requires introspection and the ability to identify and challenge dysfunctional cognitions; the latter is assumed to be the primary mechanism of action in CBT (Beck, 1993; Anderson & Morris, 2006). Involvement in a cognitive–behavioural approach emphasises using various cognitive skills, such as self-reflection, perspective taking, causal reasoning, meta-cognition (thinking about thinking) and emotion regulation; consequently, immature or deficient cognitive skills may hinder participation in this type of treatment (Kinney, 1991; Grave & Blissett, 2004). Thus, there has been some debate as to whether CBT is appropriate for ASD, given the difficulty people with the condition have with introspection and given that CBT relies on certain cognitive abilities (Attwood, 2004; Sturmey, 2005; Anderson & Morris, 2006; Lickel *et al*, 2012). Furthermore, many of the adaptations that have been made to CBT programmes for individuals with ASD have emphasised the use of behavioural versus cognitive techniques, which calls into question the mechanism of action that leads to a positive therapeutic outcome (Lang *et al*, 2010). A study examining the cognitive skills needed to participate in a cognitive–behavioural intervention found that children with ASD performed comparably to typically developing children on tasks requiring cognitive mediation and discrimination among thoughts, feelings and behaviours, but not emotion recognition (Lickel *et al*, 2012). The authors recommended providing the children with affective education before the start of CBT, given that emotion recognition was challenging. Thus, this study provides preliminary evidence that children with ASD are able to engage in the cognitive tasks required in CBT and are likely to benefit from cognitive–behavioural interventions.

A number of modifications and adaptations have been recommended when using cognitive–behavioural techniques with children and adolescents with ASD (Attwood, 2004; Anderson & Morris, 2006; Moree & Davis, 2010; Donoghue *et al*, 2011). Moree & Davis (2010) conducted a review that summarises four predominant CBT modification trends for anxious individuals with ASD, which include the use of: (1) disorder-specific hierarchies (e.g. targeting social skills, communication, independence skills); (2) concrete, visual tactics (e.g. less abstract language, visual worksheets); (3) child-specific interests (e.g. use child's preferred language); and (4) parent involvement (e.g. encourage role as coach, increase awareness of and impact of parenting factors or style) (see Table 11.4). Donoghue *et al* (2011) propose a framework, based on clinical practice, not empirical evidence, to follow when adapting and modifying specific CBT techniques that considers the unique needs of individuals with ASD and helps support the therapeutic relationship. The framework is captured in the acronym PRECISE: Partnership working (e.g. setting clear expectations about therapy and roles); Right developmental level (e.g. visual and concrete materials, incorporating child interests, parental involvement); Empathy (e.g. recognising that the child may not readily understand non-verbal instruction and presenting information more clearly); Creative (e.g. use of various media such as computers, pictures, cartoons, puppets, stories); Investigation and experimentation (e.g. use of Socratic questioning); Self-discovery and efficacy (e.g. highlight skills the child is already using); and Enjoyable (e.g. use of various materials, shorter sessions, use of humour). Many of these PRECISE components are consistent with modification trends that had appeared in previous studies.

Thus, a number of modifications have been used to tailor CBT treatments to be more appropriate for children and youths with ASD, and evidence suggests that CBT is a potentially helpful treatment option when suitably adapted. Although these modifications appear to be useful, more research is needed to determine which modifications are most effective for which individuals and at what developmental stage (Tables 11.3 and 11.4).

Table 11.4 Examples of modifications to cognitive–behavioural therapy (CBT) programmes for children with autism spectrum disorder (ASD)

Modification	Example of activities/strategies	Reported benefits
Disorder-specific hierarchies	Module that targets disorder-related problems (e.g. social skills, communication, independence)	Helps overall improvement and increases effectiveness of exposures and generalisation
Concrete, visual tactics	Use of less abstract language/concepts Visual worksheets/tactics (e.g. choice lists, thought bubbles, list of emotion/coping statements) Creating a video; role-play; narratives; stories; cartoons Toolbox that contains strategies as reminders Written schedule, routine, structure and careful pacing of the sessions Use of developmentally appropriate materials Repetition and practice	
Child-specific interests	Use child's preferred language when describing emotions, symptoms or fear ratings, although may need to introduce age-appropriate language Include child's interests (e.g. in worksheets) but being mindful of reinforcing problematic obsessions Expand child's areas of interest	Increases motivation/engagement in therapy
Parent involvement	Provide psychoeducation Encourage role as a coach/co-therapist Acknowledge and address family/parent stress Encouraging positive interactions with child/adolescent Increasing awareness of parenting factors Encourage parents to implement strategies, and promote generalisation of skills and coping strategies across settings	Preliminary research shows that outcomes are better when parents are involved

Sources of information: Reaven & Hepburn (2003, 2006); Sofronoff *et al* (2005); Chalfant *et al* (2007); Sze & Wood (2007, 2008); Lehmkuhl *et al* (2008); Reaven *et al* (2009); Wood *et al* (2009); Moree & Davis (2010); Reaven (2011).

Summary and next steps

Research evidence supports the use of ABA for treatment for children and adults with ASD and particularly the use of IBI as an early intervention for young children with ASD. There is also exciting and emerging research evidence for the use of CBT for children and youths with ASD. Together, this evidence indicates that psychological treatments are effective in modifying ASD symptoms, including social communication skills, and for treating associated difficulties such as cognitive, communication, social and self-care deficits, as well as problem behaviours and mental health issues such as anxiety.

Treatments for ASD will be strengthened by further translation of research knowledge into accessible community-based treatments. Further research is needed, including controlled comparison studies of different treatment approaches, and evaluations of treatment programmes such as IBI. Additional research is needed to understand the active ingredients in psychological treatments for ASD and, specifically, the family factors in relation to IBI and CBT treatment outcomes. Further study of adaptations to IBI and CBT for persons with ASD and intellectual disability is needed.

Finally, adults are too often forgotten. There is a desperate need for psychological treatment research for adults with ASD and for expansion of intervention services to provide behavioural and mental health treatments. There is a need to increase the range of evidence-based psychological treatments to build a more robust continuum of care across the life span.

References

American Psychiatric Association (2000) *Diagnostic and Statistical Manual of Mental Disorders* (4th edn, Text Revision) (DSM-IV-TR). APA.

American Psychiatric Association (2013) *Diagnostic and Statistical Manual of Mental Disorders* (5th edn) (DSM-5). APA.

Anagnostou E, Zwaigenbaum l, Szatmari P, et al (2014) Autism spectrum disorder: advances in evidence-based practice. *Canadian Medical Association Journal*, **186**: 509–19.

Anderson S, Morris J (2006) Cognitive behavioral therapy for people with Asperger's syndrome. *Behavioral and Cognitive Psychotherapy*, **34**: 293–303.

Antshell KM, Polacek C, McMahon M, et al (2011) Comorbid ADHD and anxiety affect social skills group intervention treatment efficacy in children with autism spectrum disorders. *Journal of Developmental and Behavioral Pediatrics*, **32**: 439–46.

Attwood T (2004) Cognitive behavioral therapy for children and adults with Asperger syndrome. *Behavior Change*, **21**: 147–61.

Attwood T (2013) Expressing and enjoying love and affection: a cognitive–behavioral program for children and adolescents with high-functioning ASD. In *CBT for Children and Adolescents with High-Functioning Autism Spectrum Disorders* (eds A Scarpa, SW White, T Attwood): pp 259–77. Guilford Press.

Axelrod S, McElrath KK, Wine B (2012) Applied behavior analysis: autism and beyond. *Behavioral Interventions*, **27**: 1–15.

Baer DM, Wolf MM, Risley TR (1968) Some current dimensions of applied behavior analysis. *Journal of Applied Behavior Analysis*, **1**: 91–7.

Baron-Cohen S, Belmonte MK (2005) Autism: a window onto the development of the social and the analytic brain. *Annual Reviews in Neuroscience*, **28**: 109–26.

Barrett P, Dadds MR, Rapee RM (1996) Family treatment of childhood anxiety: a controlled trial. *Journal of Consulting and Clinical Psychology*, **64**: 333–42.

Bauminger-Zviely N (2013) Cognitive–behavioral–ecological intervention to facilitate social–emotional understanding and social interaction in youth with high-functioning ASD. In *CBT for Children and Adolescents with High-Functioning Autism Spectrum Disorders* (eds A Scarpa, SW White, T Attwood): pp 226–55. Guilford Press.

Beck AT (1993) Cognitive therapy: past, present and future. *Journal of Consulting and Clinical Psychology*, **61**: 194–8.

Benjamin CL, Puleo CM, Settipani CA, *et al* (2011) History of cognitive–behavioral therapy (CBT) in youth. *Child and Adolescent Psychiatric Clinics of North America*, **20**: 179–89.

Bennett KD, Gutierrez A, Honsberger T (2013) A comparison of video prompting with and without voice over narration on the clerical skills of adolescents with autism. *Research in Autism Spectrum Disorders*, **7**: 1273–81.

Billstedt E, Gillberg C, Gillberg C (2005) Autism after adolescents: population-based 13- to 22-year follow-up study of 120 individuals with autism diagnosed in childhood. *Journal of Autism and Developmental Disorders*, **35**: 351–60.

Binnie J, Blainey S (2013) The use of cognitive behavioral therapy for adults with autism spectrum disorders: a review of the evidence. *Mental Health Review Journal*, **18**: 93–104.

Bondy A, Frost L (1994) The Picture Exchange Communication System. *Focus on Autistic Behavior*, **9**: 1–9.

Bondy A, Frost L (2001) The Picture Exchange Communication System. *Behavior Modification*, **25**: 725–44.

Cannella-Malone HI, Fleming C, Chung Y-C, *et al* (2011) Teaching daily living skills to seven individuals with severe intellectual disabilities: a comparison of video prompting to video modeling. *Journal of Positive Behavior Interventions*, **13**: 144–53.

Carr EG (1977) The motivation of self-injurious behavior: a review of some hypotheses. *Psychological Bulletin*, **84**: 800–16.

Carr EG, Durand VM (1985) Reducing behavior problems through functional communication training. *Journal of Applied Behavior Analysis*, **18**: 111–26.

Chalfant AM, Rapee R, Carroll L (2007) Treating anxiety disorders in children with high functioning autism spectrum disorders: a controlled trial. *Journal of Autism and Developmental Disorders*, **37**: 1842–57.

Charlop-Christy MH, LeBlanc LA, Carpenter MH (1999) Naturalistic teaching strategies (NaTS) to teach speech to children with autism: historical perspective, development, and current practice. *California School Psychologist*, **4**: 30–46.

Cohen H, Amerine-Dickens M, Smith T (2006) Early intensive behavioral treatment: replication of the UCLA model in a community setting. *Developmental and Behavioral Pediatrics*, **27**: S145–55.

Davis TE, Fodstad JC, Jenkins WS, *et al* (2010) Anxiety and avoidance and toddlers with autism spectrum disorders: evidence for differing symptom severity presentation. *Research in Autism Spectrum Disorders*, **4**: 305–13.

Dawson G, Osterling J (1997) Early intervention in autism. In *The Effectiveness of Early Intervention* (ed MJ Guralnick): pp 307–26. Brookes.

Dawson G, Rogers S, Munson J, *et al* (2009) Randomized, controlled trial of an intervention for toddlers with autism: the early start Denver model. *Pediatrics*, **125**: e17–23.

Delprato DJ (2001) Comparisons of discrete-trial and normalized behavioral language intervention for young children with autism. *Journal of Autism and Developmental Disorders*, **31**: 315–25.

DeMatteo FJ, Arter PS, Sworen-Parise C, *et al* (2012) Social skills training for young adults with autism spectrum disorder: overview and implications for practice. *National Teacher Education Journal*, **5**: 57–65.

Developmental Disabilities Monitoring Network Surveillance Year 2010 Principal Investigators (2014) Prevalence of autism spectrum disorder among children aged 8 years: Autism and Developmental Disabilities Monitoring Network, 11 Sites, United States, 2010. *MMWR Surveillance Summaries*, **63** (suppl 2): 1–21.

Dillenburger K, Keenan M (2009) None of the As in ABA stand for autism: dispelling the myths. *Journal of Intellectual and Developmental Disability*, **34**: 193–5.

Doehring P, Reichow B, Palka T, *et al* (2014) Behavioral approaches to managing severe problem behaviors in children with autism spectrum and related developmental disorders. *Child and Adolescent Psychiatric Clinics of North America*, **23**: 25–40.

Donoghue K, Stallard P, Kucia J (2011) The clinical practice of cognitive behavioral therapy for children and young people with a diagnosis of Asperger's syndrome. *Clinical Child Psychology*, **16**: 89–102.

Drmic IE, Szatmari P (2014) Emotional dysregulation and comorbidity in autism spectrum disorder (ASD). *Cutting Edge Psychiatry in Practice*, **1**: 119–31.

Dunlap G, Fox L (1999) A demonstration of behavioral support for young children with autism. *Journal of Positive Behavior Interventions*, **1**: 77–87.

Eaves LC, Ho HH (2008) Young adult outcomes of autism spectrum disorders. *Journal of Autism and Developmental Disorders*, **38**: 739–47.

Eikeseth S, Smith T, Jahr E, *et al* (2007) Outcome for children with autism who began intensive behavioral treatment between ages 4 and 7: a comparison controlled study. *Behavior Modification*, **31**: 264–78.

Eldevik S, Eikeseth S, Jahr E, *et al* (2006) Effects of low intensity behavioral treatment for children with autism and mental retardation. *Journal of Autism and Developmental Disorders*, **36**: 211–24.

Eldevik S, Hastings RP, Hughes JC, *et al* (2009) Meta-analysis of early intensive behavioral intervention for children with autism. *Journal of Clinical Child and Adolescent Psychology*, **38**: 439–50.

Evans DW, Canavera K, Kleinpeter FL, *et al* (2005) The fears, phobias, and anxieties of children with autism spectrum disorders and Down syndrome: comparisons with developmentally and chronologically aged matched children. *Child Psychiatry and Human Development*, **36**: 3–26.

Farley MA, McMahon WM, Fombonne E, *et al* (2009) Twenty-year outcome for individuals with autism and average or near-average cognitive abilities. *Autism Research*, **2**: 109–18.

Farrugia S, Hudson J (2006) Anxiety in adolescents with Asperger syndrome: negative thoughts, behavioral problems, and life interference. *Focus on Autism and Other Developmental Disabilities*, **21**: 25–35.

Frazier TW, Youngstrom EA, Haycook T, *et al* (2010) Effectiveness of medication combined with intensive behavioral intervention for reducing aggression in youth with autisms disorder. *Journal of Child and Adolescent Psychopharmacology*, **20**: 167–77.

Friedburg R, McClure J (2002) *Clinical Practice of Cognitive Therapy with Children and Adolescents: The Nuts and Bolts*. Guilford Press.

Frost L, Bondy A (2002) *The Picture Exchange Communication System Training Manual*. Pyramid Educational Products.

Gadow KD, DeVincent CJ, Pomeroy J, *et al* (2004) Psychiatric symptoms in preschool children with PDD and clinic and comparison samples. *Journal of Autism and Developmental Disorders*, **34**: 379–93.

Georgiades S, Szatmari P, Boyle M (2013) Importance of studying heterogeneity in autism. *Neuropsychiatry*, **3**: 123–5.

Ghezzi PM (2007) Discrete trials teaching. *Psychology in the Schools*, **44**: 667–79.

Goldstein H (2002) Communication intervention for children with autism: a review of treatment efficacy. *Journal of Autism and Developmental Disorders*, **32**: 373–96.

Grave J, Blissett J (2004) Is cognitive behavior therapy developmentally appropriate for young children? A critical review of the evidence. *Clinical Psychology Review*, **24**: 399–420.

Gray K, Keating C, Taffe J, *et al* (2012) Trajectory of behavior and emotional problems in autism. *American Journal on Intellectual and Developmental Disabilities*, **117**: 121–33.

Green J, Gilchrist A, Burton D, *et al* (2000) Social and psychiatric functioning in adolescents with Asperger syndrome compared with conduct disorder. *Journal of Autism and Developmental Disorders*, **30**: 279–93.

Hagopian LP, Jennett HK (2008) Behavioral assessment and treatment of anxiety in individuals with intellectual disabilities and autism. *Journal of Developmental and Physical Disabilities*, **20**: 467–83.

Haring TG, Kennedy CH, Adams MJ, *et al* (1987) Teaching generalization of purchasing skills across community settings to autistic youth using videotape modeling. *Journal of Applied Behavior Analysis*, **20**: 89–96.

Hayward D, Eikeseth S, Gale C, *et al* (2009) Assessing progress during treatment for young children with autism receiving intensive behavioral intervention. *Autism*, **18**: 613–33.

Hermans H, van der Pas FH, Evenhuis HM (2011) Instruments assessing anxiety in adults with intellectual disabilities: a systematic review. *Research in Developmental Disabilities*, **32**: 861–70.

Hoch H, Taylor BA, Rodriguez A (2009) Teaching teenagers with autism to answer cell phones and seek assistance when lost. *Behavior Analysis in Practice*, **2**: 14–20.

Hofmann SG, Smits JAJ (2008) Cognitive–behavioral therapy for adult anxiety disorders: a meta-analysis of randomized placebo-controlled trials. *Journal of Clinical Psychiatry*, **69**: 621–32.

Howard JS, Sparkman CR, Cohen HG, *et al* (2005) A comparison of intensive behavior analytic and eclectic treatments for young children with autism. *Research in Developmental Disabilities*, **26**: 359–83.

Howlin P, Goode S, Hutton J, *et al* (2004) Adult outcome for children with autism. *Journal of Child Psychology and Psychiatry*, **45**: 212–29.

Iwata BA, Dorsey MF, Slifer KJ, *et al* (1982) Toward a functional analysis of self-injury. *Analysis and Intervention in Developmental Disabilities*, **2**: 3–20.

James AC, James G, Cowdry FA, *et al* (2013) Cognitive behavioural therapy for anxiety disorders in children and adolescents. *Cochrane Database of Systematic Reviews*, **6**: CD004690.

Jennett HK, Hagopian LP (2008) Identifying empirically supported treatments for phobic avoidance in individuals with intellectual disabilities. *Behavioral Therapy*, **39**: 151–61.

Johnson CP, Myers SM (2007) Identification and evaluation of children with autism spectrum disorders. *Pediatrics*, **120**: 1183–215.

Kaat AJ, Lecavalier L (2014) Group-based social skills treatment: a methodological review. *Research in Autism Spectrum Disorders*, **8**: 15–24.

Kagohara DM, van der Meer L, Ramdoss S, *et al* (2013) Using iPods® and iPads® in teaching programs for individuals with developmental disabilities: a systematic review. *Research in Developmental Disabilities*, **34**: 147–56.

Kendall PC (1994) Treating anxiety disorders in children: results of a randomized clinical trial. *Journal of Consulting and Clinical Psychology*, **62**: 100–10.

Kendall PC (ed) (2000) *Child and Adolescent Therapy: Cognitive–Behavioral Procedures* (2nd edn). Guilford Press.

Kendall PC, Gosch EA (1994) Cognitive–behavioral interventions. In *International Handbook of Phobic and Anxiety Disorders in Children and Adolescents* (eds TH Ollendick, K Neville, W Yule): pp 415–38. Plenum Press.

Kendall PC, Panichelli-Mindel SM (1995) Cognitive behavioral treatment. *Journal of Abnormal Psychology*, **23**: 107–24.

Kendall PC, Hudson JL, Gosch E, *et al* (2008) Cognitive–behavioral therapy for anxiety-disordered youth: a randomized clinical trial evaluating child and family modalities. *Journal of Consulting and Clinical Psychology*, **76**: 282–97.

Kim J, Szatmari P, Bryson SE, *et al* (2000) Prevalence of anxiety and mood problems among children with autism and Asperger syndrome. *Autism*, **4**: 117–32.

Kinney A (1991) Cognitive–behavior therapy with children: developmental reconsiderations. *Journal of Rational–Emotive and Cognitive–Behavior Therapy*, **9**: 52–61.

Kodak T, Grow LL (2011) Behavioral treatment of autism. In *Handbook of Applied Behavior Analysis* (eds WW Fisher, CC Piazza, HS Sloane): pp 402–16. Guilford Press.

Koegel LK, Koegel RL, Harrower JK, *et al* (1999) Pivotal response intervention I: overview of approach. *Journal of the Association for Persons with Severe Handicap*, **24**: 174–85.

Kurtz PF, Boelter EW, Jarmolowicz DP, *et al* (2011) An analysis of functional communication training as an empirically supported treatment for problem behavior displayed by individuals with developmental disabilities. *Research in Developmental Disabilities,* **32**: 2935–42.

Lang R, Regester A, Lauderdale S, *et al* (2010) Treatment of anxiety in autism spectrum disorders using cognitive behaviour therapy: a systematic review. *Developmental Neurorehabilitation,* **13**: 53–63.

Lehmkuhl HD, Storch EA, Bodfish JW, *et al* (2008) Exposure and response prevention for obsessive compulsive disorder in a 12-year-old with autism. *Journal of Autism and Developmental Disorders,* **38**: 977–81.

Leyfer OT, Folstein SE, Bacalman S, *et al* (2006) Comorbid psychiatric disorders in children with autism: interview development and rates of disorders. *Journal of Autism and Developmental Disorders,* **36**: 849–61.

Lickel A, MacLean WE, Blakeley-Smith A, *et al* (2012) Assessment and prerequisite skills for cognitive behavioral therapy in children with and without autism spectrum disorders. *Journal of Autism and Developmental Disorders,* **42**: 992–1000.

Lovaas OI (1987) Behavioral treatment and normal educational and intellectual functioning in young autistic children. *Journal of Consulting and Clinical Psychology,* **55**: 3–9.

Luiselli JK, Cannon BOM, Ellis JT, *et al* (2000) Home-based behavioral intervention for young children with autism/pervasive developmental disorder: a preliminary evaluation of outcome in relation to child age and intensity of service delivery. *Autism,* **4**: 426–38.

MacNeil BM, Lopes VA, Minnes PM (2009) Anxiety in children and adolescents with autism spectrum disorders. *Research in Autism Spectrum Disorders,* **3**: 1–21.

Magiati I, Charman T, Howlin P (2007) A two-year prospective follow-up study of community-based early intensive behavioural intervention and specialist nursery provision for children with autism spectrum disorders. *Journal of Child Psychology and Psychiatry,* **48**: 803–12.

Maglione MA, Gans D, Das L, *et al* (2012) Nonmedical interventions for children with ASD: recommended guidelines and further research needs. *Pediatrics,* **130** (suppl 2): S169–78.

Makrygianni MK, Reed P (2010) A meta-analytic review of the effectiveness of behavioural early intervention programs for children with autistic spectrum disorders. *Research in Autism Spectrum Disorders,* **4**: 577–93.

Matson JL, Matson ML, Rivet TT (2007) Social-skills treatments for children with autism spectrum disorders: an overview. *Behavior Modification,* **31**: 682–707.

Matson JL, Hattier MA, Belva B (2012a) Treating adaptive living skills of persons with autism using applied behavior analysis: a review. *Research in Autism Spectrum Disorders,* **6**: 217–76.

Matson JL, Turygin NC, Beighley J, *et al* (2012b) Applied behavior analysis in autism spectrum disorders: recent developments, strengths and pitfalls. *Research in Autism Spectrum Disorders,* **6**: 144–50.

Matilla M-L, Hurtig T, Haapsamo H, *et al* (2010) Comorbid psychiatric disorders associated with Asperger syndrome/high functioning autism: a community and clinic-based study. *Journal of Autism and Developmental Disorders,* **40**: 1080–93.

Maurice C, Green G, Foxx R (eds) (2001) *Making a Difference: Behavioral Intervention for Autism.* Pro-Ed.

Mays NM, Heflin LJ (2011) Increasing independence in self-care tasks for children with autism using self-operated auditory prompts. *Research in Autism Spectrum Disorders,* **5**: 1351–7.

McGuinty E, Armstrong D, Nelson J, *et al* (2011) Externalizing metaphors: anxiety and high-functioning autism. *Journal of Child and Adolescent Psychiatric Nursing,* **25**: 9–16.

McNally Keehn RH, Lincoln AJ, Brown MZ, *et al* (2013) The coping cat program for children with anxiety and autism spectrum disorder: a pilot randomized controlled trial. *Journal of Autism and Developmental Disorders,* **43**: 57–67.

Mechling LC, Ayres KM, Foster AL, *et al* (2013) Comparing the effects of commercially available and custom-made video prompting for teaching cooking skills to high school students with autism. *Remedial and Special Education*, **34**: 371–83.

Memari AH, Ziaee V, Mirfazeli FS, *et al* (2012) Investigation of autism comorbidities and associations in a school-based community sample. *Journal of Child and Adolescent Nursing*, **25**: 84–90.

Minshawi NH, Ashby I, Swiezy N (2009) Adaptive and self-help skills. In *Applied Behavior Analysis for Children with Autism Spectrum Disorders* (ed JL Matson): pp 189–206. Springer.

Moree BN, Davis TE III (2010) Cognitive behavior therapy for anxiety in children diagnosed with autism spectrum disorders: modification trends. *Research in Autism Spectrum Disorders*, **4**: 346–54.

Munoz-Solomando A, Kendall T, Whittington CJ (2008) Cognitive behavioural therapy for children and adolescents. *Current Opinion in Psychiatry*, **21**: 332–7.

NAC (2009) *The National Standards Project – Addressing the Need for Evidence-Based Practice Guidelines for Autism Spectrum Disorders*. National ASD Center.

National Research Council (2001) *Educating Children with Autism (Committee on Education and Interventions for Children with Autism)*. National Academy Press.

NICE (2011) *Autism Diagnosis in Children and Young People: Recognition, Referral and Diagnosis of Children and Young People on the Autism Spectrum* (Clinical Guideline 128). National Institute for Health and Clinical Excellence.

NICE (2012) *Autism: Recognition, Referral, Diagnosis and Management of Adults on the Autism Spectrum* (Clinical Guideline 142). National Institute for Health and Clinical Excellence.

NICE (2013) *Autism: The Management and Support of Children and Young People on the Autism Spectrum* (CG170). National Institute for Health and Care Excellence.

NICE (2014) *Autism* (NICE Quality Standard QS51). National Institute for Health and Care Excellence.

Norton PJ (2012) A randomized clinical trial of transdiagnostic cognitive-behavioral treatments for anxiety disorder by comparison to relaxation training. *Behavior Therapy*, **43**: 506–17.

Norton PJ, Barrera TL (2012) Transdiagnostic versus diagnosis-specific CBT for anxiety disorders: a preliminary randomized controlled noninferiority trial. *Depression and Anxiety*, **29**: 874–82.

O'Neil RE, Horner RH, Albin RW, *et al* (1990) *Functional Analysis of Problem Behavior: A Practical Assessment Guide*. Sycamore Publishing.

Osborne L, McHugh L, Saunders J, *et al* (2008) Parenting stress reduces the effectiveness of early teaching interventions for autistic spectrum disorders. *Journal of Autism and Developmental Disorders*, **38**: 1092–103.

Partington JW (2006) *The Assessment of Basic Language and Learning Skills: An Assessment, Curriculum Guide, and Tracking System for Children with Autism or Other Developmental Disabilities*. Behavior Analysts.

Partington JW, Mueller MM (2012) *Assessment of Functional Living Skills*. Behaviour Analysts.

Perry A, Cummings A, Dunn Geier J, *et al* (2008) Effectiveness of intensive behavioral intervention in a large, community-based program. *Research in Autism Spectrum Disorders*, **2**: 621–42.

Perry A, Cummings A, Dunn Geier J, *et al* (2011) Predictors of outcome for children receiving Intensive Behavioral Intervention in a large, community-based program. *Research in Autism Spectrum Disorders*, **5**: 592–603.

Preston D, Carter M (2009) A review of the efficacy of the Picture Exchange System intervention. *Journal of Autism and Developmental Disorders*, **39**: 1471–86.

RAPON (2012) *Clinical Decision Making Guidelines for Continuation in Intensive Behavioural Intervention*. Unpublished manuscript.

Reaven J (2011) The treatment of anxiety symptoms in youth with high-functioning autism spectrum disorders: developmental considerations for parents. *Brain Research*, **1380**: 255–63.

Reaven J, Hepburn S (2003) Cognitive–behavioral treatment of obsessive–compulsive disorder in a child with Asperger syndrome: a case report. *Autism*, **7**: 145–64.

Reaven J, Hepburn S (2006) The parent's role in the treatment of anxiety symptoms in children with high-functioning autism spectrum disorders. *Mental Health Aspects of Developmental Disabilities*, **9**: 73–80.

Reaven J, Blakeley-Smith A, Nichols S, *et al* (2009) Cognitive–behavioral group treatment for anxiety symptoms in children with high functioning autism spectrum disorders: a pilot study. *Focus on Autism and Other Developmental Disabilities*, **24**: 27–37.

Reaven J, Blakeley-Smith A, Culhane-Shelburne K, *et al* (2012*a*) Group cognitive behavior therapy for children with high-functioning autism spectrum disorders and anxiety: a randomized trial. *Journal of Child Psychology and Psychiatry*, **53**: 410–9.

Reaven J, Blakeley-Smith A, Leuthe E, *et al* (2012*b*) Facing your fears in adolescents: cognitive–behavioral therapy for high-functioning autism spectrum disorders and anxiety. *Autism Research and Treatment*, article ID 423905. doi:10.1155/2012/423905 (Epub 3 Oct 2012).

Reichow B, Wolery M (2009) Comprehensive synthesis of early intensive behavioral interventions for young children with autism based on the UCLA Young Autism Project Model. *Journal of Autism and Developmental Disorders*, **39**: 23–41.

Reichow B, Steiner A, Volkmar F (2012) Social skills groups for people aged 6 to 21 with autism spectrum disorders (ASD). *Cochrane Database of Systematic Reviews*, **7**: CD008511.

Reitzel J, Summers J, Lorv B, *et al* (2013) Pilot randomized controlled trial of a Functional Behavior Skills Training program for young children with autism spectrum disorder who have significant early learning skills impairments and their families. *Research in Autism Spectrum Disorders*, **7**: 1418–32.

Remington B, Hastings RP, Kovshoff H, *et al* (2007) Early intensive behavioral intervention: outcomes for children with autism and their parents after two years. *American Journal on Mental Retardation*, **112**: 418–38.

Reynolds S, Wilson C, Austin J, *et al* (2012) Effects of psychotherapy for anxiety in children and adolescents: a meta-analytic review. *Clinical Psychology Review*, **32**: 251–62.

Ringdahl JE, Kopelman T, Falcomata TS (2009) Applied behavior analysis and its application to autism and autism related disorders. In *Applied Behavior Analysis for Children with Autism Spectrum Disorders* (ed JL Matson): pp 15–32. Springer.

Rogers SJ, Vismara LA (2008) Evidence-based comprehensive treatments for early autism. *Journal of Clinical Child and Adolescent Psychology*, **37**: 8–38.

Rutter M (2005) Incidence of autism spectrum disorders: changes over time and their meaning. *Acta Paediatrica*, **94**: 2–15.

Safren SA (2006) Cognitive–behavioral approaches to ADHD treatment in adulthood. *Journal of Clinical Psychiatry*, **67** (suppl 8): 46–50.

Sallows G, Graupner T (2005) Intensive behavioral treatment for children with autism: four-year outcome and predictors. *American Journal on Mental Retardation*, **110**: 417–38.

Scarpa A, Lorenzi J (2013) Cognitive–behavioral therapy with children and adolescents: history and principles. In *CBT for Children and Adolescents with High-Functioning Autism Spectrum Disorders* (eds A Scarpa , SW White, T Attwood): pp 3–26. Guilford Press.

Scarpa A Reyes NM (2011) Improving emotion regulation with CBT in young children with high functioning autism spectrum disorders: a pilot study. *Behavioural and Cognitive Psychotherapy*, **39**: 495–500.

Schlosser RW, Wendt O (2008) Effects of augmentative and alternative communication intervention on speech production in children with autism: a systematic review. *American Journal of Speech-Language Pathology*, **17**: 212–30.

Sheinkopf SJ, Siegel B (1998) Home-based behavioral treatment of young children with autism. *Journal of Autism and Developmental Disorders*, **28**: 15–23.

Shipley-Benamou R, Lutzker JR, Taubman M (2002) Teaching daily living skills to children with autism through instructional video modeling. *Journal of Positive Behavioral Intervention*, **4**: 166–77.

Simonoff E, Pickles A, Charman T, *et al* (2008) Psychiatric disorders in children with autism spectrum disorders: prevalence, comorbidity, and associated factors in a population-derived sample. *Journal of the American Academy of Child and Adolescent Psychiatry*, **47**: 921–9.

Simonoff E, Jones CRG, Baird G, *et al* (2013) The persistence and stability of psychiatric problems in adolescents with autism spectrum disorders. *Journal of Child Psychology and Psychiatry*, **54**: 186–94.

Singh NN, Lancioni GE, Manikam R, *et al* (2011) A mindfulness-based strategy for self-management of aggressive behavior in adolescents with autism. *Research in Autism Spectrum Disorders*, **5**: 1153–8.

Skokauskas N, Gallagher L (2010) Psychosis, affective disorders, and anxiety in autistic spectrum disorder: prevalence and nosological considerations. *Psychopathology*, **43**: 8–16.

Smith T (2001) Discrete trial training in the treatment of autism. *Focus on Autism and Other Developmental Disabilities*, **16**: 86–92.

Smith T, Eikeseth S (2011) O. Ivar Lovaas: pioneer of applied behavior analysis and intervention for children with autism. *Journal of Autism and Developmental Disorders*, **41**: 375–8.

Smith T, Eikeseth S, Klevstrand M, *et al* (1997) Intensive behavioral treatment for preschoolers with severe mental retardation and pervasive developmental disorder. *American Journal on Mental Retardation*, **102**: 238–49.

Smith T, Groen AD, Wynn JW (2000) Randomized trial of intensive early intervention for children with pervasive developmental disorder. *American Journal on Mental Retardation*, **105**: 269–85.

Sofronoff K, Attwood T, Hinton SA (2005) A randomized controlled trial of a CBT intervention for anxiety in children with Asperger syndrome. *Journal of Child Psychology and Psychiatry*, **46**: 1152–60.

Sofronoff K, Attwood T, Hinton S, *et al* (2007) A randomized controlled trial of a cognitive behavioural intervention for anger management in children diagnosed with Asperger syndrome. *Journal of Autism and Developmental Disorders*, **37**: 1203–14.

Sofronoff K, Eloff J, Sheffield J, (2011) Increasing the understanding and demonstration of appropriate affection in children with Asperger syndrome: a pilot trial. *Autism Research and Treatment*, article 214317. doi:10.1155/2011/214317 (Epub 24 Nov 2011).

Spek AA, van Ham NC, Nyklíček I (2013) Mindfulness-based therapy in adults with an autism spectrum disorder: a randomized controlled trial. *Research in Developmental Disabilities*, **34**: 246–53.

Stavropoulos KKM, Carver LJ (2013) Research review: social motivation and oxytocin in autism – implications for joint attention development and intervention. *Journal of Child Psychology and Psychiatry*, **54**: 603–18.

Stokes TF, Baer DM (1977) An implicit technology of generalization. *Journal of Applied Behavioral Analysis*, **10**: 349–67.

Storch EA, Arnold EB, Lewin AB, *et al* (2013) The effect of cognitive–behavioral therapy versus treatment as usual for anxiety in children with autism spectrum disorders: a randomized controlled trial. *Journal of the American Academy of Child and Adolescent Psychiatry*, **52**:132–42.

Strauss K (2011) Parent inclusion in early intensive behavioral intervention: the influence of parental stress, parent treatment fidelity and parent-mediated generalization of behavior targets on child outcomes. *Research in Developmental Disabilities*, **33**: 688–703.

Strauss K, Vicari S, Valeri G, *et al* (2012) Parent inclusion in early intensive behavioral intervention: the influence of parental stress, parent treatment fidelity and parent-mediated generalization of behavior targets on child outcomes. *Research in Developmental Disabilities*, **33**: 688–703.

Sturmey P (2005) Against psychotherapy with people who have mental retardation. *Mental Retardation*, **43**: 55–7.

Sturmey P (2012) Treatment of psychopathology in people with intellectual and other disabilities. *Canadian Journal of Psychiatry*, **57**: 593–600.

Summers J, Reitzel J, Szatmari P, *et al* (2012) The early learning measure as a predictor for 12-month adaptive behavior outcomes for children with autism and intellectual disabilities. Poster presentation at IMFAR: Toronto, ON. International Society for Autism Research. Available at https://imfar.confex.com/imfar/2012/webprogram/Paper11705.html (accessed April 2015).

Sundberg ML (2008) *The Verbal Behavior Milestones Assessment and Placement Program: The VB MAPP*. AVB Press.

Sung M, Ooi YP, Goh TJ, *et al* (2011) Effects of cognitive–behavioral therapy on anxiety in children with autism spectrum disorders: a randomized controlled trial. *Child Psychiatry and Human Development*, **42**: 634–49.

Szatmari P, McConnell B (2011) Anxiety and mood disorders in individuals with autism spectrum disorder. In *Autism Spectrum Disorders* (eds DG Amaral, G Dawson, DH Geschwind): pp 330–8. Oxford University Press.

Sze KM, Wood JJ (2007) Cognitive behavioral treatment of comorbid anxiety disorders and social difficulties in children with high-functioning autism: a case report. *Journal of Contemporary Psychotherapy*, **3**: 133–43.

Sze KM, Wood JJ (2008) Enhancing CBT for the treatment of autism spectrum disorders and concurrent anxiety. *Behavioural and Cognitive Psychotherapy*, **36**: 403–9.

Tantum D (2000) Psychological disorders in adolescents and adults with Asperger's syndrome. *Autism*, **4**: 47–62.

Teaford P (2010) *Hawaii Early Learning Profile HELP 3-6: Curriculum Guide* (2nd edn). VORT.

Thomson K, Walters K, Martin GL, *et al* (2011) Teaching adaptive and social skills to individuals with autism spectrum disorders. In *International Handbook of Autism and Pervasive Developmental Disorders* (eds JL Matson, P Sturmey): pp 339–54. Springer.

Totsika V, Hastings RP, Emerson E, *et al* (2011*a*) Behavior problems at 5 years of age and maternal mental health in autism and intellectual disability. *Journal of Abnormal Child Psychology*, **39**: 1137–47.

Totsika V, Hastings RP, Emerson,E, *et al* (2011*b*) A population-based investigation of behavioral and emotional problems and maternal mental health: associations with autism spectrum disorder and intellectual disability. *Journal of Child Psychology and Psychiatry*, **52**: 91–9.

Tureck K, Matson JL, May A, *et al* (2014) Comorbid symptoms in children with anxiety disorders compared to children with autism spectrum disorders. *Journal of Developmental and Physical Disabilities*, **26**: 23–33.

Van Laarhoven T, Kraus E, Karpman K, *et al* (2010) A comparison of picture and video prompts to teach daily living skills to individuals with autism. *Focus on Autism and Other Developmental Disabilities*, **25**: 195–208.

Vismara LA, Rogers SJ (2010) Behavioral treatments in autism spectrum disorder: what do we know? *Annual Review of Clinical Psychology*, **6**: 447–68.

Walkup JT, Albano AM, Piacentini JC, *et al* (2008) Cognitive behavioral therapy, sertraline, or a combination in childhood anxiety. *New England Journal of Medicine*, **359**: 2753–66.

Walton KM, Ingersoll BR (2013) Improving social skills in adolescents and adults with autism and severe to profound intellectual disability: a review of the literature. *Journal of Autism and Developmental Disorders*, **43**: 594–615.

Wang S-Y, Parilla R, Cui Y (2013) Meta-analysis of social skills interventions of single-case research for individuals with autism spectrum disorders: results from three-level HLM. *Journal of Autism and Developmental Disabilities*, **43**: 1701–16.

Ward-Horner J, Seiverling LJ, Sturmey P (2011) Functional behavioral assessment and analysis. In *International Handbook of Autism and Pervasive Developmental Disorders* (eds JL Matson, P Sturmey): pp 271–86. Springer.

Warren Z, McPheeters ML, Sathe N, *et al* (2011) A systematic review of early intensive intervention for autism spectrum disorders. *Pediatrics*, **127**: e1303–11.

Weiss MJ (1999) Differential rates of skill acquisition and outcomes of early intensive behavioral intervention for autism. *Behavioral Interventions*, **14**: 3–22.

Weiss JA (2014) Transdiagnostic case conceptualization of emotional problems in youth with ASD: an emotion regulation approach. *Clinical Psychology: Science and Practice*, doi: 10.1111/cpsp.12084 (Epub 15 Dec 2014).

Weiss, M.J, Harris, S (2001) Teaching social skills to people with autism. *Behavior Modification*, **25**: 785–802.

Werner S, Stawski M (2012) Mental health: knowledge, attitudes, and training of professionals on dual diagnosis of intellectual disability and psychiatric disorder. *Journal of Intellectual Disability Research*, **56**: 291–304.

White S, Oswald D, Ollendick T, *et al* (2009) Anxiety in children and adolescents with ASD. *Clinical Psychology Review*, **29**: 216–29.

Wilson A, Arnold M, Rowland ST, *et al* (1997) Promoting recreation and leisure activities for individuals with disabilities: a collaborative effort. *Journal of Instructional Psychology*, **23**: 76–9.

Wood JJ, Drahota A (2005) *Behavioral Intervention for Anxiety in Children with Autism.* University of California.

Wood JJ, Drahota A, Sze K, *et al* (2009) Cognitive behavioral therapy for anxiety in children with autism spectrum disorders: a randomized, controlled trial. *Journal of Child Psychology and Psychiatry*, **50**: 224–34.

Zwaigenbaum L, Bryson S, Garon N (2013) Early identification of autism spectrum disorders. *Behavioural Brain Research*, **251**: 133–46.

Part 4
Service provision

Improving the general health of people with disorders of intellectual development

Mike Kerr and Penny Blake

People with disorders of intellectual development (DID) have higher rates of common morbidity, communication difficulties and serious conditions such as epilepsy; they also have specific patterns of health needs associated with the aetiology of their disability. Unfortunately, this combination of need is mirrored by a consistent picture of poor uptake of health promotion initiatives, inadequate care for serious morbidity, unrecognised health needs and poor access to healthcare. Consequently, there is a disparity between the health of people with DID and that of the general population. Psychiatrists can address this disparity in clinical practice by focusing on these patients' mental health, epilepsy management and the impact of behaviour on health. They can also influence health planning and service development.

Inequalities in health status

The achievement of good health is an appropriate goal for all, including, of course, people with DID. This brings particular challenges, as this is a heterogeneous population with varying needs, who receive a similarly complex array of healthcare provision. Furthermore, the impact of societal and environmental factors on health status is arguably greater in this group. The imperative to remove the disparity between the health of people with DID and that of the general population is strong, because improved health is likely to improve quality of life, both of individuals and of their families. In this chapter we make the premise that the general health of people with DID can be improved by addressing those areas in which disparities in health and in healthcare provision are evident. These include:

- a difference in health because of
  - increased mortality
  - increased morbidity
  - more commonly experienced negative determinants of health such as poverty;

- a difference in healthcare because of
  - unequal access to services
  - inequality of services.

To focus on how health improvements can be made, we consider here the following five areas: the disparity in health; health needs; barriers to healthcare; healthcare provision in primary care; and addressing the disparity.

The disparity in health

If an appropriate aim for this population is to reach at least the same level of health and access to healthcare as that enjoyed by the general population, then it is necessary to address the issue of disparity in health. In the past, the concept of health disparity has mainly been applied to minority ethnic or other special groups (such as those facing social deprivation) to show inequality in health status and health access between such groups and the general population. More recently, interest has focused on the disparity for people with DID when they receive healthcare. There have been several nationally published reports which demonstrate the scale of this disparity and its devastating consequences. *Death by Indifference* (Mencap, 2009) was a key example; that report highlighted the death of six people with intellectual disabilities whose deaths in hospital could have been prevented. Important themes from these deaths were: the need to provide appropriate nutrition in hospital; the need to listen to carer concern; the need to access cancer treatment pathways; and the risk of assessing physical illness as behavioural. Since that report was published, there have been several further investigations looking at the care of people with DID and inequalities are still being found.

The knowledge gained from these reports is important and can add a focus to the planning of services. Direct comparisons between people with

Table 12.1 Health disparity in people with disorders of intellectual development

Area of disparity	Example in disorders of intellectual development
Increased mortality	Lower life expectancy
Increased morbidity	High levels of epilepsy, sensory impairment and behavioural disorder
Increase in negative determinants of health	High levels of obesity and underweight; low rates of employment; fewer social connections and meaningful relationships
Access to services	Low rates of uptake of health promotion initiatives
Quality of services	High prescription rate of antipsychotic medication to people with no evidence of psychosis; high rates of unrecognised disease identified on health screening

DID and the general population can, however, present some difficulties, particularly when trying to allow for the impact of the aetiology of the individual's disability on any apparent disparity. Examples of this would be the reduced life expectancy of people with profound DID and the reduced life expectancy in Down syndrome that is associated with Alzheimer's disease. To address this problem, comparison within groups who share the same disability may be needed. This is not to say that some aspects of mortality in the different groups are not preventable. For example, continued advances in accident prevention and in the treatment of swallowing abnormalities and epilepsy may well reduce the disparity in some groups. Table 12.1 highlights key disparity issues.

Health needs

People with DID have both general and special health needs. General health needs include the treatment of acute and chronic illness, health promotion, health screening and appropriate hospital or other referral. These should be met within a primary healthcare setting.

Specialist health needs can be divided into common morbidities that occur at a greater frequency and patterns of health need associated with specific medical conditions. These conditions are not unique to people with DID, but their high prevalence in this population means that they are an important part of any assessment. Sensory deficit, epilepsy and behavioural and psychological disturbance in particular are more common in people with DID.

Sensory deficit: vision and hearing

An institutional survey of vision (McCulloch *et al*, 1996) showed that 12% of people with a mild level of disability, more than 40% of those with a severe level and 100% of those with a profound level had poor visual acuity. The prevalence of ocular health problems ranged from 25% in the group with a mild level of disability to 60% in the group with profound disability. These sensory deficits need assessment and where possible treatment or the provision of specialised sensory aids. If these deficits are neglected, this may impact on the interaction and feedback given by the person when they see any healthcare professional.

Epilepsy

The association between the severity of DID and the prevalence of epilepsy is reflected in the wide variation of prevalence figures in the literature and it is established that the prevalence of epilepsy increases with increasing severity of intellectual disability (see Chapter 6). Prevalence figures also vary with the particular population. Recent community estimates for the prevalence of epilepsy in the population with intellectual disabilities suggest a point prevalence of approximately 18% (Matthews *et al*, 2008), whereas in the general population the prevalence of epilepsy is less than 1% (Linehan *et al*, 2010).

Syndrome-specific conditions

Certain syndromes that cause DID are particularly associated with an increased risk of specific morbidity. Down syndrome, for example, is associated with increased risks of cardiovascular disease, respiratory disease, eye disorders, leukaemia, Alzheimer's disease and hypothyroidism. People with fragile-X syndrome have increased connective tissue disease, leading to joint laxity and cardiac abnormalities. Major disorders in the control of satiety have been recognised in Prader–Willi syndrome, with an associated risk of obesity-related pathology.

Mortality and intellectual disability

There is a higher mortality rate (seen in both standardised mortality ratios and reduced life expectancy) in people with DID compared with the general population (Morgan *et al*, 2001). Glover & Ayub (2010) found that people with intellectual disabilities die on average 15 years younger than the general population. Predictors of mortality include the severity of the intellectual disability, reduced mobility, feeding difficulties and Down syndrome (Strauss *et al*, 1998; Van Allen *et al*, 1999). Additionally, people with epilepsy have increased mortality and are at greater risk of sudden unexplained death in epilepsy (SUDEP) (Shorvon & Tomson, 2011).

Barriers to healthcare

A potential cause of the disparity between the health of people with DID and that of the general population are what may be conceptualised as barriers to care. Several such barriers have been suggested (Table 12.2) and it is likely that all of these, often interacting, play a role in disparity. Certainly, the clinician will need to recognise the potential existence of these barriers and minimise them where possible.

Mobility

When the accessibility of services to people with a disability was assessed, a great variation was found across healthcare settings in whether they could be accessed by people with mobility problems (Bachman *et al*, 2007).

Sensory impairment

Sensory impairment may reduce the ability of patients to attend appointments unaccompanied. It can also increase their distress during consultations and physical examinations, as communication and comprehension are reduced.

Table 12.2 Barriers to healthcare for people with disorders of intellectual development

Domain	Effect
Mobility	Difficulty accessing health services
Sensory impairment	Reduced communication and comprehension of health processes
Behaviour problems	Difficulty in examination and investigation of disease
Communication	Reduced comprehension of health processes; difficulty in presenting disease owing to poor communication skills; poor communication skills of health professionals
Knowledge and attitudes	Poor professional knowledge; attitudinal barriers to accessing care; accessibility of specialist services

A reliance on signs and notices in health centres make the experience difficult for people with DID who also have a visual impairment or who are unable to read (Alborz *et al*, 2005)

Behavioural problems

In the USA, Minihan & Dean (1990) found that 20% of patients with an intellectual disability could be examined or treated only after measures such as pre-medication or pre-visits for desensitisation had been taken. Only one in five primary care physicians reported that they felt well prepared to handle a patient who refused to cooperate with an examination or treatment (Minihan *et al*, 1993).

Behavioural problems may hinder the diagnosis of conditions if investigations such as electroencephalography (EEG) are needed. In rare cases of epilepsy, doubt may exist as to whether a behavioural outburst does in fact represent a seizure (IASSID Guidelines Group, 2001).

The parents of children with DID may be reluctant to attend appointments if the child is likely to be disruptive in waiting areas (Alborz *et al*, 2005).

Communication

DID often affect people's ability to recognise and communicate health problems and needs, and they therefore rely on carers to do this for them. The reliance on carers to communicate health needs has been cited as a major barrier to healthcare. Carers are often central to recognising and facilitating access to healthcare for people with DID and are heavily involved in the communication and negotiation that occur in health appointments (Alborz *et al*, 2005).

Knowledge and attitudes and access to specialist services

Lennox *et al* (1997) found that Australian primary care physicians listed lack of knowledge of conditions and illnesses specific to DID as among the top five barriers to care. These included: communication difficulties, problems with history taking, lack of compliance with management plans, lack of knowledge and time constraints.

Does primary care meet the health needs of people with DID?

Three key areas of health needs for people with DID can be identified:

- untreated, yet treatable, medical conditions
- untreated specific health issues related to the individual's disability
- a lack of uptake of generic health promotion such as blood-pressure screening.

Research has found that despite the increased frequency of health problems in people with DID, they access general practice less frequently than the general population (Alborz et al, 2005).

The health of people with DID is worse than that of the general population, although it has improved over the past two decades. People with DID are now living longer than before, although they still do not on average live as long as their peers without DID.

Studies indicate a lack of uptake of health promotion initiatives in people with DID. This is unlikely to be due to lower levels of contact with primary care teams. Research in the UK, the USA and Australia suggests that people with DID visit their general practitioners at least as regularly as do the general population (Jacobson et al, 1989; Beange et al, 1995; Kerr et al, 1996a; Welsh Office, 1996). Furthermore, they have been shown to use specialist services and to be hospitalised more frequently than the general population (Beange et al, 1995; Kerr et al, 1996b).

Also in Australia, Beange et al (1995) found that 74% of 202 individuals with DID had conditions for which specialist care was needed. This care had, however, not always been received, and half of the identified conditions were found to be inadequately managed.

Specific issues in relation to primary care are elaborated in Chapter 13.

Addressing the disparity

To decrease the disparity between the health of people with DID and that of the general population, two separate key areas need to be discussed: first, primary care; and second, specialist psychiatric care.

Primary care

Primary care provision is central to improving the health of people with DID. The barriers as discussed above need to be overcome in order to provide effective primary care.

Assessment

Assessment should enable a physician to recognise the potential morbidities and likely problems that might be seen in clinical practice. As individuals with DID often present vague symptoms compounded by communication difficulties, clinicians should follow a structured assessment comprising:

- assessment of the initial complaint
- recognition and assessment of comorbidity
- recognition of health promotion status.

Probably the biggest change within the UK in the 21st century has been the implementation of centrally funded annual health checks for people with DID. This is provided through a direct enhanced service; general practitioners provide structured health screening using a tool like the Welsh Health Check (Fraser *et al*, 1998), which covers health promotion, physical examination and morbidity specific to people with DID, such as epilepsy and behavioural disturbance. It is optional for general practitioners to provide this service, however, and so there is marked geographical variation as to which patients receive this. Baxter *et al* (2006) emphasised that health checks are a mechanism for identifying illness in this population. Until this is mandatory, however, there will continue to be many patients who miss out on this service and hence may be missing healthcare that they require.

Practice organisation

Following the recent papers, mentioned above, which demonstrated increased morbidity and mortality in people with DID, the Department of Health in England published *Valuing People Now* in 2009 which was a strategy to improve the care of people with DID. It advocates their right to access the same facilities as people without a disability. The aim of the proposal is to bridge the gap between the inequalities in healthcare received by the DID population compared with the general population. *Valuing People Now* recommended the following:

- *Practice registers*. Practices need to identify all individuals with DID on their lists, and this requires a comprehensive practice register. Identification from existing lists can be performed using keyword searches for common conditions such as Down syndrome, and also by asking practice staff. Once the register is established, the recording of names should be proactive.
- *Recall and audit*. Recall is necessary to assess the uptake of health promotion initiatives. The presence of health action plans may be an appropriate audit topic. It is likely that recall is best served by a 'one-stop shop' annual health check, such as the Welsh Health Check.
- *Contact with other services*. Practices will need to ensure that the number of contacts with and patterns of referral to disability services and health facilitators are clearly established and recorded.

Clinical competencies

Primary care teams need skills specific to the care of people with DID: health assessment, health promotion, communication and ethics, assessment of need and referral patterns for complex pathology, and specific skills such as epilepsy management.

Melville *et al* (2006) tested the effectiveness of education and training on intellectual disability for primary care staff, in particular practice nurses. They found it had a positive impact on the staffs' knowledge, understanding and clinical practice for their patients.

Specialist psychiatric care

A specialist multidisciplinary psychiatric care team can provide specific psychiatric assessment and treatment. The team's broader function as an organiser of and conduit to general healthcare services is equally important, though less well defined. In both of these areas, key clinical competencies

Table 12.3 Functions of psychiatric practice in delivering healthcare to people with disorders of intellectual development

Function	Health improvement	Clinical competencies
Psychiatric illness		
Treatment and assessment of all psychiatric illness	Reduced morbidity in individuals and carers	Knowledge of presentation of mental illness in those with communication deficits
Treatment and assessment of challenging behaviour		Assessment of behaviour disorder
		Knowledge of use of treatment modalities (pharmacological, behavioral and psychotherapeutic)
Interface between epilepsy and psychiatric illness		
Diagnostic assessment	Reduced seizure-related morbidity and mortality	Knowledge of seizure types and their presentation as behaviour disorder or mental illness
Treatment of epilepsy		
Treatment of mental illness coexistent with epilepsy	Reduced inaccurate diagnosis	Knowledge of epilepsy treatment
	Identify and treat mental illness when a comorbidity	Knowledge of diagnostic standards for epilepsy
		Knowledge of behavioural assessment
Healthcare organisation		
Recognition of psychiatric symptoms as presentation of physical morbidity	Reduction in inappropriate psychiatric diagnosis and treatment	Knowledge of patterns of unrecognised physical ill health
Appropriate referral to healthcare specialty through general practitioner	Decrease in physical ill health	Knowledge of appropriate referral pathways

are required, particularly when medical and psychiatric needs combine, for example in issues relating to the treatment of epilepsy in people with DID. Table 12.3 identifies these functions and necessary competencies. Of particular importance in DID services is the presentation of physical disease through psychiatric symptoms. This is commonly seen when pain presents as agitation. The chronic pain and anorexia associated with reflux oesophagitis and gastric ulcer disease mimic depressive symptoms. There should be particular diagnostic caution with patients with DID whose 'depression' is associated with sleep disturbance and agitation.

Conclusion

Considerable evidence points to a disparity between the health of people with DID and that of the general population. Psychiatric practice can be central to ameliorating this situation. Psychiatric interventions for common mental illnesses and complex behavioural problems in DID can have a direct impact on health status. Perhaps the most important function of psychiatric practitioners in this area is to act as catalysts and drivers of general health improvement by facilitating patients' access to the appropriate pathways to care.

References

Alborz A, McNally R, Glendinning C (2005) Access to healthcare for people with learning disabilities in the UK: mapping the issues and reviewing the evidence. *Journal of Health Services Research and Policy*, **10**: 173–82.

Bachman SS, Vedrani M, Drainoni ML, *et al* (2007) Variations in provider capacity to offer accessible health care for people with disabilities. *Journal of Social Work in Disability and Rehabilitation*, **6**: 47–63.

Baxter H, Lowe K, Houston H, *et al* (2006) Previously unidentified morbidity in patients with intellectual disability. *British Journal of General Practice*, **56**: 93–8.

Beange H, McElduff A, Baker W (1995) Medical disorders of adults with mental retardation. A population study. *American Journal of Mental Retardation*, **99**: 595–604.

Department of Health (2009) *Valuing People Now: A New Three-Year Strategy for People with Learning Disabilities*. TSO (The Stationery Office).

Fraser W, Sines D, Kerr M (eds) (1998) *The Care of People with Intellectual Disabilities* (9th edn). Oxford: Butterworth-Heinemann.

Glover G, Ayub M (2010) *How people with learning disabilities die*. Improving Health & Lives: Learning Disabilities Observatory, Department of Health.

IASSID Guidelines Group (2001) IASSID clinical guidelines for the management of epilepsy in adults with an intellectual disability. *Seizure*, **10**: 401–9.

Jacobson JW, Janicki MP, Ackerman LJ (1989) Health care service usage by older persons with developmental disabilities living in community settings. *Adult Residential Care Journal*, **3**: 181–91.

Kerr M, Richards D, Glover G (1996a) Primary care for people with an intellectual disability – a group practice study. *Journal of Applied Research in Intellectual Disabilities*, **9**: 347–52.

Kerr M, Thapar A, Dunstan F (1996b) Attitudes of general practitioners to people with a learning disability. *British Journal of General Practice*, **46**: 92–4.

Lennox NG, Diggens JN, Ugoni AM (1997) The general practice care of people with intellectual disability: barriers and solutions. *Journal of Intellectual Disability Research*, **41**: 380–90.

Linehan C, Kerr MP, Walsh PN, *et al* (2010) Examining the prevalence of epilepsy and delivery of epilepsy care in Ireland. *Epilepsy*, **51**: 845–52.

Matthews T, Weston N, Baxter H, *et al* (2008) A general practice-based prevalence study of epilepsy among adults with intellectual disabilities and of its association with psychiatric disorder, behavioural disturbance and carer stress. *Journal of Intellectual Disability Research*, **52**: 1635–73.

McCulloch DL, Sludden PA, McKeon K, *et al* (1996) Vision care requirements among intellectually disabled adults. *Journal of Intellectual Disability Research*, **40**: 140–50.

Melville CA, Cooper SA, Morrison J, *et al* (2006) The outcomes of an intervention study to reduce the barriers experienced by people with intellectual disabilities accessing primary health care services. *Journal of Intellectual Disabilities Research*, **50**: 115–17.

Mencap (2009) *Death by Indifference*. Mencap.

Minihan PM, Dean DH (1990) Meeting the needs for health services of persons with mental retardation living in the community. *American Journal of Public Health*, **80**: 1043–8.

Minihan PM, Dean DH, Lyons CM (1993) Managing the care of patients with mental retardation: a survey of physicians. *Mental Retardation*, **31**: 239–46.

Morgan CL, Scheepers MIA, Kerr MP (2001) Mortality in patients with intellectual disability and epilepsy. *Current Opinion in Psychiatry*, **14**: 471–5.

Shorvon S, Tomson T (2011) Sudden unexpected death in epilepsy. *Lancet*, **378**: 2028–38.

Strauss D, Anderson TW, Shavelle R, *et al* (1998) Causes of deaths of persons with developmental disabilities. Comparison of institutional and community residents. *Mental Retardation*, **36**: 386–91.

Van Allen MI, Fung J, Jurenka SB (1999) Health care concerns and guidelines for adults with Down syndrome. *American Journal of Medical Genetics*, **89**: 100–10.

Welsh Office (1996) *Welsh Health Survey, 1996*. Welsh Office.

CHAPTER 13

Bridging the gap: linking primary and secondary care for people with disorders of intellectual development

Neill J. Simpson and Neil Arnott

Do words matter?

Different definitions and descriptions may be required for different purposes (Fryers, 1991). Teachers identifying learning difficulties require a different definition from that required by policy makers describing eligibility for services for adults who need support or welfare benefits. The needs of epidemiologists are different to the needs of criminal prosecutors. The definition (of mental retardation) the World Health Organization (WHO) used in ICD-10 is 'a condition of arrested or incomplete development of the mind, which is especially characterized by impairment of skills manifested during the developmental period, skills which contribute to the overall level of intelligence, i.e. cognitive, language, motor, and social abilities' (World Health Organization, 1992). Neurodevelopmental disabilities may occur that do not include significant intellectual impairment but which affect language, mobility, learning, self-help and independent living.

All definitions of what ICD-11 is due to call disorders of intellectual development (DID) have three elements:

- cognitive impairment that affects intelligence
- impairment of social functioning (due to cognitive impairment) to a degree that requires support
- the impairments originated in the developmental period.

At the time of writing, 'learning disability' was the term most frequently used by professional services for people with intellectual and developmental disabilities; it was adopted in the UK in 1991 by the Department of Health to replace the term 'mental handicap'. Over the years, the Royal College of Psychiatrists has changed the title of the Faculty (formerly the Section) specialising in the mental health of people with DID: 'mental deficiency', 'mental handicap', 'learning disability' and from 2012 'intellectual disability'. DSM-5 uses the term 'intellectual disability (intellectual developmental

Box 13.1   Telling parents that their child has a disability

Preparation
- Be aware of the family dynamics, environment and understanding of their child.
- Wherever possible, access the shared knowledge of the multidisciplinary team.
- Ensure there is appropriate generic training in communication skills, and that there is full information and confidence in the diagnosis.

The consultation

Timing:
- Allocate sufficient time.
- Ensure that the appointment is made as soon as possible after diagnostic investigation and that all relevant information is available.
- Give parents realistic timescales as to when investigation results will be available.
- Ensure that the timing allows for a prompt follow-up appointment.
- There should be no interruptions.

Personnel present:
- Try to see parents together and be aware that other family members or friends may want to attend initial or subsequent consultation.
- The number of staff present should be kept to a minimum; however, a key professional, such as a community nurse or therapist, should be present to advocate for the family, prompt appropriate questions and clarify medical information.
- Where an interpreter is required, this should be arranged professionally; a family member or friend is not appropriate. Take extra care about confidentiality if the interpreter is part of the family's cultural community.

Style and content of information shared:
- Seek to convey empathy, sensitivity and honesty during the consultation through verbal and non-verbal communication.
- Check concerns, expectations and understanding of ideas.
- Use plain, understandable language and frequently check understanding by summarising and giving opportunities to ask questions.
- Refer to the child by name as an individual (not a diagnosis) and always remain positive but realistic.
- Depending on age and level of cognition, try to keep the child with the parents throughout the consultation. Where this is inappropriate, for example where the child is older, ensure provision for supervision of the child outside the consultation is available and ensure that at least some explanation is given to the child as soon as possible.
- When disclosing a diagnosis to an older child consider the following:
  - the timing and amount of information disclosed should be decided in discussion with the parents
  - a suitable member of the team should be selected
  - the child should be allowed to have further follow-up discussions with or without parents (they may wish to select their own friend or professional to discuss issues with).

Based on Kisler & McConachie (2010)

disorder)' (American Psychiatric Association, 2013). Other official terms have included 'mental subnormality' and 'mental impairment'. This process of repeatedly changing terminology has been described as 'the euphemism treadmill' (Pinker, 1994). In recent years, the terms 'learning disability' and 'learning difficulty' were regarded as descriptive and sufficiently respectful; it remains to be seen whether 'disorders of intellectual development' is meaningful to families. As throughout the present volume, the term disorder of intellectual development (DID) is used in this chapter unless the context requires otherwise.

Cognitive impairment is associated with social disadvantage and with behaviour that is socially devalued or disapproved. Doctors need to communicate with patients and families about conditions for which the words may sound like insults. Reynolds (2003) found that the acceptability of population-based antenatal screening (linked to a decision about possibly terminating pregnancy) may be influenced by the words used to describe the features of Down syndrome. Words to describe disability with cognitive impairment become pejorative, and it appears that technical words (e.g. 'spastic') become derogatory more rapidly than plain English. Advice is available on how best to tell parents that their child has a disability (Kisler & McConachie, 2010) (see Box 13.1), but the processes of diagnosis and planning continue to be extremely stressful for parents (Keenan et al, 2010). The staff of health and education services should learn how to improve their approach (Bartolo, 2002). Similar principles apply whenever a doctor discusses disability with patients and families.

Do people benefit from having their disabilities identified?

Some educational theorists assert that 'labelling' children with developmental disorders results in stigma and other social disadvantages, so that identification is alleged to be harmful, but classifying, categorising and labelling children are often essential to ensuring equal opportunity in the allocation of education and social services (Florian et al, 2006).

It has been estimated that one child with severe intellectual disability is born in 10 years on the list of a general practitioner (GP) serving 2000 patients (including 400 children) (British Paediatric Association, 1994). The proportion of patients of all ages with any type of intellectual impairment is low in primary care (less than 3%) until old age. It is not feasible for a GP to know all of the overlapping definitions and labels and to become expert in assessment and diagnosis.

In secondary care, the proportion is also low for most specialties, and recognition of DID is very low. Consequently, there are often difficulties ensuring that the person's ongoing needs for support are met; risks associated with the disability may be overlooked (such as the risk of choking) and capacity to consent may not be assessed. GPs making referrals

---

Box 13.2 Examples of health needs of individuals with disorders of intellectual development

- Advice on diet and eating (e.g. weight problems, constipation)
- Advice on dental hygiene and dental problems
- Advice on menstrual hygiene and menstrual problems
- Advice about lifestyle risks (e.g. smoking, alcohol misuse, less safe sexual activity)
- Advice about contraception
- Support to access to health programmes in primary care – immunisation, screening for breast, cervical and bowel cancer
- Detecting and responding to additional needs (e.g. communication problems, mobility problems, sensory problems, emotional and behavioural problems)
- Access to screening and monitoring for problems associated with the cause of DID (e.g. thyroid disease for those with Down syndrome)
- Detecting, diagnosing and treating illness – and awareness of common conditions such as epilepsy, respiratory problems and mental ill health
- Access to good practice in prescribing (e.g. undertaking blood tests for people taking anti-epileptic or antipsychotic medication; reviewing polypharmacy and long-term repeat prescriptions)

---

to secondary care could improve this by highlighting DID and key issues for the individual (such as whether the person has impaired capacity to consent). If a person with DID needs to be admitted to hospital, it is very useful to provide a copy of the care plan, so that it can be continued. The General Medical Council (2013) provides useful advice on its website.

People with DID have increased likelihood of having difficulty maintaining their health and responding appropriately to health needs that could affect anyone; and they may have increased risks of some health problems (van Schrojenstein Lantman-de Valk & Noonan Walsh, 2008) (see Box 13.2). Without identification they are unlikely to receive appropriate support for personal development.

It is not always possible for doctors to identify disabling conditions in early infancy, and disability may emerge over several years. Parents may become concerned about their child's development and then approach their GP; or teachers may alert the community child health service; or a problem may be detected through developmental screening. In the UK, the National Screening Committee has advised against developmental screening of the population (Public Health England, 2005). McDonald *et al* (2006) have produced guidelines on the referral of children for investigation of global developmental delay.

There are complex reasons why people with DID have difficulty accessing good healthcare (Box 13.3). Evidence is growing to show that improved identification of DID and improved access to general healthcare results in better health (Robertson *et al*, 2010).

Box 13.3 Barriers to good healthcare for people with disorders of intellectual development

The person with DID may not:

- Recognise symptoms as indicators of ill health
- Report their symptoms to anyone
- Be aware of the possibility of help from a doctor
- Be able to describe symptoms clearly to a doctor
- Be able to provide additional information that a doctor needs (such as timing of symptoms)
- Understand the need for examination
- Cooperate with examination and investigations
- Understand information about diagnosis and prognosis
- Understand advice about treatment
- Follow instructions about treatment, including when to stop

Families and carers may not:

- Realise that a person is describing symptoms of ill health
- Feel that symptoms warrant medical attention
- Provide support that a person needs to consult a doctor
- Give the doctor an accurate history with their observations (i.e. they may give only their own interpretation)
- Understand the risks of ill health and the risks of treatment

The doctor may not:

- Recognise the significance of signs and symptoms of ill health because of their unfamiliarity with the person's usual disabilities ('diagnostic overshadowing')
- Recognise the need to obtain information from the person with DID as well as from an informant
- Distinguish distress due to emotion from distress due to pain in a person with poor language skills
- Feel confident assessing a person with multiple disabilities
- Be aware of availability of additional support for accessing general healthcare via local specialist services
- Consider the context of behavioural change, to recognise causes other than ill health
- Give information in a way the patient understands
- Obtain consent
- Prescribe optimum treatment (e.g. avoid using antipsychotics for problem behaviour)

Specialist services aim to help people with DID to use mainstream services if possible, and to provide additional services for those who require them (Box 13.4). These specialist services focus on severe and profound DID and do not have the capacity to screen the population to identify people whose social impairments may be related to mild cognitive impairment. Fortunately, schools sometimes assess performance related to intelligence, so it is extremely useful if GPs obtain information about educational

Box 13.4 How to meet the needs of people with intellectual disabilities in healthcare settings

Mild DID
- Show respect (e.g. by explaining your duty of confidentiality)
- Interview the patient to obtain the history, and ask for a collateral history from an informant who knows the person well
- Provide assistance with new or complex information (e.g. ask pharmacy to provide drug information in a way that the patient understands)
- Allow additional time to explain and check understanding
- Assess capacity to consent (while presuming capacity) and make a record of the assessment; ensure the forms are completed if the person lacks capacity
- Give active attention to the need for support to obtain healthcare (e.g. ask if there is a 'health action plan', 'health passport' or similar)
- Be aware of the need in healthcare settings for support in some aspects of social functioning, such as maintaining a healthy lifestyle
- Provide (or facilitate) support to cope with crises and life events such as onset of illness and bereavement
- Be aware of possible vulnerability to abuse, coercion or neglect (and ensure that discharge arrangements do not expose the person to harm)

Moderate DID

All of the above, plus:
- Identify the main carer
- Request consent from the patient to share information with the main carer
- Coordinate the healthcare plan with the existing support plan, if possible; refer for assessment if the support plan is inadequate
- Assess capacity to consent to processes of healthcare such as discharge and after-care

Severe DID

All of the above, plus:
- Be aware that families and carers may be able to help you to understand the person and vice versa, acting as interpreters
- Be aware of health problems associated with DID
- Be aware of causes of reduced life expectancy associated with DID
- Be aware of health problems associated with common causes of DID (e.g. Down syndrome)
- Actively plan the processes of healthcare (e.g. ensure there is support to attend follow-up appointments)

Profound DID

All of the above, plus:
- Recognise that the person may be unable to give a history but can still provide some information – for example, ask the main carer about how the person shows pain and how the person shows emotional distress, then observe for those indicators
- Recognise that there may be increased risk of avoidable death such as choking or uncontrolled epilepsy and ensure the care plan provides protection

attainment and use it when making referrals to specialist services. If a school has not assessed the reason why a child has 'learning difficulties' and the GP wishes to make a referral to specialist services in adulthood, it may be necessary for an assessment of intellectual ability to be undertaken (perhaps by a psychologist) before a decision can be made about eligibility for adult services. Depending on local arrangements, a referral that lacks evidence for DID may be routed to a psychologist in an adult mental health service. This is a source of delay and frustration, which can be avoided by positively identifying people with DID before making a referral. In the UK, contractual arrangements with primary care have invited practices to produce registers of patients with DID under the Quality Outcomes Framework and to provide health checks for people with DID as 'Enhanced Services'. This has improved the identification of DID in primary care in participating practices.

Several types of neurodevelopmental disability are associated with cognitive impairment. Access to appropriate treatment and services depends on doctors and carers being aware of these conditions and the availability of help (see Table 13.1). Psychiatrists are often involved in the process of diagnosing developmental disabilities such as autism spectrum disorder or attention-deficit hyperactivity disorder (hyperkinetic syndrome).

Do we know which models of service work best?

In the past, doctors may have assumed that people with DID were living in institutions and that their general medical care was the responsibility of someone else (Barker & Howells, 1990), although the majority always lived in the community. There is no basis for assuming that people with DID received better general healthcare in institutions. Plans for closure of institutions typically assumed that the numbers of people registering with any GP would be so small as to make no difference. Resettlement plans rarely included primary care, yet studies of the effects of resettlement showed that GPs became the professionals in contact with the highest proportion of resettled people (De Paiva & Lowe, 1991).

Health systems based on primary healthcare principles (Box 13.5) achieve better health and greater equity in health than systems with a specialty care orientation (Starfield, 2009).

Consultation rates of people with DID in general practice have been low in the past (Wilson & Haire, 1990) and it is believed that this is still the case (Royal College of General Practitioners, 2013). There is increasing recognition of the benefits of good primary care for people with DID (Lindsay, 2011). These benefits are dependent on universal access to those primary care services. Because people with DID are less likely to initiate contact than are others in the population, there is a risk of inequity unless GPs are proactive in making contact, so comprehensive systematic annual 'health checks' using one of the standardised approaches

Table 13.1 Some neurodevelopmental disabilities that should be detected in primary care

	Key features	Benefits of identification
Cerebral palsy	Impairment of movement, sometimes causing severe expressive communication problems (http://www.nhs.uk/conditions/cerebral-palsy/pages/diagnosis.aspx)	Access to physiotherapy and pharmaceutical treatment Awareness that the person may have normal intellectual development Awareness of risks for people with cerebral palsy and DID (http://www.improvinghealthandlives.org.uk/projects/deaths)
Autism spectrum disorder	Impairment of reciprocal social interaction, language development, imaginative play (http://www.nhs.uk/conditions/autistic-spectrum-disorder/pages/introduction.aspx)	Access to suitable education and therapeutic programmes Awareness of association with epilepsy, depression and behavioural problems Awareness that the person may have normal intellectual development
Attention-deficit hyperactivity disorder/ hyperkinetic syndrome	Impulsiveness, distractibility, lack of persistence with tasks requiring attention, impaired emotional regulation, short duration of sleep, motor overactivity (http://www.nhs.uk/conditions/attention-deficit-hyperactivity-disorder/pages/introduction.aspx)	Access to psychological and pharmaceutical treatment and suitable education Awareness of association with other neurodevelopmental problems Awareness that the person may have normal intellectual development
Tourette syndrome	Multiple tics and involuntary vocalisations (http://www.nhs.uk/conditions/tourette-syndrome/pages/introduction.aspx)	Access to psychological and pharmaceutical treatment Awareness of association with obsessive–compulsive features Awareness that the person may have normal intellectual development
Specific developmental disorders (e.g. dyslexia, dyspraxia)	Impairment of specified aspects of development (http://www.nhs.uk/conditions/dyslexia/pages/introduction.aspx, http://www.nhs.uk/Conditions/Dyspraxia-%28childhood%29/Pages/Introduction.aspx)	Access to suitable education and technology Awareness that the person may have normal intellectual development

now available (Royal College of General Practitioners, 2013) represent a reasonable adjustment to usual care provision. The Royal College of General Practitioners is addressing the issue of reduced access in DID, and its publications endorse such health checks (Hoghton, 2010).

Comorbidity and complexity create a challenge for achieving high-quality healthcare for people with DID, especially for those with profound

---

Box 13.5   Good primary healthcare: attributes and threats

Attributes of good primary healthcare
- Provision of access to all groups in the community
- Promoting health
- Identifying conditions early and preventing unnecessary hospital admission
- Focusing on the patient, not the disease
- Managing comorbidities which do not fit disease guidelines
- Protection from unnecessary overinvestigation in low-prevalence settings

Threats to achieving the benefits of primary healthcare
- Reduced continuity in larger teams
- Reduced comprehensiveness in relation to less common conditions that require shared care with specialists
- Difficulties coordinating care when multiple referrals are made
- Focus on health risks (e.g. smoking, alcohol misuse) that are important for the general population may result in failure to identify hidden needs for people with DID, resulting in inequity

---

multiple disability. A service response to these may be summarised as requiring:

- a comprehensive systematic approach
- teamwork
- coordination
- continuity of care
- communication of clinical information within teams and between teams
- clarity about decision-making if the patient lacks capacity to consent.

A comprehensive systematic approach involves managing comorbidity and coordinating care of acute illness, chronic illness, health promotion and disease prevention (Royal College of General Practitioners, 2010*b*).

The key concept of teamwork is that there is a shared set of goals, which team members work towards by filling a set of complementary roles. Modern health services have focused on multidisciplinary teams in both primary and secondary care, with benefits to patients and staff. GPs fill several roles, defined in the document *Being a General Practitioner* (Royal College of General Practitioners, 2010*a*). In addition to consultation, they provide professional advocacy, and act as mentors to patients and carers through complex health systems.

There is still a challenge to achieve the benefits of teamwork across the organisational gap between primary and secondary care. Close working with carers and members of multidisciplinary teams is sometimes achieved through identifying an individual to coordinate care and support, and to ensure all services agreed are delivered. This person may be a trained nurse, such as an intellectual disabilities nurse, or be in a social care role, with a title such as 'key worker'; in a hospital setting the title may be 'liaison nurse'. It is not yet known whether any model of achieving teamwork is superior to others.

Coordination of specialist health services (together with social care services) is complex. For example, a neurologist, a specialist epilepsy nurse and a psychiatrist specialising in DID may be involved in assessing and managing epilepsy; and sometimes the GP may have a special interest in epilepsy. The family or support workers need to be clear whom to approach if a problem arises. Some GPs prefer to make all referrals to specialists, while some expect that a psychiatrist specialising in DID will make additional referrals if they detect a condition needing specialist advice. The problem may then arise that the specialist may ask the referrer to undertake some interventions that require competence in primary care. Single-point coordination of inter-specialty referrals may enhance the overall appropriateness of referrals for an individual (Watson *et al*, 2005). Non-medical professionals (such as community DID nurses) make some referrals directly (e.g. to podiatry), notifying the GP about the referral. In any case, the GP should be informed to ensure the patient record is updated.

The Royal College of General Practitioners' curriculum statement includes 'Demonstrate an understanding of the importance of continuity of care in this group' (Royal College of General Practitioners, 2010*b*). It describes three main types: personal continuity (seeing the same doctor); episodic continuity (ensuring that information is always available when taking over or referring); and the continuity provided by the discipline (which guarantees organised 24-hour care).

Communication within teams, between teams and with carers is frequently identified as a factor in incidents of serious harm (e.g. Scottish Courts, 2007). Methods for improving communication include the use of an Immediate Discharge Document from hospitals (Scottish Intercollegiate Guidelines Network, 2012) and the Emergency Care Summary (see NHS

Box 13.6   Prescribing issues for individuals with DID

- Careful assessment of the underlying reason for distress and challenging behaviour before prescribing
- Acknowledging diagnostic uncertainty
- Consideration of how prescriptions may be used or misused
- Prescribing variable-dosage and temporary medication (first aid, rescue and as required)
- Assessing and recording consent or incapacity
- Issues after signing the prescription (dispensing, storage and prompting)
- Thinking ahead to next time

Adapted from Simpson & Douglas (2011).

24, 2007). Coordination of prescribing between hospital and community is vital for patient safety (see Box 13.6).

The legal authority to provide healthcare for a person who lacks capacity to consent derives from a certificate issued by a doctor. Assessment of competence to make healthcare decisions requires the doctor to ensure that the person can understand, appreciate, reason about and express a choice about the treatment. This involves asking the person to explain what the effects (desired and undesired) of the treatment and the alternatives are expected to be, so it is sometimes helpful to arrange for another professional, such as a pharmacist, to provide the information in the most accessible format. The legal concept of capacity includes retaining and communicating the decision (by any means). A failure at any part of the assessment suggests incapacity at that point in time, and has been shown to affect 13% of patients in acute hospitals and 39% in psychiatric hospitals (Owen *et al*, 2013). Key workers and community DID nurses will often have a record of whether a proxy decision maker has legal authority to give consent to medical treatment if the person lacks capacity (i.e. power of attorney and guardianship), and in all cases the local authority social work department should have this information. A copy of this information, along with certificates as necessary, should be updated annually at health checks.

Mental ill health has raised prevalence among people with DID (Smiley *et al*, 2007). In the UK, the most frequently used model for meeting mental health needs is to have a psychiatrist specialising in mental health of people with DID working as a member of local specialist health teams for people with DID. Other models have been advocated, including attaching psychiatrists with specialist skills to local mental health teams, or 'mainstreaming' the mental health service by having no specialisation. There is a shortage of evidence to recommend any particular model. Professionals who have experienced more than one service model can describe advantages and disadvantages of each. A key factor is the accessibility of additional services when risks escalate. The Royal College of Psychiatrists (2013) has described the need for access to a range of in-patient facilities and (jointly with Royal College of General Practitioners and Public Health England) the standards required to commission a quality service (Royal College of General Practitioners, 2012).

Acute hospitals also have difficulty in recognising and responding to the needs of people with DID (Healthcare Improvement Scotland, 2009). Referrals from primary care should include information about the person's disabilities, support needs and existing support plan. Hospitals may not readily have access to this information for emergency admissions, although transferable key information summaries are now sometimes used (Scottish Information Management in Practice, 2013) and potentially could link with 'need to know' information from health check electronic templates. It is desirable that ward nursing staff identify each person with DID every day at their daily briefing, so that support needs and risks are accurately identified. Models of liaison between hospitals and specialist support services have been developed (Bradbury-Jones *et al*, 2013) and have some evidence of benefit. Utilisation of 'triggers' to highlight the need for a holistic reassessment of health needs after a certain number of unplanned admissions or attendances at an emergency department have been shown to reduce further admissions (Scottish Government, 2013).

Does education of doctors bridge the gap?

Attitudes towards disability are formed before and during the early years of medical education, when doctors may not yet have decided on their career path – into hospital medicine or general practice. Medical students typically have strong regard for patients who have disabilities but may develop negative attitudes in the course of training. This may be due to a lack of appropriate training and the use of inappropriate interventions (Boyle *et al*, 2010). Doctors recognise that patients with DID receive a lower standard of medical care (Lawrence, 2013). Gill *et al* (2002) suggested that they have not been prepared to spend more time or complete necessary training to manage such patients more effectively.

Students benefit from spending time with users of DID services and their carers rather than simply didactic teaching (Sinai *et al*, 2013). Collaborative initiatives for healthcare students (such as the website http://www.intellectualdisability.info) have produced excellent resources for learning about DID. Training could use excerpts from positive cultural references. Examples might include the 1988 film *Rain Man* (with Tom Cruise and

Table 13.2 Legal framework

	Scotland	England and Wales
Equality	Equality Act 2010 (http://www.legislation.gov.uk/ukpga/2010/15/contents)	
Disability discrimination	Disability Discrimination Act 2005 (http://www.legislation.gov.uk/ukpga/2005/13/contents)	
Mental health	Mental Health (Care & Treatment) (Scotland) Act 2003 (http://www.scotland.gov.uk/Topics/Health/Services/Mental-Health/Law)	Mental Health Act 2007 (http://www.legislation.gov.uk/ukpga/2007/12/contents)
Adults with incapacity	Adults with Incapacity (Scotland) Act 2000 (http://www.legislation.gov.uk/asp/2000/4/contents)	Mental Capacity Act 2005 (http://www.legislation.gov.uk/ukpga/2005/9/contents)
Vulnerable adults	Adult Support and Protection (Scotland) Act 2007 (http://www.legislation.gov.uk/asp/2007/10/contents)	Adult safeguarding (policy guidance) 2012 (https://www.gov.uk/government/publications/adult-safeguarding-statement-of-government-policy)

Dustin Hoffman), the novel *The Curious Case of the Dog in the Night-time* (Haddon, 2003) and the 1993 film *What's Eating Gilbert Grape* (with Johnny Depp and Leonardo DiCaprio). The General Medical Council (2009) has recognised the need for medical schools to provide human rights education and training on DID. However more still needs to be done to foster awareness training for medical students on the subject of DID to meet the needs of these patients (Hall, 2013). Enhanced standards may come to pass after the General Medical Council's ongoing review of 'tomorrow's doctors'.

Table 13.2 shows examples of important developments in the legal framework for providing services for people with DID, which might form part of a curriculum for healthcare students and professionals.

The Royal College of General Practitioners (2010*a*) is addressing DID education needs in the published curriculum for membership, but postgraduate training programmes do not universally include competency statements on DID. Doctors in training may be offered few opportunities to develop their skills and knowledge in working with people with DID, perhaps because trainers lack confidence in demonstrating their own expertise. One recently described framework to teach students and doctors about the factors important in communication with patients who have DID, to aid earlier diagnosis, uses the acronym FASTER CARE (Heslop *et al*, 2013). Patients with DID should be seen as an educational 'gift' for a doctor to develop advanced communication and problem-solving skills.

Conclusion

The use of the correct terminology does matter. It can influence attitudes, improve understanding between primary and secondary care and leave a lasting impression on patients and carers. The early identification of DID allows for appropriate interventions to be coordinated between primary and secondary care and delivery of care in communities, coordinated over the long term by general practices centred around defined populations. This reduces gaps in care and creates safety nets for residual gaps in care. Learning on issues relating to DID from an early stage in medical training ensures a generic understanding of the needs of patients with DID, irrespective of medical specialty.

References

American Psychiatric Association (2013) *Diagnostic and Statistical Manual of Mental Disorders* (5th edn) (DSM-5). APA.

Barker M, Howells G (1990) The medical needs of adults. In *Primary Care for People with a Mental Handicap* (Occasional Paper 47): pp 6–8. Royal College of General Practitioners.

Bartolo PA (2002) Communicating a diagnosis of developmental disability to parents: multiprofessional negotiation frameworks. *Child Care, Health and Development*, **28**: 1, 65–71.

Boyle M, Williams B, Brown T, *et al* (2010) Attitudes of undergraduate health science students towards patients with intellectual disability, substance abuse, and acute mental illness: a cross-sectional study. *BMC Medical Education*, **10**: 71.

Bradbury-Jones C, Rattray J, Jones M, *et al* (2013) Promoting the health, safety and welfare of adults with learning disabilities in acute care settings: a structured literature review. *Journal of Clinical Nursing*, **22**: 1497–509.

British Paediatric Association (1994) *Services for Children and Adolescents with Learning Disability (Mental Handicap)* (report of a working party). British Paediatric Association.

De Paiva S, Lowe K (1991) *NIMROD – An Overview: A Summary Report of a 5-Year Research Study of Community-Based Service Provision for People with Learning Difficulties*. TSO (The Stationery Office).

Florian L, Hollenweger J, Simeonsson RJ, *et al* (2006) Cross-cultural perspectives on the classification of children with disabilities. *Journal of Special Education*, **40**: 36–45.

Fryers T (1991) Recent epidemiological studies in mental retardation. *Current Opinion in Psychiatry*, **4**: 662–6.

General Medical Council (2009). Tomorrow's doctors: outcomes 3 – the doctor as a professional. At http://www.gmc-uk.org/education/undergraduate/tomorrows_doctors_2009_outcomes3.asp (accessed April 2015).

General Medical Council (2013) Learning disabilities. At http://www.gmc-uk.org/learningdisabilities (accessed April 2015).

Gill F, Stenfert-Kroese B, Rose J (2002) General practitioners' attitudes to patients who have learning disabilities. *Psychological Medicine*, **32**: 1445–55.

Haddon M (2003) *The Curious Case of the Dog in the Night-time*. Jonathan Cape.

Hall PL (2013) Meeting the needs of patients with learning disabilities. *BMJ*, **346**: f3421.

Healthcare Improvement Scotland (2009) Tackling indifference: healthcare services for people with learning disabilities. National overview. At http://www.healthcareimprovementscotland.org/previous_resources/performance_review/tackling_indifference.aspx (accessed April 2015).

Heslop P, Hoghton M, Blair P, *et al* (2013) The need for FASTER CARE in the diagnosis of illness in people with intellectual disabilities. *British Journal of General Practice*, **63**: 661–2.

Hoghton M (2010) *A Step by Step Guide for GP Practices: Annual Health Checks for People with a Learning Disability*. Royal College of General Practitioners. At http://www.rcgp.org.uk/clinical-andresearch/clinicalresources/~/media/Files/CIRC/CIRC-76-80/CIRCA%20StepbyStepGuideforPracticesOctober%2010.ashx (accessed April 2015).

Keenan M, Dillenburger K, Doherty A, *et al* (2010) The experiences of parents during diagnosis and forward planning for children with autism spectrum disorder. *Journal of Applied Research in Intellectual Disabilities*, **23**: 390–7.

Kisler J, McConachie H (2010) Parental reaction to disability. *Paediatrics and Child Health*, **20**: 309–14.

Lawrence P (2013) Human rights should be taught in medical school to ensure proper care for people with learning disabilities. *BMJ*, **346**: f4047.

Lindsay P (ed) (2011) *Care of the Adult with Intellectual Disability in Primary Care*. Radcliffe Press.

McDonald L, Rennie A, Tolmie J, *et al* (2006) Investigation of global developmental delay. *Archives of Diseases of Childhood*, **91**: 701–705.

NHS 24 (2007) Emergency Care Summary – What is it? At http://www.nhs24.com/explained/myinfonhs24/ecs/ (accessed April 2015).

Owen GS, Szmukler G, Richardson G, *et al* (2013) Decision-making capacity for treatment in psychiatric and medical in-patients: cross-sectional, comparative study. *British Journal of Psychiatry*, **203**: 461–7.

Pinker S (1994) The game of the name. *New York Times*, 3 April.

Public Health England (2005) The UK NSC recommendation on Developmental and behavioural problems screening in children. At http://www.screening.nhs.uk/developmentbehaviour (accessed September 2013).

Reynolds TM (2003) Down's syndrome screening is unethical: views of today's research ethics committees. *Journal of Clinical Pathology*, **56**: 268–70.

Robertson J, Roberts H, Emerson E (2010) *Health Checks for People with Learning Disabilities: A Systematic Review of Evidence*. Learning Disabilities Observatory, Department of Health.

Royal College of General Practitioners (2010a) *Being a General Practitioner*. Available at http://www.rcgp.org.uk/gp-training-and-exams/~/media/Files/GP-training-and-exams/Curriculum-2012/RCGP-Curriculum-1-Being-a-GP.ashx (accessed April 2015).

Royal College of General Practitioners (2010b) Care of people with intellectual disability At http://www.rcgp.org.uk/gp-training-and-exams/~/media/Files/GP-training-and-exams/Curriculum-2012/RCGP-Curriculum-3-11-People-With-Intellectual-Disability. ashx (accessed April 2015).

Royal College of General Practitioners (2012) *Improving the Health and Wellbeing of People with Learning Disabilities: An Evidence-Based Commissioning Guide for Clinical Commissioning Groups* RCGP. Available at http://www.rcgp.org.uk/revalidation-and-cpd/centre-for-commissioning/~/media/Files/CIRC/LD%20Commissioning/RCGP%20LD%20Commissioning%20Guide%20v1%200%202012%2009%2024%20FINAL%20pdf.ashx (accessed April 2015).

Royal College of General Practitioners (2013) Learning disabilities. At http://www.rcgp. org.uk/learningdisabilities (accessed April 2015).

Royal College of Psychiatrists (2013) *People with Learning Disability and Mental Health, Behavioural or Forensic Problems: The Role of In-Patient Services* (FR/ID/03). Royal College of Psychiatrists. Available at http://www.rcpsych.ac.uk/pdf/FR%20ID%2003%20for%20 website.pdf (accessed April 2015).

Scottish Courts (2007) Fatal accident inquiry into the death of Roderick McIntosh Donnet. At http://www.scotcourts.gov.uk/opinions/donnet.html (accessed April 2015).

Scottish Government (2013) The keys to life. At http://www.scotland.gov.uk/ Publications/2013/06/1123/7 (accessed April 2015).

Scottish Information Management in Practice (2013) Key information summary. At http://www.scimp.scot.nhs.uk/key-information-summary(accessed April 2015).

Scottish Intercollegiate Guidelines Network (2012) *The SIGN Discharge Document* (Guideline 128). SIGN. At http://www.sign.ac.uk/guidelines/fulltext/128/index.html (accessed April 2015).

Simpson N, Douglas J (2011) Recommended prescribing for people with learning disabilities. *Prescriber*, **22**: 33–8.

Sinai A, Strydom A, Hassiotis A (2013) Evaluation of medical students' attitudes towards people with intellectual disabilities: a naturalistic study in one medical school. *Advances in Mental Health and Intellectual Disabilities*, **7**: 18–26.

Smiley E, Cooper S-A, Finlayson J, *et al* (2007) The incidence, and predictors of mental ill-health in adults with intellectual disabilities. *British Journal of Psychiatry*, **191**: 313–19.

Starfield B (2009) Primary care and equity in health: the importance to effectiveness and equity of responsiveness to people's needs. *Humanity and Society*, **33**: 56–73.

van Schrojenstein Lantman-de Valk H, Noonan Walsh P (2008) Managing health problems in people with intellectual disabilities. *BMJ*, **337**: 1408–12.

Watson JM, McDonnell V, Bhaumik S (2005) Valuing people: evaluating referral systems. A study of multidisciplinary single point of referral system to dedicated adult learning disability health services in Leicester, UK. *British Journal of Developmental Disabilities*, **51**: 155–70.

Wilson D, Haire A (1990) Health care screening for people with mental handicap living in the community. *BMJ*, **301**: 1379–81.

World Health Organization (1992) *International Statistical Classification of Diseases and Related Health Problems* (10th revision) (ICD-10). WHO.

CHAPTER 14

Ageing in people with disorders of intellectual development

Gregory O'Brien and Paul White

Until very recently the notion that there might be a population of older adults with serious intellectual and developmental disabilities was not widely considered. Most efforts in care, treatment, service development and planning were focused on children and 'early intervention'. Now there is a growing population of elderly adults with developmental disabilities because of innovations in health and social care. This chapter focuses on health and general care needs of those with disorders of intellectual development (DID), with a particular focus on comorbid dementia.

Increasing longevity

People are living longer. The life expectancy of 'three score years and ten' has not only been replaced by a much older age but has also been steadily increasing. Recent figures for England and Wales quote a life expectancy for boys born in England and Wales in 2009–11 of 78.7 years and 82.6 years for girls. This rising life expectancy is largely due to advances in nutrition and in medical services.

The overall severity of intellectual disability is a strong determinant of life expectancy among people with DID. Recent estimates are framed for high-income countries, given that life expectancy is so inextricably linked to the availability of healthcare. It is estimated that in the year 2000, life expectancy for adults with mild intellectual disability was 70 years, while life expectancy for adults with severe intellectual disability was 60 years (Bittles & Glasson, 2004). In the UK, *Valuing People*, the official government policy document, estimated that there were over 200 000 people over the age of 60 years with DID in 2000 (Department of Health, 2001). It was further estimated therein that this will increase by 1% per year for at least the next 15 years, due to further increased longevity. In the USA, the American Association for Intellectual Disability estimated that at the turn of the century there were between 600 000 and 1.6 million adults over the age of 60 years with intellectual disabilities and other similarly disabling developmental disabilities (Braddock *et al*, 2008). The most recent US estimate for the average life expectancy of adults with DID is 66 years and rising (Fisher & Ketti, 2005).

Longevity among people with DID will continue to increase for the foreseeable future, with certain caveats. First of all, just as this current trend is the result of improvements in healthcare and indeed of basic care, so will the trend continue only if such improvements continue. For individual patients – and in service planning – the interested clinician may need to highlight this from time to time. Secondly, any figures produced in respect of life expectancy or longevity are necessarily average ones, behind which lies a wide range of individual variation – importantly, among people with DID that individual variation is far wider than within the general population. This latter observation reflects the wide heterogeneity of serious health problems and disabilities which figures so highly in this population, in which are found numerous high-profile important genetic disorders, many of which feature major health problems and disabling conditions. Moreover, some of these genetic syndromes result in progressive deterioration in neurological and other functioning, such that survival into old age is not possible. These metabolic and other disorders may be individually quite rare, but there is such a multitude of them that, taken together, they represent a significant number. Until gene therapy or other advances alter the course of any or all of these disorders, it has to be assumed that such outliers to the means will remain.

There is a further and in some ways more fundamentally important issue – *avoidable mortality*. This occurs wherever a treatable medical problem goes unrecognised or untreated, and ultimately death occurs. The extent to which this is a major issue among people with DID was emphasised in the UK by the Disability Rights Commission (2006), which carried out a careful investigation into health inequalities among people with DID and reported that their avoidable mortality may be as high as ten times that of the general population.

Ageing and treatable morbidity among people with DID

The clinician attending to the healthcare needs of older adults with DID faces an important challenge – to anticipate and recognise deteriorating functioning where it occurs, while being alert to the need to identify and treat remediable health problems. Systematic healthcare screening is of proven benefit among people with DID (Cooper *et al*, 2006).

Take as an example the adult with Down syndrome, and the common morbidities which may arise over middle age and later life. This is the most common genetic cause of intellectual disability. It demonstrates age-associated problems that run throughout the wider population of people with DID, while showing certain problems unique to the syndrome itself. For people with Down syndrome, the dominant concern for most carers and informed families is the occurrence of dementia. This is estimated to present in around 10% of those aged 40–49 years, 36% aged 50–59 years and 55% aged 60 years and over (Prasher, 1995). Consequently, any report of deteriorating function or confusion in a middle-aged adult with Down syndrome typically prompts a request for diagnostic assessment for possible dementia. Rather than accepting these as features of dementia or even of the premature ageing, which is common in the condition, the clinician needs to be alert to the possibility of remediable problems. When approaching this common problem, the following steps are recommended.

A strategy of proactive planned health screening

First of all, in the face of the impaired intelligence, self-organisation and communication skills that characterise the adult with Down syndrome, health screening checks must be offered on a planned and proactive basis. This is particularly because the person themselves is most unlikely to come forward and request such crucial health screening.

Standard health checks

It must be remembered that the same conditions which compromise the health and functioning of the general population in later life are at least as prevalent among older people with DID (Holland, 2000). Importantly, if the person leads a more sedentary life, or has other health risk factors such as smoking, then the risk of a number of common cardiovascular, respiratory and gastrointestinal conditions may be raised. Among adults with Down syndrome, all of the established health checks now standard in the general population for men and for women must therefore be applied, including the various age-specific and gender-specific protocols for health checks sensitive to the health needs of men and women of different ages.

Syndrome-specific screening for treatable health conditions

The principal treatable health conditions of adulthood in Down syndrome that should be the specific targets for routine clinical assessment include the following:

- *Premature cataract formation.* This typically presents in the third or fourth decade in life. The gradually increasing blindness of cataract development can present as the person becoming lost or less independent for self-care. Being readily treated surgically, it is of considerable importance. Examination of the eyes, by light reflex, is a brief but essential part of the clinical assessment.
- *Hypothyroidism.* Hypothyroidism is very common in Down syndrome, presenting at some time in 30% of those with the condition (Bhaumik et al, 1991). Hypothyroidism is part of a wider set of autoimmune characteristics of Down syndrome, which most notably include the lifelong susceptibility to infections noted next. Hypothyroidism can present at any age in Down syndrome, and the clinical picture of general motor slowing, loss of drive and dryness of the skin and hair can be very similar to dementia or depression. Being easily treated, testing for this condition should be a routine matter.

- *Infections.* Throughout life, people with Down syndrome have very high rates of infection, especially chest and ear, nose and throat (ENT) infections. This is due to a deficiency of both cell- and antibody-mediated immunity, compounded by the anatomy of the Eustachian tubes, which by their more horizontal orientation and narrower gauge are very prone to becoming blocked and infected. This set of problems typically first presents in childhood, but is likely to re-emerge in middle age and beyond, when the impact of pyrexia can result in both confusion and malaise. Examination of the respiratory and ENT systems should therefore be routine in the assessment of adults of all ages with Down syndrome, and especially when acute or subacute confusion presents.
- *Muscle hypotonia and joint laxity.* Low muscle tone and lax joints are lifelong features of Down syndrome, and are part of a generalised disorder of the connective tissue in the syndrome. In middle age and later life, these problems can become significantly worse, with some deterioration in gait and motor functioning. Arthritic and structural degenerative changes in the joints compound advanced cases. These clinical changes are readily distinguished and identified, and should be the target of physiotherapy and occupational therapy and assessment for aids for living.
- *Congenital heart disease.* Congenital heart disease affects some 50% of people with Down syndrome. Routinely, these disorders are corrected surgically in childhood. However, among middle-aged and elderly people with the syndrome, and closely linked to the general laxity of the connective tissues noted above, decompensation of cardiac function may occur, through mitral valve regurgitation or aortic valve prolapse. The presentation here is likely to be dominated by lethargy, tiredness, breathlessness and increasing withdrawal from accustomed activities. Any findings on clinical examination which suggest such changes should prompt specialist referral.
- *Depression.* Depression is common in Down syndrome (Cooper, 1997a), although recent evidence suggests that it may be no more common than in other syndromes of disability matched for intellectual level (Walker *et al*, 2011).
- *Epilepsy.* Epilepsy is no more or less prevalent in Down syndrome than in the wider population of people with a similar degree or severity of intellectual disability. For many people with epilepsy, constancy of health needs predominates their treatment and care. Also, often, there is an element of predictability over time in any one person regarding episodic changes in seizure occurrence and pattern. However, among older people, epilepsy control and the seizures themselves can change. This can result from other health problems, and notably as a result of drug interactions. In addition, whether or not there is a history of seizures in any one person, the onset of new major seizures, or

a worsening of seizure control, are common accompaniments of dementia, in its more advanced stages. Any change in epilepsy control or of seizure occurrence or frequency should therefore meet prompt and careful clinical assessment.

The treatment of depression

The drug treatment of depression among elderly people with Down syndrome – and indeed among all elderly people with DID – should follow the approach to psychopharmacological therapy for the population outlined by Deb in Chapter 7. The proviso to this is that the caution advised therein is all the more important in the drug treatment of the elderly patient with DID, who is even more prone to side-effects affecting the central nervous system (CNS) and to be in receipt of treatment for other health conditions. Consequently, the clinician must:

- start treatment with a lower dose
- space out any incremental increase slowly
- be particularly careful to minimise polypharmacy
- be alert to the possibility of drug interactions if any comorbid conditions are being treated.

Being a treatable, common condition, which may mimic some of the features of dementia, depression should be borne in mind in clinical assessment, as part of the differential diagnosis of dementia.

Dementia among people with DID

Dementia is characterised by progressive and irreversible decline in cognitive and adaptive functioning. Consciousness is preserved, at least until the very late stages. Dementia has multiple causes, all of which feature diffuse degenerative changes in the brain. The progressively worsening cognitive impairments that result include, *inter alia*, deterioration of memory, orientation, language, praxis and executive functioning. Non-cognitive common accompaniments of these changes in cognitive functioning include changes in overall personality, and in certain aspects of mood and behaviour.

Dementia is primarily a disease of older people and so one result of the greater longevity now manifest among people with DID is a new population of people with dementia in the context of other premorbid complex disabilities.

Epidemiology

In the general population, dementia is mainly a disease of later life, although it is not unknown earlier in life. The general population rates of dementia are 1–2% among people aged 65–69 years, rising to 16–25% in those aged 80 years and over (American Psychiatric Association, 2000, 2013). In the population of people with DID, dementia is more common, and more often appears earlier in life. The best available community-based studies of the prevalence of dementia in this population have demonstrated rates of around 14% at aged 60 years and over, and of 22% at age 65 years and over (Cooper, 1997*b*). The overall rate and especially the rate among younger adults is higher in Down syndrome, as stated above.

Diagnostic criteria

The standard systems for the classification of mental disorder, notably DSM-5 (American Psychiatric Association, 2013) and ICD-10 (World Health Organization, 1992), cite four cardinal criteria for the diagnosis of dementia:

* progressive memory loss
* decline in at least one other aspect of cognitive functioning (language, praxis, executive functioning, etc.)
* these cognitive deficits result in some impairment(s) in adaptive functioning for daily living
* the overall progressive decline is not accompanied by disturbed or loss of consciousness.

As these criteria have been developed for dementia in the general population, assessing them and thereby diagnosing dementia among people with DID poses significant challenges.

First, the standard schedules and instruments measure change against an index of normal population functioning, which in cognitive and adaptive behavioural functioning is quite at variance with that of people with DID. This severely limits their use, and increasingly so at the more severe end of the intellectual disability spectrum. This has resulted in the need for diagnostic and assessment instruments developed specifically for use in that population. Furthermore, the premorbid, 'normal', baseline of cognitive and adaptive functioning in the index population varies enormously across the spectrum of mild to profound intellectual disability – far more than in the general population. The approach to diagnosis and assessment of dementia therefore needs to take account of this, with great care being taken to establish a premorbid baseline in clinical, adaptive and behavioural functioning.

Equally importantly, the inherent impairments in cognitive and adaptive functioning of the index population, coupled with the proneness to emotional and behavioural problems therein, result in changes in overall adaptive functioning being quite common, both in younger and in older people. This can result in the early, more subtle changes of dementia being easily missed among people with DID. Also, certain specific features of dementia, although common, can be particularly difficult to identify in this group, notably dysphasia, dyspraxia and agnosia. These clinical problems are therefore not routinely included in some of the dementia diagnostic and assessment measurements which have been developed for the index population.

Faced with these challenges, while significant progress has been made in the development of diagnostic and assessment schedules for use in dementia in the index population, there is as yet no agreed standardised approach. The IASSID (International Association for the Scientific Study of Intellectual Disabilities) made a significant contribution through its Working Group for the Establishment of Criteria for the Diagnosis of Dementia in Individuals with Intellectual Disability (Burt & Aylward, 2000). These criteria follow the approach of ICD-10, in placing more emphasis on non-cognitive features than DSM-5. By this approach, the four cardinal criteria to be applied are:

- memory decline
- decline in at least one other aspect of cognitive functioning (language, praxis, executive functioning, etc.)
- these cognitive deficits result in some impairment(s) in adaptive functioning for daily living
- changes in emotional/motivational functioning.

With this approach, dementia is diagnosed only when there are longitudinal data that show significant deterioration in functioning in the domains cited. Notably, also, if not all criteria are met, but the clinical impression is still suggestive of dementia, the label 'possible dementia' can be ascribed, this being an indication for further longitudinal observation and reassessment. This Working Group has also supplied a list of recommended measurement schedules for use in the assessment of dementia among people with DID. The recommended measurement schedules are selected to provide the maximal clinical assessment, in face of the widely varying clinical picture with which dementia presents in the index population. These schedules are summarised in Box 14.1, which also incorporates insights from Deb *et al* (2001), and is adapted from Nagdee & O'Brien (2009). The schedules are listed according to their applicability to the four cardinal criteria of dementia in intellectual disability as recognised by the IASSID Working Group, namely, memory and cognition, adaptive and maladaptive behaviour, and emotional functioning and psychopathology.

Classification

The most widely used classification is according to neurological localisation (see Box 14.2). The alternative classification systems for dementia, namely 'association with medical or neurological illness' and 'treatability and reversibility of dementia' are of interest, but are of less direct practical relevance to the present population. When adopting neurological localisation for the classification of dementia in the present population, three main types emerge: cortical dementia, subcortical dementia and mixed dementia.

Box 14.1 Instruments recommended for assessment of dementia in people with disorders of intellectual development

Criteria 1 and 2: memory and cognition

- Autobiographical Memory Test
- Boston Naming Test (modified)*
- Clifton Assessment Procedure for the Elderly (CAPE)
- Dementia Questionnaire for Mentally Retarded Persons (DMR)*
- Dementia Rating Scale (DRS)*
- Informant Questionnaire on Cognitive Decline in the Elderly (IQOCDE)*
- McCarthy Verbal Fluency Test
- Modified Mini Mental State (3MS) Examination*
- Purdue Pegboard Test (modified)*
- Simple Command Test (modified)*
- Spatial Recognition Span
- Standford Binet Sentences
- Test for Severe Impairment (modified)*

Criterion 3: adaptive and maladaptive behaviour

- Aberrant Behaviour Checklist (ABC)
- Adaptive Behaviour Scale (ABS) – Residential and Community
- Disability Assessment Schedule (DAS)
- Handicaps, Behaviour and Skills Schedule (HBS)
- Past Behavioural History Inventory (PBHI)
- Reiss Screen for Maladaptive Behaviour
- Scales of Independent Behaviour – Revised (SIB-R)
- Vineland Adaptive Behaviour Scales

Criterion 4: emotional functioning and psychopathology

- Diagnostic Assessment for the Severely Handicapped (DASH)
- Emotional Problems Scale
- Psychiatric Assessment Schedule for Adults with Developmental Disability (PAS-ADD)
- Psychopathology Inventory for Mentally Retarded Adults (PIMRA)
- Reiss Screen for Maladaptive Behaviour

*Denotes schedule designed or modified for use in assessment of dementia among people with disorders of intellectual development. Other schedules, while not having been designed, developed or modified specifically for this purpose, have been found to be of utility in assessment of the criteria/domains cited.

Adapted from Nagdee & O'Brien (2009)

The archetypal form of *cortical dementia* is Alzheimer's disease. By its localisation, and especially its onset in the cerebral cortex, cortical dementia initially presents with impairments in complex cognitive functioning, notably in memory, language, praxis and other higher cognitive functions.

Box 14.2 Classification of dementia among people with disorders of intellectual development according to neurological localisation

Cortical
- Alzheimer's disease
- Frontotemporal dementia

Subcortical
- Huntington's disease
- Parkinson's disease
- Wilson's disease

Mixed
- Vascular dementia
- Lewy body dementia
- Neoplastic
- Traumatic

The impact of such changes depends critically on the premorbid level of higher cortical functioning, and so varies substantially over the spectrum of intellectual disability. Behavioural and psychiatric changes may also appear relatively early in cortical dementia, with mood lability, general disinhibition, motor restlessness and temper control problems being common. Importantly, these latter features of the presentation do not typically respond to psychopharmacological interventions.

In *subcortical dementia*, the early presentation varies according to the actual structures of damage and deterioration: motor disorder is common, often accompanied by early loss of orientation and attention, while memory loss is typically of retrieval, and the other complex cognitive cortical functions cited above are initially preserved.

Mixed dementia, as its name implies, carries features of both cortical and subcortical dementia. Vascular dementia and Lewy body dementia are the two types most often seen in clinical practice with the present population. Also notable is traumatic dementia, which can come into the picture where the cause of the intellectual disability is acquired brain damage.

Investigation

The clinical assessment of dementia among the index population entails a thorough clinical evaluation and set of investigations. This includes, but is not limited to:

- investigation of factors that may be underlying, predisposing to or directly causing the dementia

- elimination of other medical disorders that may be mimicking dementia, in exploration of the differential diagnoses
- investigation of other comorbid medical disorders
- monitoring of health as dementia progresses.

The investigation set in the individual case will be determined by the individual clinical picture and history and examination. As regards specific investigations, neuroimaging, where readily available, is now part of the norm. This contributes to the differential diagnosis, and can clarify the location and extent of disease. Computerised tomography (CT) is often sufficient where structural information is required – investigation of local functional activity requires functional neuroimaging, such as single photon emission computerised tomography (SPECT). Electroencephalography (EEG) should be carried out where there is either recent onset or change in seizure activity (see the above section 'Ageing and treatable morbidity among people with DID'). The full set of routine haematological investigations should be carried out, as would be employed in any investigation of unexplained lethargy and progressive malaise in an elderly person, supplemented in the individual case according to need. Toxicology levels may be particularly important when investigating the possible role of concurrent drug treatment as a causal or complicating factor in the clinical presentation. Box 14.3 (after Nagdee & O'Brien, 2009) summarises the more commonly used investigations of dementia in the index population.

Natural history of dementia among people with DID

The clinical course of dementia varies considerably within the index population. This is both because of the varying aetiologies (see Box 14.2) with their variable clinical features and patterns of progression, and also because of the very variable level and pattern of premorbid cognitive and adaptive behavioural functioning. That said, most authorities support the use of a three-stage model to describe the natural history of all dementia, including that among people with DID (American Psychiatric Association, 2013).

Stage 1

The clinical features in the early stages of dementia, being changes against the baseline level of functioning, may be overlooked or difficult to detect in the individual case. In most cases, there is some early memory loss, coupled with deterioration in some aspect of cognitive functioning – according to the type of dementia – and some loss of adaptive functioning. Some change in emotional and/or behavioural functioning is also common.

Stage 2

Stage 2 is characterised by progression of the features of stage 1, with cognitive decline becoming more generalised, affecting a wide range of

---

Box 14.3 Investigation of dementia among people with disorders of intellectual development

Haematological

- Full blood count
- Urea and electrolytes
- Blood glucose
- Liver function tests
- Thyroid function tests
- Serum vitamin B12 and red-cell folate
- Erythrocyte sedimentation rate
- C-reactive protein
- Serum toxicology screen
- Calcium, magnesium and phosphate levels
- Autoimmune screen
- Lipid profile
- Caeruloplasmin

Radiological

- Chest radiograph
- Computerised tomography (CT)
- Functional neuroimaging (e.g. functional MRI, PET, SPECT)

Electrophysiological

- Electroencephalography (EEG)
- Electrocardiography (ECG)

Other medical

- Urine testing (for microscopy, culture and serology, toxicology)
- Lumbar puncture (LP)

---

domains, such that adaptive functioning and especially self-care and orientation become markedly impaired. Mood and emotional functioning often become more disturbed, with marked mood lability, emotional fragility and disinhibition. The affected individual is characteristically increasingly dependent on carers for everyday needs.

Stage 3

In the late stages of dementia, there is impairment of all domains of functioning – memory, other cognitive, adaptive behavioural and psychiatric. Gross disorientation, profound amnesia, motor withdrawal, loss of language and loss of all organised functions of self-care result. Concurrently, medical problems such as seizures, incontinence, frequent infections, weight loss and muscle contractures may all figure. Death is often from infection or a cardiovascular event.

The prognosis, in common with all aspects of dementia, is highly variable. While it is not possible to individualise from the established general patterns, the following factors tend towards a poorer prognosis:

- family history of dementia
- Down syndrome
- onset at an early age
- delay in diagnosis and treatment
- greater premorbid intellectual disability and developmental disability
- more severe early pattern of cognitive and/or adaptive behavioural impairment
- any comorbid significant medical and especially neurological illness
- poor psychosocial support.

Conclusion

The improved life expectancy of people with DID is to be welcomed and extended further, through ongoing improvements in health and other care. Sadly, one result of this is a growing population of older people with increased healthcare needs. Prompt, proactive recognition and attention to treatable health problems in this population can have a major impact, resulting in improved overall health, functioning and self-care. Where dementia is suspected, careful assessment is required to exclude other differential diagnoses – especially treatable ones. Dementia being diagnosed is not just an end-stage label, but entry into a new care pathway, which must be informed by ongoing assessment and targeted intervention.

References

American Psychiatric Association (2000) *Diagnostic and Statistical Manual of Mental Disorders* (4th edn, Text Revision) (DSM-IV-TR). APA.

American Psychiatric Association (2013) *Diagnostic and Statistical Manual of Mental Disorders* (5th edn) (DSM-5). APA.

Bhaumik S, Collacott RA, Garrick P, *et al* (1991) Effect of thyroid stimulating hormone on adaptive behaviour in Down syndrome. *Journal of Mental Deficiency Research*, **35**: 512–20.

Bittles AH, Glasson EH (2004) Clinical, social, and ethical implications of changing life expectancy in Down syndrome. *Developmental Medicine and Child Neurology*, **46**: 282–6.

Braddock D, Hemp R, Rizzolo MK (2008) *State of the States in Developmental Disabilities*. American Association for Intellectual Disability.

Burt DB, Aylward EH (2000) Test battery for the diagnosis of dementia in individuals with intellectual disability. Working group for the establishment of criteria for the diagnosis of dementia in individuals with intellectual disability. *Journal of Intellectual Disability Research*, **44**: 175–80.

Cooper SA (1997a) Epidemiology of psychiatric disorders in elderly compared with younger adults with learning disabilities. *British Journal of Psychiatry*, **170**: 375–80.

Cooper SA (1997b) High prevalence of dementia among people with learning disabilities not attributable to Down's syndrome. *Psychological Medicine*, **27**: 609–16.

Cooper SA, Morrison J, Melville C, *et al* (2006) Improving the health of people with intellectual disabilities: outcomes of a health screening programme after 1 year. *Journal of Intellectual Disability Research*, **50**: 667–77.

Deb S, Matthews T, Holt G, *et al* (2001) *Practice Guidelines for the Assessment and Diagnosis of Mental Health Problems in Adults with Intellectual Disability*. Pavilion.

Department of Health (2001) *Valuing People – A New Strategy for Learning Disability for the 21st Century*. Department of Health.

Disability Rights Commission (2006) *Equal Treatment: Closing the Gap. A Formal Investigation into Physical Health Inequalities Experienced by People with Learning Disabilities and/or Mental Health Problems*. DRC.

Fisher K, Ketti P (2005) Aging with mental retardation: Increasing population of older adults with MR require health interventions and prevention strategies. *Geriatrics*, **60**: 26–9.

Holland AJ (2000) Ageing and learning disability. *British Journal of Psychiatry*, **176**: 26–31.

Nagdee M, O'Brien G (2009) Dementia in developmental disability. In *Developmental Disability and Ageing* (eds G O'Brien, L Rosenbloom): pp 10–30. MacKeith Press.

Prasher V (1995) Age specific prevalence, thyroid dysfunction and depressive symptomatology in adults with Down syndrome and dementia. *International Journal of Geriatric Psychiatry*, **10**: 25–31.

Walker JC, Dosen A, Buitelaar JK, *et al* (2011) Depression in Down syndrome: a review of the literature. *Research in Developmental Disabilities*, **32**: 1432–40.

World Health Organization (1992) *International Statistical Classification of Diseases and Related Health Problems* (10th revision) (ICD-10). WHO.

CHAPTER 15

Services for children with disorders of intellectual development and mental health needs

Asif Zia and Anagha Sardesai

Disorders of intellectual development (DID) are, by definition, global impairments of cognitive function with onset in the developmental years (i.e. before 18 years of age). As a lifelong condition, the specific health and social care needs of this population are different at different ages. Increasingly, there has been an emphasis on the social as opposed to medical model of disability. The social model of disability focuses on the barriers experienced by people with a disability that impede their full participation in family, community and society. In defining disability it is no longer sufficient to look only at the individual impairments or conditions without reference to the wider social environment.

This chapter focuses on mental health needs during childhood. It describes the epidemiology, aetiology, assessment and treatment of mental health problems, and models of service provision. In this chapter, DID is used synonymously with 'learning disability' and 'intellectual disability'.

Epidemiology of mental health problems in DID

Various research studies and service development projects have estimated that at least 2.5% of the general population in Great Britain has a DID of such severity that, at some point in their childhood, they will need specialist services (Emerson & Hatton, 2008). Within this group, over one in three (36%) children and adolescents with a DID in Britain will have a diagnosable psychiatric disorder, compared with less than 10% of those of normal ability (Emerson, 2003; Emerson & Hatton, 2007).

Higher rates of psychiatric morbidity have been consistently reported in children with DID (Rutter *et al*, 1976; Corbett, 1979). Rutter *et al* (1976) reported that 30% of 10- to 12-year-old children with DID had a mental health disorder, compared with just 7% of children without. A more recent UK-wide enquiry by the Foundation for People with Learning Disabilities

(2002) stated that approximately 40% of children and adolescents with DID are likely to have a diagnosable mental health problem. Emerson (2003) analysed data that had been collected by the Office for National Statistics in 1999 in a survey of the mental health of children and adolescents in Great Britain and found that in a sample of just over 10 000 children, 39% of 5- to 15-year-old children with DID had a diagnosable mental health problem (compared with 8% among children who did not have DID). This would suggest that there has been no dramatic shift in the incidence or prevalence of mental health problems in children with DID over the decades.

There is evidence that the prevalence of mental health problems increases as children grow older. Mental disorders affect 10.4% of boys aged 5–10 years, rising to 12.8% of boys aged 11–15 years, and 5.9% of girls aged 5–10 years, rising to 9.6% of girls aged 11–15 years (Joint Commissioning Panel for Mental Health, 2013).

The combination of biological, psychological and social factors contributes towards greatly increased prevalence rates of mental health problems in children with DID. Moreover, confounding the diagnosis of mental health problems is the common comorbidity with epilepsy (see Chapter 6), autism spectrum disorder (ASD) (see Chapter 8), cerebral palsy and sensory impairments. The prevalence of ASD and epilepsy increases as the level of disability increases (Deb & Prasad, 1994; Emerson, 2012). Where one or more of these conditions are present, the risks are cumulative. Crucially, the level of disability seems to have a significant impact on the presentation and prevalence of mental health problems in children with DID.

Aetiology of mental health problems in DID

Allington-Smith (2006) and Emerson & Hatton (2007) described a number of factors that have been consistently demonstrated to have an association with risk of mental health problems among children with DID. They can be divided into categories, individual and environmental, as follows:

- individual –
  - communication vulnerabilities
  - sensory disability
  - epilepsy
  - physical illness
  - limited range of coping strategies
  - side-effects of medication used to treat physical disorders
  - the 'behavioural phenotypes' of particular genetic disorders (see Chapter 2);

- environmental –
  - socioeconomic deprivation
  - inadequate support services
  - poor educational provision

- • a lack of local residential projects
- • abuse (physical, sexual, emotional or neglect)
- • a remote rural population
- parental mental health problems.

The impact that the DID has on an individual is dependent on the complex interaction between the biological and environmental factors. Up to a point, level of disability dictates how much independence an individual is capable of, but modifying the physical environment can considerably reduce the level of support needed; for example, providing a mobility aid or a hearing aid can significantly improve quality of life and reduce the support needed at home and at school.

Comorbidities associated with DID

Younger children with DID frequently present with comorbid ASD, attention-deficit hyperactivity disorder (ADHD), emotional and behavioural disorders, sleep and eating problems and conduct disorder (Emerson & Baines, 2010; Enfield *et al*, 2011). On the other hand, older children are more likely to present with emotional difficulties. It is important to bear in mind that conduct and attentional problems are diagnosed only if the difficulties are beyond what would be expected for the developmental age of the child and not just the chronological age. Particular expertise is needed when dealing with ASD, which is associated with high rates of behavioural and psychiatric problems, especially in children who have moderate or severe DID. These children represent the vast majority of those with severe challenging behaviours (Allington-Smith, 2006). Interestingly, children with specific intellectual difficulties (i.e. without global intellectual impairment) also have higher comorbidity for ADHD, conduct disorder and emotional difficulties.

Vulnerability

Children and young people with disabilities form a heterogeneous group, accessing a range of services provided by both health and social care. Children with DID will be affected where services are not well 'joined up' in their policies, procedures and delivery. Under the National Service Framework for Children, Young People and Maternity Services, local authorities and National Health Service (NHS) trusts are expected to ensure that there are 'arrangements to encourage multi-agency strategic planning of services for disabled children' (Department of Health, 2004: p. 39). Emerson & Hatton (2007) compiled a report on the mental health of children and adolescents with DID in Britain based on the experiences of over 18 000 children aged between 5 and 15 years. They found that there were some important differences between the children with and without

DID. In particular, children with DID were significantly more likely:

- to be boys
- to have poor general health
- to have been exposed to a greater variety of adverse life events (e.g. abuse, serious accidents, bereavement, domestic violence)
- to be brought up by a single parent (nearly always a single mother)
- to live in poverty (47% reported this)
- to live in a poorly functioning family (e.g. one characterised by disharmony)
- to have a mother in poor health
- to have a mother with mental health needs (33% reported this)
- to live in a family with lower educational attainments and higher rates of unemployment
- to have fewer friends.

They also found that children with DID were:

- 33 times more likely to have ASD
- 8 times more likely to have ADHD
- 6 times more likely to have a conduct disorder
- 4 times more likely to have an emotional disorder
- 0.7 times more likely to have a depressive disorder
- significantly more likely to have multiple psychiatric disorders.

These differences are consistent with previous and subsequent research (Emerson & Baines, 2010; Emerson *et al*, 2011) that has documented the considerable social disadvantage faced by children with DID and their families. All the above factors have been identified as risk factors for mental health problems among children and adolescents generally. What this means is that we would expect children with DID to have more mental health problems, not necessarily as an inevitable consequence of their DID, but simply because of their increased chances of being exposed to poverty, social exclusion and more challenging family environments. However, we also now know that specific genetic syndromes are associated with particular patterns of behavioural and psychiatric morbidity, and, therefore, an additional 'layer' of aetiology (i.e. genetic) needs to be considered in this population (for a more in-depth discussion of behavioural phenotypes see Chapter 2).

Assessment

Many professionals are involved in the diagnosis of DID. These include psychologists, educational specialists and other professionals who work in specialised fields, such as occupational therapy and speech and language therapy. Each has a unique role to play in the comprehensive assessment of an individual with DID. Establishing a diagnosis of DID usually involves four primary types of assessment:

- testing of intellectual capacity or cognitive potential
- testing information processing skills and sensory and motor abilities
- assessment of current educational attainment
- assessment of adaptive functioning.

These assessments are carried out by various professionals in a multi-disciplinary team. In addition to the assessment of DID, professionals, particularly psychiatrists, are asked to be involved in the assessment of associated behaviour difficulties, mental health problems such as depression, psychosis and obsessive–compulsive disorder, and neurodevelopmental disorders such as ADHD and ASD.

Assessment involves a systematic approach that starts with history taking (including collateral history from parents and carers), mental state and physical examination, and with psychometric tests and other investigations conducted as needed. Paediatricians and neurologists are often involved in the assessment, particularly in the context of medical complications. In contrast, a psychiatrist is principally involved in assessing and managing the mental health needs of an individual with DID.

When taking a history, it is particularly important to consider the following:

- *Presenting complaint and history of presenting complaints, with onset, duration and progress of the presenting complaint, along with any precipitating or ameliorating factors.* The more common presenting complaints include change in functioning, behavioural disturbance (e.g. aggression towards peers, siblings, parents or carers), withdrawal from activities and loss of skills. This information may also form the basis of applied behaviour analysis (see Chapter 11). Occasionally patients present with more unusual behaviours that typically indicate an underlying genetic aetiology (such as severe self-mutilation in Lesch–Nyhan syndrome or hyperphagia in Prader–Willi syndrome).
- *Psychiatric history.* This often identifies a similar pattern of difficulties in the past, which may point towards aetiology. For example, a child who is not able to express himself verbally may present with agitation or aggression in times of pain or when constipated.
- *Family history of psychiatric illness or developmental disorder.*
- *Detailed developmental history.* This will help to ascertain the individual's level of function and ability, as well as identifying any loss of acquired skills that may point towards a specific diagnosis (e.g. depression or Rett syndrome). The developmental history can also uniquely shed light on the aetiology of the DID as well as whether there is any associated ADHD, ASD or other specific learning difficulty (e.g. apraxia).
- *Social history.* This should include any changes to routine, stability in the provision of carers, the availability of social networks, as well

as any losses of relationships. Individuals with DID may struggle to verbalise and express their sadness, anxiety or anger at these changes, or may not fully understand why, for example, a carer is no longer visiting them, and may consequently present with agitation or withdrawal.

- *Biological functions, particularly sleep, appetite, menstrual abnormalities and bowel function.* These may be indicators of underlying problems such as hypothyroidism, which is relatively common in Down syndrome.
- *Medical history.* This should include any current medication, previous medication, and allergies.

Physical examination is also important, with particular focus on physical markers of underlying genetic or chromosomal conditions. For example, the presence of cafe-au-lait spots, adenoma sebaceum, shagreen patches or periungual fibromas may suggest tuberous sclerosis. It is also important to look for signs suggestive of physical trauma such as bruises, though they may of course indicate an underlying medical problem, and to look for evidence of infection or constipation.

Investigations should attempt to identify the cause of the presentation as well as to establish a baseline. Blood tests, including blood count, electrolytes and liver and renal function, are important to identify possible infections or anaemia (which may cause lethargy), as well as ensuring the vital organs are able to metabolise medication if this is prescribed. As indicated above, thyroid function is sometimes abnormal in patients with Down syndrome, who are known to have a greater risk of hypothyroidism. A magnetic resonance imaging scan may be indicated, particularly in late-onset epilepsy (discrete periods of focal difficulties, loss of consciousness, episodic confusion or agitation), in the presence of focal neurological signs or in suspected neurofibromatosis. A computerised tomography scan may be more efficient (and tolerated better) in cases of suspected brain trauma (e.g. in cases of repeated head banging).

In cases of behavioural difficulties it is often helpful to carry out an observation by a skilled professional that looks at antecedents, behaviour and consequences in relation to the difficulty. Additionally, a communication assessment can be helpful in terms of facilitating interaction between the child and those around them. Psychometric assessments such as the Wechsler Intelligence Scale for Children (WISC-IV UK; Wechsler, 2004) can give a better idea of the child's intellectual abilities and may identify discrepancies in verbal and perceptual skills which may lead to educational non-attainment or behaviour difficulties at school or home when demands are placed on the child. They also provide information regarding the overall functioning of the child and may indicate the need for further tests, for example if there is evidence of attentional vulnerabilities or executive dysfunction.

Treatment

The most common treatment approach draws on a wide range of specialist skills in order to reduce vulnerability and maximise potential. The child's educational milieu is crucial in affording the child the opportunity to learn academic and more general adaptive skills. A full consideration of this important topic is beyond the scope of this chapter and the interested reader is referred to Frederickson & Cline (2009).

Mental health problems in children with DID are treated using medication, either alone or in combination with psychological treatment. When using medication the old adage 'start low and go slow' is invaluable, as not only are children with DID more sensitive to the effects of medication, but also they may not be able to report unwanted effects if they occur. Moreover, many children with DID are taking more than one medication, and it is therefore important to take into account potential drug interactions. The evidence base for drug use in DID is limited. Evidence is therefore drawn from the literature on the general population. A further complication is that children with DID may not be able to self-reflect and hence evaluate the benefits and side-effects of medication. Hence, direct observation and third-party corroboration are crucial.

The National Institute for Health and Care Excellence (NICE) has recommended a combination of psychological therapies (e.g. cognitive–behavioural therapy) and medication for the treatment of mild and moderate depression in children (NICE, 2005). For severe and enduring symptoms, selective serotonin reuptake inhibitors (SSRIs) such as fluoxetine or citalopram can be extremely beneficial (Bramble, 2011). For the treatment of unipolar depression, standard doses of SSRIs may be used. Similarly, children with anxiety symptoms may also require treatment with SSRIs. Higher doses of SSRIs may be required to treat obsessional and compulsive symptoms, as well as stereotypies. Situational anxiety symptoms (e.g. that arise when travelling by plane) can be managed with small doses of benzodiazepines, although caution is needed owing to the risk of paradoxical disinhibition (Bramble, 2011). Common side-effects of SSRIs include mild gastrointestinal disturbance, sleep difficulties and agitation, but these are generally transient. Less commonly, activation symptoms may occur within the first week or so of treatment. SSRIs can also increase agitation in the early stages of treatment of depression, resulting in higher risk of suicide. In view of these potential adverse effects, a test dose may be a useful strategy. Where physiological symptoms of anxiety are prominent, a beta-blocker, such as propranolol, may be given. A proposed dosage schedule for antidepressants and anxiolytics is set out by Bramble (2011).

Stimulant medication such as methylphenidate can be beneficial in helping to manage attention and concentration problems in some patients with DID. It is important to remember that these problems need to be assessed in relation to the developmental age of the child rather than the chronological age. It is also important to monitor the patient very closely for side-effects, particularly hypertension and retardation of growth (on account of appetite suppression). As with the general population, atomoxetine can be used as a second-line and clonidine as a third-line treatment.

Behaviour problems are often treated by a combination of psycho-education of carers, modifying the environment to decrease demands on the child, and, if needed, low doses of antipsychotics such as risperidone or aripiprazole. Risperidone and aripiprazole continue to be licensed for this use in ASD by the US Food and Drug Administration. It is particularly important to monitor for metabolic side-effects of these drugs.

There is a range psychological therapies available to children with DID. These can include music, art, cognitive–behavioural therapy and more recently brief therapies (NHS, 2012). These are particularly helpful in very young children with DID who are either not able to communicate or who have suffered significant life events and psychological trauma.

Service provision for children with DID

Service needs

In the UK, the Disability Discrimination Act 2005 and Equality Act 2010 require all service providers to make 'reasonable adjustments' to ensure people with disabilities can access services. The Equality Act 2010 sets out the legal framework under which such people have rights. It identifies people as having a disability if they have 'a physical or mental impairment which has a substantial and long-term adverse effect on their ability to carry out normal day-to-day activities'.

Children with DID vary widely in the level of their intellectual impairment, their ability to communicate and the presence or absence of additional sensory, physical or social disabilities. Work with young people with DID therefore differs substantially from mainstream child psychiatry in important ways. In treating children with DID, the presence or absence of epilepsy, ASD and sensory impairments makes the diagnostic formulation challenging, as there may be significant interaction between organic, behavioural and environmental factors. Close liaison with parents, education, paediatricians, social care and other support agencies poses particular challenges, as information generally does not sit in one place. There is also a difference in the terminology and criteria used to describe disability between different professional groups, especially when describing children with borderline and mild DID.

Professionals' involvement also differs between mainstream child psychiatry and child DID services. For example, speech and language therapy, occupational therapy, physiotherapy and other specialist therapies, such as art and music, play an important part in the multidisciplinary team's formulation for a child with DID. It is this combination of organic, dynamic and systemic factors that necessitates community teamwork (Berney, 2006). In addition to the competencies required for mainstream child and adolescent psychiatry, professionals working with children and young people with DID should have particular expertise in the following areas (Royal College of Psychiatrists, 2010):

- diagnosis and assessment of DID and other neurodevelopmental disorders
- counselling services
- other family work
- specialised individual therapies
- pharmacological therapy for children
- liaison and joint working with other agencies
- expert witness in legal cases.

UK government policy has affected the way the services for children (and adults) with DID are provided (Department of Health, 2010; NICE, 2012). Current government policy, set out in standards 8 ('disabled child') and 9 ('child and adolescent mental health') of the National Service Framework for Children, Young People and Maternity Services (Department of Health, 2004) stipulates that every local area in England should offer a psychiatric service for children with DID. However this is only a recommendation, not a legal requirement. To compound the problem, there are often huge hurdles that families have to leap in order to receive help from psychiatric services. In many areas of Britain services exclude children who have DID. In 2005, the Department of Health's mapping exercise for child and adolescent mental health services (CAMHS) found that only about half of the services had specialist provision for intellectual disability (see Royal College of Psychiatrists, 2010). The increased demand on services, coupled with limited resources, meant that in many areas young people with DID found themselves in limbo and looked to community paediatrics to bridge the gap. In such cases it is often left to paediatricians to deal with very complex behavioural issues. In regions where specialist service provision exists, it may be provided by child psychiatrists or by intellectual disability psychiatrists.

Despite the evidence that early intervention has a significant impact on the outcome for children with DID (Berney, 2006), delay in referrals, lack of understanding and knowledge among professionals (at the primary care level, tier 1 and 2 – see below) and lack of training among psychiatrists all contribute towards relatively poor outcomes for children with DID. Owing to these limitations, children with complex needs are often placed out of area or in specialist placements (Allington-Smith, 2006). This lack of understanding of the needs of these individuals makes it very difficult for them to access adult services when they return to their local area later on in their lives. Transitional services were set up in various parts of the UK to plan better for the transition from child to adult services. These transition services met with limited and variable success, on account of economic, workforce, policy and planning issues. If the transitions policy were properly implemented, it would help to bring together and plan for a joint approach towards health, social care, education and the criminal justice system, to prevent out-of-area placement and to ensure safe transfer of care from child to adult services.

The number of patients with DID on the list of an average general practitioner (GP) has been estimated as 30–40 with mild disability and 6–8 with severe disability, across the age range, including 2–3 people still living in hospital (Livingstone, 1990). Psychiatric services for children and young people with moderate and severe intellectual disabilities require 0.5 whole-time equivalent psychiatrists per 100 000 total population aged 0–18 years (Royal College of Psychiatrists, 2004). The Children's Act 2004 places responsibility on the local authority to provide these services for children with DID. In the UK, the CAMHS provides assessment and treatment to children and young people up to the age of 18 years where there are concerns about their behaviour or emotional well-being. This service does not exclude children with a DID. Indeed, in several parts of the UK there is a smaller team within the service that is dedicated to the needs of children and young people with DID, but it is difficult to judge the quality of this specialist provision (Royal College of Psychiatrist, 2010).

Tier model of services

Children's services can be broken down into three main areas:

- *universal services* (tier 1), which work with all children and young people
- *targeted services* (tier 2), which provide early interventions for vulnerable children and young people
- *specialist services* (tiers 3 and 4), which work with children and young people with complex, severe and/or persistent needs.

Universal services are those that are provided to, or are routinely available to, all children, young people and their families. They are designed to meet more general needs and include early-years provision and mainstream schools, and health services provided by GPs, midwives and health visitors. These are tier 1 services, provided by non-specialist mental health professionals in primary care and by other front-line services, for example GPs or associated health professionals such as school nurses and health visitors who may work with, for instance, common problems of childhood such as sleeping difficulties or feeding problems. The interventions at this stage include early identification, general advice for mild–moderate problems, and mental health promotion and prevention. The Healthy Child Programme (HCP) is the universal clinical and public health programme for children and families from pregnancy to 19 years of age. The HCP, led by health visitors and their teams, offers every child a schedule of health and development reviews, screening tests, immunisations, health promotion guidance and support for parents tailored to their needs, with additional support when needed and at key times. There is strong evidence supporting delivery of all aspects of the HCP, which is based on Health for All Children, the recommendations of the National Screening Committee, guidance from NICE and a review of health-led parenting programmes by the University of Warwick (Department of Health, 2009).

Tier 2 consists of specialised primary mental health workers (PMHWs), who can offer support around assessment (which may result in further referral within their team) and treatment of problems in primary care, such as family work, bereavement and parenting groups. This tier also includes substance misuse and counselling services. These services are a functional interface between tier 1 and multidisciplinary specialist services, and may be defined as a level of service provided by specialist CAMH professionals working on their own who relate to others through a network rather than through a team (Audit Commission, 1999). Tier 2 represents the first line of specialist services, and is clearly distinguished from the work of multi-disciplinary specialist teams who provide secondary-level (tier 3) and tertiary-level (tier 4) care for children with severe, complex and persistent disorders (Appleton, 2000).

Government policy states that targeted support (i.e. tier 2), such as services aimed at particular groups of children and young people and their families, should be embedded within universal settings wherever possible:

> 'Embedding targeted services within universal settings can ensure more rapid support without the delay of formal referral, and enable frontline practitioners to seek help and advice. Developing networks across universal and specialist professionals can strengthen inter-professional relationships and trust.' (Department for Education, 2004: p 63)

Tier 3 services consist of specialist multidisciplinary teams based in a local clinic. They deal with more complex cases, such as assessment of developmental problems, ASD, inattentive and hyperactive behaviour, depression or early-onset psychosis. Some services for DID are seen in tier 3 clinics. Issues these teams are often called on to help with include:

- behavioural difficulties
- anxiety and depression
- self-harm
- emotional difficulties
- attention or overactivity problems
- family relationships
- sleep or toileting problems where other agencies have not been able to help
- liaising with professionals from other agencies, such as school or social workers to help resolve issues.

The development of the National Service Framework (Department of Health, 2004) included an external working group for young people with

DID. It recommended that a community team (including psychiatrists) should comprise 5–6 whole-time equivalent members for a population of 100000 (Royal College of Psychiatrists, 2010). For psychiatry, the Royal College of Psychiatrists (2010) suggests that a community service for young people with severe DID requires a minimum of two sessions of consultant clinical time per 100000 total population, whereas the inclusion of young people with mild DID will require a further three clinical sessions; these sessions do not include time for administration and training.

Essential components of a children's community DID team include (Allington-Smith, 2006):

- one or more psychiatrists
- community nurses trained in DID (registered nurses in learning disability) and/or mental health (registered nurses in mental health)
- clinical psychologists
- behavioural specialists, who may have clinical psychology, nursing or even social work backgrounds
- speech and language therapists
- occupational therapists trained in sensory integration
- community dietician.

Tier 4 services are in-patient units, highly specialised out-patient units and day units. They may include secure forensic adolescent units, eating disorders units or specialist neuropsychiatric teams.

It should be noted that these definitions are not inflexible, and practitioners may be working across tiers. There are a limited number of such teams for children with DID across the UK. Children with DID requiring specialist in-patient care are also seen within these services. The Royal College of Psychiatrists (2004) recommends for a population of 1 million 3–4 beds for young people with severe DID and 2–3 beds for those with moderate DID, plus 1 bed for those who require low-secure provision.

Future service development

Increasingly, services have become dedicated to the management of the young person in the home and at school. The associated curtailment of NHS hospital resources has encouraged the retention of young people in their community and has also led to the development of other institutions, particularly in the independent sector. There is a shortage of in-patient places, 40% of which are provided by the private sector (O'Herlihy et al, 2001). Residential schools continue to flourish, some providing care for up to 52 weeks per year, but not always with good access to appropriate healthcare. In recent years integrated pathways have been developed; for instance, ASD and ADHD may coexist in the same child, and care pathways work best if aligned as much as possible. Indeed, the term 'children with troublesome behaviour' is a good catch-all.

Most of the new investment in the UK is around a project to transform the CAMHS project, the Increased Access to Psychological Therapies (IAPT) programme. The changes involve improved access, more precise categorisation of the nature and severity of the difficulties on presentation, a recognition of complexity (such as being subject to a care order or protection plan) and the effect on the child's or young person's education, employment or training (EET). There will be a greater emphasis on recording measures of recovery, change and satisfaction with treatment (Department for Education, 2012; Department of Health, 2012),

Conclusion

Children and young people with DID are likely to face mental health problems and considerable social adversity. There is also some tentative evidence that the more hard pressed a family is, the less likely it is to have easy access to formal means of support. In addressing the difficulties faced by this group, it is crucial for services to work together across a plethora of areas, not the least of which are medical, social and educational.

References

Allington-Smith P (2006) Mental health of children with learning disabilities. *Advances in Psychiatric Treatment,* **12**: 130–40.

Appleton P (2000) Tier 2 CAMHS and its interface with primary care. *Advances in Psychiatric Treatment,* **6**: 388–96.

Audit Commission (1999) *Children in Mind: Child and Adolescent Mental Health Services* (Briefing). Audit Commission.

Berney T (2006) The new developmental psychiatry. Invited commentary on mental health of children with learning disabilities. *Advances in Psychiatric Treatment,* **12**: 138–40.

Bramble D (2011) Psychopharmacology in children with intellectual disability. *Advances in Psychiatric Treatment,* **17**: 32–40.

Corbett J (1979) Psychiatric morbidity and mental retardation. In *Psychiatric Illness and Mental Handicap* (eds FE James, RP Snaith): pp 11–25. Gaskell.

Deb S, Prasad KB (1994) Prevalence of autistic disorder among children with a learning disability. *British Journal of Psychiatry,* **165**: 395–9.

Department for Education (2004) *Every Child Matters: Change for Children.* Available at http://www.dcsf.gov.uk/everychildmatters (accessed 3 March 2014).

Department for Education (2012) *Support and Aspiration: A New Approach to Special Educational Needs and Disability – Progress and Next Steps. Increasing Options and Improving Provision for Children with Special Educational Needs (SEN).* Department for Education.

Department of Health (2004) *The National Service Framework for Children, Young People and Maternity Services: Disabled Children and Young People and Those with Complex Health Needs.* Department of Health.

Department of Health (2009) *Healthy Child Programme. Pregnancy and the First Five Years of Life.* Department of Health. Available at https://www.gov.uk/government/uploads/system/uploads/attachment_data/file/167998/Health_Child_Programme.pdf (accessed May 2015).

Department of Health (2010) *Fulfilling and Rewarding Lives: The Strategy for Adults with Autism in England.* Department of Health.

Department of Health (2012) *Children and Young People's Improving Access to Psychological Therapies Project – Applying to Join an Existing Learning Collaborative in 2012–13*. Department of Health.

Emerson E (2003) Prevalence of psychiatric disorders in children and adolescents with and without intellectual disability. *Journal of Intellectual Disability Research*, **47**: 51–8.

Emerson E (2012) Deprivation, ethnicity and the prevalence of intellectual and developmental disabilities. *Journal of Epidemiology and Community Health*, **66**: 218.

Emerson E, Baines S (2010) *The Estimated Prevalence of Autism Among Adults with Learning Disabilities in England: Improving Health and Lives*. Learning Disabilities Observatory. Available at http://www.improvinghealthandlives.org.uk/uploads/doc/vid_8731_IHAL2010-05Autism.pdf (accessed 3 March 2014).

Emerson E, Hatton C (2007) The mental health of children and adolescents with learning disabilities in Britain. *British Journal of Psychiatry*, **191**: 493–9.

Emerson E, Hatton C (2008) *Estimating Future Need for Adult Social Care Services for People with Learning Disabilities in England*. Centre for Disability Research (CeDR) Research Report 2008:6.

Emerson E, Baines S, Allerton L, *et al* (2011) *Health Inequalities and People with Learning Disabilities in the UK*. Public Health England.

Enfield S, Ellis L, Emerson E (2011) Co-morbidity of intellectual disability and mental disorder in children and adolescents: a systematic review. *Journal of Intellectual and Developmental Disability*, 36: 137–43.

Foundation for People with Learning Disabilities (2002) *Count Us In. The Report of the Committee of Inquiry into Meeting the Mental Health Needs of Young People with Learning Disabilities*. Foundation for People with Learning Disabilities.

Frederickson N, Cline T (2009) *Special Educational Needs, Inclusion and Diversity: A Textbook (2nd edn)*. Open University Press.

Joint Commissioning Panel for Mental Health (2013) *Guidance for Commissioners of Child and Adolescent Mental Health Services*. Joint Commissioning Panel for Mental Health. Available at http://www.jcpmh.info (accessed 3 March 2014).

Livingstone D (1990) Mentally handicapped people, community care and the general practitioner. In *Primary Care for People with a Mental Handicap* (Occasional Paper 47): pp 2–3. Royal College of General Practitioners.

NHS (2012) *Children and Young People's Improving Access to Psychological Therapies Project – Applying to Join an Existing Learning Collaborative in 2012–13*. Department of Health. Available at http://www.iapt.nhs.uk/silo/files/cyp-iapt-applying-to-become-a-learning-collaborative-in-201213.pdf (accessed April 2015).

NICE (2005) *Depression in Children and Young People: Identification and Management in Primary, Community and Secondary Care* (Clinical Guideline 28). National Collaborating Centre for Mental Health.

NICE (2012) *Autism: Recognition, Referral, Diagnosis and Management of Adults on the Autism Spectrum* (Clinical Guideline 142). National Institute for Health and Clinical Excellence.

O'Herlihy A, Worrall A, Banerjee S, *et al* (2001) *National In-patient Child and Adolescent Psychiatry Study (NICAPS)*. Royal College of Psychiatrists.

Royal College of Psychiatrists (2004) *Psychiatric Services for Children and Adolescents with Learning Disabilities* (CR123). Royal College of Psychiatrists.

Royal College of Psychiatrists (2010) *Psychiatric Services for Children and Adolescents with Intellectual Disabilities* (CR163). Royal College of Psychiatrists.

Rutter M, Tizard J, Yule W, *et al* (1976) Isle of Wight Studies, 1964–74 research report. *Psychological Medicine*, **6**: 313–32.

Wechsler D (2004) *Wechsler Intelligence Scale for Children* (4th edn) (WISC-IV UK). Pearson Clinical.

CHAPTER 16

Forensic psychiatry for people with disorders of intellectual development: a personal reflection

Simon Martin Halstead

The invitation to contribute a chapter to this volume has been a welcome, but somewhat intimidating, opportunity to review the opinions I had expressed almost two decades ago (Halstead, 1996). At that time I was a newly appointed consultant psychiatrist at St Andrew's Hospital, Northampton, for a 15-bed locked ward for patients with what may now be termed disorders of intellectual development (DID). I was an enthusiast for compulsory treatment under the Mental Health Act 1983 (MHA), using a rich therapeutic milieu, such was available at St Andrew's Hospital at that time. I had boundless therapeutic optimism. In the era of the Reed report (Department of Health & Home Office, 1992) and a relatively enlightened Department of Health, the message was very clearly to provide liberal and scientific treatment for offenders with mental disorders (and others with similar needs), in secure hospital settings, diverting them from prison and from the criminal justice system in general.

In the mid-1990s I certainly did not anticipate the massive increase in the provision of secure beds for people with DID, within the independent and charitable sectors, which would occur from approximately 1997, led by companies such as Care Principles (of which I was medical director between 2001 and 2007), Partnerships in Care, St Andrew's Healthcare, Castlebeck, The Huntercombe Group, Priory Group and several smaller providers.

I now work as an independent consultant psychiatrist and the vast majority of my work involves, in one way or another, the defence of patients' rights within the context of the criminal justice system, the MHA and the Mental Capacity Act 2005 (MCA). This is therefore something of a 'gamekeeper turned poacher' story. I ask for the reader's indulgence, but I think I should be open, from the outset, concerning the perspective from which I am writing.

The Royal College of Psychiatrists has recently published an excellent review of forensic DID services, *Forensic Care Pathways for Adults with Intellectual Disability Involved with the Criminal Justice System* (Royal College of Psychiatrists, 2014), which is available on the internet and which I would strongly recommend. I can only hope that this chapter is a humble complement to this document rather than a restatement of the facts and opinions that it contains.

Historical and philosophical issues

The first legislation concerning 'idiots' in England was *de prerogativa regis* ('concerning the prerogative of the king'), which dates to the reign of the ill-fated Edward II, in 1324. The lands of the 'idiot' reverted to the king, whereas those of the 'lunatic' were held in trust, pending the recovery of his wits. I have argued elsewhere (Halstead, 1997) that there is a tension, or dichotomy, in society's attitudes to people with mental disorder, and DID in particular, in respect of whether it is the disordered individual who presents a risk to society, or vice versa.

Conflicting humanitarian and eugenic concerns led to the establishment of the Royal Commission on the Care and Control of the Feeble-Minded in 1904 (which reported in 1908) and its very title betrays the conflict. The report in turn led to the Mental Deficiency Act 1913, which correspondingly contained coercive and liberal measures.

We have seen similar contradictions in the move from 'de-institutionalisation' to 'safeguarding'. To what extend should people with DID be free, coerced or protected? I recall watching in the early 1990s a video of two gay men with Down syndrome living in a flat in East London as an exemplar. Today, I can see me being asked to do assessments of capacity to consent to sexual relations, in accordance with the bewilderingly complex contemporary legal test for capacity to have sexual relations (which no person with a DID could possibly understand), for the purposes of safeguarding.

Moreover, I consider that the very title of this chapter bears further investigation and scrutiny. Is there a 'forensic psychiatry for people with DID' at all? Let us examine each term separately.

What is psychiatry?

Psychiatry is the medical approach to the diagnosis and treatment of mental disorder. Diagnosis on its own is not enough. As with any branch of medicine, the very least the doctors can do is to tell patients what will happen to them and what they can best do to ameliorate their condition (if at all). The injunction of Hippocrates to 'first, do no harm' (ἐπὶ δηλήσει δὲ καὶ ἀδικίῃ εἴρξειν)[1] has been woefully ignored in the history of medicine (with bleeding, etc.) up to the 19th century and the origins of scientific medicine. It can be argued that in the era of scientific and 'evidence-based medicine' we continue to do harm (the doling out of antidepressants,

---

1. For some bizarre reason usually quoted in Latin: *primum non nocere*.

hospital-acquired infections, etc.). Maybe we do harm in the present age by detaining patients in conditions of excessive security, for want of appropriate community facilities, and overmedicating them.

The 'alienists'[2] of the 19th century would not have recognised the diversity of modern mental health disciplines which have been historically created and arbitrarily divided from one another. My personal lament is the division between psychiatry and psychology, which seems to me to have no basis in science whatsoever. We tend to do what we do within our professional boundaries, which may not meet the needs of people with DID (to name but a few).

In the mid-20th century, the advent of psychosurgery, electroconvulsive therapy, antipsychotics and antidepressants gave psychiatry some prestige and raised the realistic prospect of effective treatments and a reversal of institutionalisation. It would take a separate chapter to debate the extent to which that dream has been fulfilled, but I think 'partially at best' would be an accurate summation.

On the other hand, having worked in this area for a full two decades, I am not aware of a single medical treatment for DID.

The closure of the tuberculosis aslya[3] resulted from a proper understanding of the aetiology, treatment and prevention of infection by the bacillus. They have not reopened. As already pointed out above, the closure of the learning disability hospitals led to a burgeoning of provision in the private sector. Ideology had trumped science and the consequences were swept under the carpet (only to come to public attention in the most dramatic way, a theme to which I shall return later).

If there is a psychiatry of DID, then it must involve other psychiatric skills (developmental understanding, treatment of epilepsy and other neuropsychiatric conditions, understanding of psychodynamics and family and clinical team dynamics) in addition to the diagnosis and treatment of superadded mental illness in order to validate itself as a subspecialty. There is a counter-argument which states that only psychiatrists trained in DID can diagnose mental disorder in people with DID (generally moderate and severe DID); however, this alone would not justify a subspecialty, namely, the forensic psychiatry of DID.

What is forensic psychiatry?

Forensic psychiatry is generally understood to be the psychiatric management of risk, predominantly to others, but also to self (particularly in the independent sector and the high-secure hospitals, where prolific self-harmers find a home). But this definition is not sufficient, as all branches of psychiatry are concerned with the management of risk. The

---

2. From the Latin *alienatus* ('estranged', i.e. from wits).
3. Asylums is the generally accepted plural. However, it is a Latin type 2 neuter noun, not a gerund like 'referendum' (which cannot have plural in Latin, like 'playing' in English).

term 'forensic' refers to the application of law[4] and so forensic psychiatry involves the interface between law and psychiatry at every level: civil, family and criminal. The forensic psychiatrist has to have skills in addressing the legal tests in medical language and in giving evidence in court.

However, there is a more fundamental question. Is there a scientific link between dangerous behaviour, mental disorder and treatment? If not, then the domain of forensic psychiatrists is confined to their courtroom skills.

The hubristic high-water mark of forensic psychiatry was, in my opinion, the Dangerous and Severe Personality Disorder (DSPD) Programme of the Blair government in the 1990s (Duggan, 2011). It has now been discredited and abandoned within hospitals, if not within prisons. Its core was idealistic. It sought to use the best science to address the most intractable of human mental disorders. Indeed, its founding text was *Personality Disorder: No Longer a Diagnosis of Exclusion* (National Institute for Mental Health for England, 2003). Surely optimism there, but there was also the mendacious public protection agenda, namely that if the 2000 'DSPDs' could be located and detained, the public would be significantly protected. I recall scornfully remarking at the time that when 1999 were detained, the hunt would be on for the last remaining 'DSPD' still at liberty.

During those dark years, in the last decade, I provided independent medical reports for many men who were sent to high-security hospitals, often on the last day of their prison sentence, to face many years of *faux* treatments in blatant contradiction of the medically informed decision of the sentencing judge. Amnesty International has used the term 'administrative detention' to describe the preventive detention of suspect individuals outwith the criminal justice system. When I first encountered the transfer of sentenced prisoners from Changi Prison to (the then) Woodbridge Hospital in Singapore for extended and indeterminate hospital sentences, in 1989, I thought that this could never happen in Britain. How very wrong I was.

High- and medium-secure hospitals in England now care for the tiny proportion of the population who suffer from the most intractable mental disorders. Noble work, indeed, but falling far short of the therapeutic optimism of the founding fathers and mothers of forensic psychiatry in the 1960s and 1970s. Few of these terribly ill individuals remotely have the ability to scale the impressive walls of the high-secure hospitals.

Moreover, I hear from my colleagues, as I visit these institutions, that the famed forensic psychodynamic psychotherapy services are dwindling in the face of funding cuts.

The other major change over the past 20 years is the doubling of the prison population in England and Wales, to around 85 000 (Ministry of Justice, 2013). 'The prison population in England and Wales, including those held in Immigration Removal Centres, was at a record high of 88,179 prisoners on 2 December 2011. In Scotland the prison population reached a

---

4. Latin: *forum, forensis.*

record high of 8,420 on 8 March 2012' (Berman & Dar, 2013). This increase has occurred despite falling levels of crime. It is argued by politicians that crime has fallen because of increased incarceration; however, there is abundant evidence that this is not the case. Crime has fallen worldwide irrespective of the flavour of the criminal justice regime in a particular country (*Economist*, 2013). Far from the ideal of diversion from the criminal justice system, people with mental disorders (including people with DID) are being managed within the penal system. Part III of the MHA contains the 'forensic sections', orders made by the courts or by the Ministry of Justice. In 2009/10 there were 159 such orders made for people with learning disability[5] in England and Wales and this had fallen, year by year, to 55 in 2012/13 (Health and Social Care Information Centre, 2013), which is approximately one a week nationwide.[6] Yet one would expect there to be approximately 2000 prisoners with DID (2.5% of 85 000) on the basis of population distribution alone. Estimates for the prevalence of DID in the prison system go as high as 20–30% (Talbot, 2008), which would equate to tens of thousands. The diversion of people with DID from the criminal justice system seems to be dwindling in the face of an expanding prison population. On the other hand, people with DID represent 8% of those detained under the MHA, which is roughly three times their prevalence in the population (Talbot, 2008).

What is DID?

As I have noted above, there has always been an awareness that certain individuals were inherently incapable of managing their own affairs. Terms have been applied that would be seen as offensive today: idiot, subnormal, mentally handicapped and, latterly, learning disabled. Indeed, the requirement of impairment of social functioning (rather than intelligence alone) remains part of the definition of intellectual disability today (Royal College of Psychiatrists, 2014).

It was only in the late 19th and early 20th centuries, with the work of Galton (a noted eugenicist), Binet and Simon, that the notion of a measurable and reliable central intelligence took hold. Today we use the various permutations of the Wechsler intelligence scales (child and adult) to measure IQ (intelligence quotient). The concept of the full-scale IQ allowed human intelligence to be plotted on a graph. As with height and weight, it follows the pattern of the Gaussian normal distribution. Unlike eye colour and sex, which are (generally) categorical, IQ is distributed according to the 'normal' distribution curve. The tests are calibrated so that the average, mean and mode coincide at a score of 100. The standard deviation is set at

---

5. The term used by the MHA and Code of Practice.
6. Intriguingly, this is not very different from the figures for 1985 (39 unrestricted, 9 restricted) which I quoted in my 1996 paper, although this did not include sections 35, 36 and 38.

15, such that 4 standard deviations (i.e. 60 points) encompass 95% of the population. Thirty points below 100 (i.e. 2 standard deviations) sets the lower threshold at 70 and the converse above 100 sets the upper threshold at 130. Therefore 2.5% of the population have an abnormally low IQ and 2.5% are blessed with an abnormally high IQ. The curve is not entirely smooth, however, as there is a little blip at the bottom which includes people with inherited and acquired conditions which impair intelligence. There are though no known conditions which 'bump' people up the scale.[7].

Eugenic theory stated that if the people at the bottom of the spectrum were allowed to breed, they would spread contamination, undermine the race and bring the whole distribution curve down. However, it is an irony that Sir Francis Galton himself discovered the answer to this, which is called the 'law of regression to the mean'. Without this, the curve would flatten over time as a result of 'assortative mating'.[8] In other words, the more intelligent would have ever more intelligent children and would zoom off to the right and the converse would happen with the less able. The centre would collapse and flatten. We now know that this is not the case. Two highly intelligent parents are statistically more likely to have children who are more intelligent than the mean, but, crucially, less intelligent than the parents are. The same correcting effect happens at the bottom of the scale; thus, offspring tend back towards the mean, not to the extremities.

The other factor of which Galton would have been unaware is the 'Flynn effect', so-called after James Flynn (Herrnstein & Murray, 1994).[9] There has been a worldwide increase in intelligence (not just measured IQ) in the past 100 years or so. The increase over the past century could be as much as 1 standard deviation (15 points). While it would be impossible to put a precise figure on it, the implication is that in 1914, a substantial proportion of the population would be considered to have a DID by comparison with their descendants today. As we shall spend the next 4 years wondering why people were willing to run onto machine guns rather than turn their rifles on their officers and go home (as recommended by Lenin and Armand), the fact that they were markedly less intelligent than we are should attract some attention. The biggest contributors to increasing intelligence, probably, are better nutrition and prevention of childhood infections. We are taller and brighter than we were a century ago, though this is likely to be due to fulfilling our genetic potential rather than a trend that will continue, upwards, indefinitely.

The use of IQ data to stigmatise racial minorities falls when social class and the variables mentioned above are controlled for. Skeletons of our hunter-gather ancestors resemble the large size of the Dutch today, but with more war wounds (however, that is another story).

---

7. Though Augustus John, the artist, is reputed to have become a genius only after hitting his head on a rock while swimming in 1897. Similar metamorphoses are surely rare.
8. Breeding with someone like oneself.
9. Referencing this book is a matter of history and does not imply any support for its racially divisive conclusion.

By tradition – and according to ICD-10 (World Health Organization, 1992) – 'mental retardation' is divided into four levels: mild, moderate, severe and profound. Mild mental retardation is classified as being between 50 and 69; however, with an error rating of 5 either way on any score, this can be 45–74. It would be extremely rare and unlikely for anyone with an IQ of below 50 to be considered to be an offender and culpable for their actions in the eyes of the law. This would not, of course preclude them from being detained in hospital under the MHA.

Therefore, historically, the forensic psychiatry of DID has been concerned only with people with an IQ between 50 and 70, or so, the mild DID or mild mental retardation group. The term 'mild' is somewhat misleading. Having an IQ in the bottom 1–2% of the population is a significant handicap in terms of coping with everyday life: it is only 'mild' when compared with more severe levels of DID.

Yet in the moderate to profound levels of DID there is an increased prevalence of genetic, physical and neuropsychiatric disorder. The 'mild' DID group, on the other hand, may not be obviously distinguishable from the normal population upon casual encounter. This applies more so to those with a borderline DID (i.e. a formal IQ of 70 or above but who can be functionally in the DID range). It is well established that forensic and prison populations have a lower average IQ than the normal population. It is therefore reasonable to ask whether or not a mild DID clinical population is sufficiently different in terms of needs and clinical vulnerability from a general forensic population to justify separate provision. I am not aware that this issue has ever been addressed scientifically.

There are some very good reviews of the epidemiology of offending within a population with DID and I have reviewed some of these in my earlier paper (Halstead, 1996). However, the area is bedevilled by methodological problems, largely around definition, culture and perception. What we label as 'challenging behaviour' in people with DID would be considered severe offending in members of the normal population; conversely, behaviours that would be considered within the expected range in members of the normal population (drug and alcohol use, sexual promiscuity) are viewed with concern in people with DID.

Johnston, in *The Handbook of Forensic Learning Disabilities*, concluded her chapter by stating:

> The factors that protect or support the complex decision making when considering aberrant behaviours as challenging or offences are as yet poorly described in the literature, although they present everyday dilemmas for clinicians, carers and criminal justice professionals. Most offenders with learning disability have mild learning disability and many comorbid health and social conditions. However, *there is little evidence to suggest that there are particular risk factors associated with learning disability per se which increase this potential.*' (Johnston, 2005: p. 27; emphasis added)

So there is no inherent propensity for people with DID to offend.

Take the statement: 'X sexually abused Y' (common enough as an entry in clinical records). However, in reality, it is euphemistic and varies greatly depending on the three elements, the verb and the two placeholders. Regarding 'Y', as recently as the 1990s, the rape of non-consenting, highly vulnerable female patients was seemingly acceptable within some long-stay institutions. A female patient with severe disabilities could return at the end of the day with a handful of cigarettes which she had obtained by giving sexual favours in the hospital grounds. It has been a huge achievement of the safeguarding movement that the consciousness of service providers has been irreversibly shifted to the position that such things are no longer tolerable, no longer something to be smiled about and indulged.

With regard to 'X' the situation is less clear. If X is a service user, with perceived low status in society, the statement may remain an entry in the notes and in the risk assessment. Police are unwilling to charge, and prosecutors unwilling to prosecute, where perpetrators with DID are concerned. They seem to be unaware of the unfitness-to-plead procedures and the powers of the courts to test facts. If 'X', on the other hand, is a member of staff, quite rightly, all hell breaks loose. Suspension and a harrowing internal and criminal investigation have to be endured. The key point about this is that the establishment of guilt or innocence is something that is at the very heart of justice. We are all jealous of our personal and professional reputations. The fact that we are prepared to 'administratively detain' service users without the right to a hearing by a court, and the possibility of defending themselves, betrays, in my view, enduring prejudices concerning their status and value as human beings.[10]

Special issues

This brief chapter cannot do justice to the many complex issues that are relevant to this area. Here are a few that I consider to be relevant.

Suggestibility

The idea that people with DID are especially vulnerable to changing their recollection of events under pressure (suggestibility) or to agreeing with the version of a powerful person (acquiescence) has been investigated (Gudjonsson *et al*, 1993). However, an intriguing book by Ian Leslie, *Born Liars: Why We Can't Live Without Deceit* (2011), reviews research over the past century which indicates that we may all be a lot more suggestible than we think, and our memories much more fallible, with huge potential implications for criminal justice across the board, not just for people with DID.

---

10. Detention under the MHA is reviewed by a mental health tribunal. This examines the grounds for detention, which do not automatically include the establishment of the facts of particular events.

Fitness to plead

Concerns about an individual's ability to stand trial have been expressed since medieval times. Positive findings of unfitness to plead are relatively uncommon in England and Wales and of these the number applying to people with DID would be in only single digits per year. This is surprising given the frequency of 'challenging' (often criminal) behaviour in people with DID and behaviour disorders. The answer probably is that there is a reluctance for the Crown Prosecution Service to prosecute people with significant DID on the one hand, unless there is an overriding public interest in a trial taking place.

Capacity

The ability to take decisions on one's own behalf has been a historic concern of the law. A huge chasm in English and Welsh law opened up with the failure of guardianship under the Mental Health Act 1959. Essentially, no one was able to consent on behalf of an incapacitated adult. In the interim, the civil courts filled the gap with 'declaratory jurisdiction' (i.e. a declaration that an action would not be illegal – a double negative). Lawyers and psychiatrists operated nimbly within this legal lacuna. The gap was closed (after an agonisingly long consultation period) by the Mental Capacity Act 2005 and the later Deprivation of Liberty Safeguards.

The result has been tortuous, complex, long and highly expensive legal cases through the Court of Protection. I have, personally, been cross-examined all afternoon by four barristers in a case which I considered pretty obvious (and said so to the judge), and how expensive is that? Not to mention the interminable delay for the client. The MHA, in comparison, offers speedy access to orders and equally speedy access to appeal to an independent tribunal. The Adults with Incapacity Act (Scotland) 2000 has a similarly good reputation for rapid access to justice.

Models of care

This is a difficult area to review, as there is no one model which will suit all individuals. A person who is aggressive because of a mental illness may settle on drug treatment alone. A person who presents with a particular propensity to arson, anger or sexual offending may require the appropriate, specific treatment. Someone presenting complex and risky behaviours in the context of mental and psychosocial disorder may benefit from a nuanced, individualised and multidisciplinary treatment plan.

However, there is a clear consensus that the term 'challenging behaviour' should not be used as a diagnosis in itself and that therapeutic approaches should seek to understand the factors within the individual, and in the environment, which maintain risky behaviours, and that responses should be positive and never punitive. This has been called positive behavioural support (Department of Health, 2014). It does seem to me to be an irony that we advocate only positive approaches to behaviour in people with DID, whereas the rest of us live in a punitive, controlling and surveillance society, in which the government is constantly 'clamping down' on one benighted and unpopular social group or another.

Hospital treatment

As the MHA is directed to hospital treatment, I think it is reasonable to start there in assessing the claim to a separate forensic psychiatry of DID. There have been few studies of the effectiveness of hospital treatment and few follow-up studies of its longer-term benefits. A recent report from the Royal College of Psychiatrists (2014) confirms that outcome studies are sparse compared with the possibly £300 million a year investment in the area in England and Wales.

The building frenzy of the early 2000s offered the ideal opportunity to set up information technology systems that would track patients' progress, both within the hospitals and after discharge. However, it is understandable that private companies, in competition with each other, and driven by the seemingly limitless funding available at that time to open beds as quickly as possible, would see the needs of science as essentially off the agenda and to be addressed *mañana*. When I worked at the Care Principles company in the early 2000s, we did not even have to advertise in order to fill beds when we opened approximately 280 of them (low and medium secure) between 1997 and 2003.

The areas which have been well researched are sex offending, anger management and arson. These are well reviewed in the standard textbooks listed under 'Recommended further reading', at the end of the chapter. However, the majority of these studies involve group therapy, for which not everyone is suitable. Moreover, sex offending and arson are behavioural topographies which cover a wide range of underlying disorders (and, of course, no disorder at all).

Despite modern examples like the Rwandan genocide, we may need to remind ourselves that the vast majority of horror in the world is carried out by perfectly normal people, living under perfectly abnormal circumstances, and being given permission to fulfil their wildest fantasies, or else being compelled to carry out atrocities which they would never have had imagined otherwise.

Anger is something fundamental, a universal experience indeed, from the moment the umbilical cord is cut, and a driver of human antisocial behaviour and violence. Most people learn to moderate and modulate their anger through a process (poorly understood) of intellectual, emotional and behavioural maturation. People who have suffered early damage and who are relatively unsophisticated in the areas mentioned may be expected to experience anger as a fundamental response to frustration and to have a relatively poor ability to express and define their feelings in language. This is indeed the case. It has always been a matter of mystery to me that we classify anxiety as a mental disorder but not anger. Maybe we remain stuck in a Kraeplinian dichotomy which limits the range of human emotion in which pathology (and therefore diagnosis) may be recognised to occur.

In terms of formal mental illness, while diagnosis can be difficult, as patients with DID may not be able to express symptoms of mental illness to a sufficient degree of precision and sophistication, essentially there is no difference between the pharmacotherapy of people with DID and those of normal intelligence. Indeed, medication is often 'piled on', layer after layer, in a vain attempt to quell challenging behaviour, resulting only in physical and mental sickness.

The evidence from my own clinical experience (which I cannot support with evidence from the literature) is that people with autism are especially vulnerable to misdiagnosis of psychotic and affective disorders because of their oddities and changeability of mood, behaviour and speech. And therefore to overmedication.

One of the roles of the hospital is to reduce, withdraw and rationalise psychotropic medication, which can be difficult in the community, owing to fear of relapse or worsening of the patient's behaviour.

During my time working in this area, hospitals have become much more secure, ostentatiously, with huge fences being erected so that they can meet the guidelines for secure care. Correspondingly, patient activities have been restricted and diminished on the grounds of risk assessment (in reality cost). Risk is everywhere, and the more you look the more you will find. Hence risk assessment, unless it is focused upon the areas of key clinical concern, will always turn up more reasons 'why not' rather than 'why should'. No one minds being searched at the airport because the metal detector has flipped, but it is hugely stigmatising to be detected as a potential sex offender or psychopath. We all too willingly accept low standards for our patients which we would reject for ourselves. Yet society has the power. In the 1990s we took detained patients on holidays to Wales and on canal holidays on the 'Warwickshire ring' of canals. Totally unthinkable today.

As compliance has become a totem, I have witnessed creativity, spontaneity and, indeed, care itself being squashed out of the hospital system, as clinicians retreat to the office, the meeting room and the computer, while patients are left sitting on the ward, waiting for something to be risk assessed so that it can happen.

On the other hand, I have never encountered a requirement of a regulator or purchaser which has been inherently unreasonable or unethical. The problem is that the minimum standard quickly becomes the maximum. There are huge sighs of relief when regulatory compliance is achieved. However, this is where we should start to build imaginative and creative services rather than where we should say 'job done'.

Forensic DID services care for some of the most disturbed and unclassifiable individuals. Often they do not fit into any particular diagnostic category. They may be truly unique human beings for whom there is no manual.

Rather than be restricted by the narrow tram lines of conventional practice, within our own disciplines, I think that we should be scouring the behavioural and brain sciences (and, indeed, the arts and social sciences) for new and innovative ways of helping these terribly disordered and unfortunate individuals. However, this may be a pipe dream in a risk-averse and financially restricted care culture.

Also, we design hospitals, in general, to be bland, overcrowded and, above all, noisy places (bells, doors slamming, telephones, walkie-talkies, alarms, etc.) where privacy, peace and, yes, asylum are rare commodities.

Winterbourne View

Winterbourne View was the game changer. Horrific abuse of patients was exposed by concealed cameras and revealed on the BBC1 current affairs programme *Panorama*.

The Department of Health review, or concordat, was published in 2012. It stated:

> 'The abuse of people at Winterbourne View hospital was horrifying. Children, young people and adults with learning disabilities or autism and who have mental health conditions or behaviour that challenges have for too long and in too many cases received poor quality and inappropriate care. We know there are examples of good practice. But we also know that too many people are ending up unnecessarily in hospital and they are staying there for too long. This must stop.
>
> We (the undersigned) commit to a programme for change to transform health and care services and improve the quality of the care offered to children, young people and adults with learning disabilities or autism who have mental health conditions or behaviour that challenges to ensure better care outcomes for them.
>
> These actions are expected to lead to a rapid reduction in hospital placements for this group of people by 1 June 2014. People should not live in hospital for long periods of time. Hospitals are not homes.' (Department of Health, 2012: p. 5)

The Department of Health had been well aware of the growth 'like Topsy' of independent sector hospital provision for people with DID. After all, it had been ultimately paying the bill. Suddenly, sincere and committed staff were being seen as potential abusers. Yet were the community facilities available to move people out of hospital? Local authorities had been stung with savage spending cuts, so it is understandable that social workers would prefer to see highly vulnerable patients languish in hospital, on the health budget, rather than being transferred to social care.

Despite working in the independent sector this long, I cannot recall a single instance when I was put under financial pressure to keep a person in hospital longer than was necessary. The attempts by the clinical team to discharge patients were always supported by the management of the companies. This is not a defence of the system, but a fact of my personal experience.

It has been implicit in what I have said so far that the explosion of beds in private secure hospitals was not sustainable and was, moreover, indefensible (although I freely admit I believed in it at the time and was a willing participant). As I write this at the end of April 2014, I see no sign that the Winterbourne Concordat's aim of reducing hospital beds is likely to happen. The investment in community care is simply not there.

Conclusion

I have deliberately not repeated the material covered in the Royal College of Psychiatrists' (2014) report but have adopted a more polemical and provocative approach.

It is not intrinsically valid to create a psychiatric subspecialty by combining two specialties. A 'child and adolescent psychiatry of old age' is a logical impossibility, whereas a 'forensic psychiatry of DID', while logically possible, does not mean that it is nosologically valid. The creation of subspecialties necessarily entails the establishment of service boundaries, which can lead patients to be excluded rather than included. I reflected upon this in my 1996 paper.

There is still no special interest group within the Royal College of Psychiatrists for forensic DID, despite efforts being started in 1994 (by me, as it happens). Providers (in general) advertise secure services for people with DID rather than forensic services. Forensic sections for learning disability (the MHA term) for England and Wales total approximately only one a week nationwide. The Department of Health has committed itself to a dramatic reduction of secure facilities for people with DID, but notably not to a corresponding increase in community facilities. We still do not know if the services that we offer are effective, let alone cost-effective. People with DID continue to be detained in hospital for lack of community options for them to move on to.

The Royal College of Psychiatrists (2014) has recommended the establishment of community forensic DID teams; this is laudable indeed, but the resources need to be there to implement the care which these teams will surely identify, while the legal framework (the MHA) is still very much hospital based.

In the introduction to the above report, Ian Hall, Chair of the Faculty of Intellectual Disability, Royal College of Psychiatrists, says:

'The report also makes clear that proper outcome-based research is required, including an economic analysis, to ensure that we make the optimum use of resources to provide services that give the best chance for people with intellectual disability to successfully address their offending behaviour.'

Without that outcome-based research, demonstrating that we make a difference (or not), the forensic psychiatry for people with DID will remain an association of convenient words.

303

Recommended further reading

Levitt SD, Dubner SJ (2014) *Think Like a Freak: How to Think Smarter about Almost Everything*. Penguin Books.

Lindsay WR, Taylor JL, Sturmey P (eds) (2004) *Offenders with Developmental Disabilities*. Wiley.

Paris J (2013) *Fads and Fallacies in Psychiatry*. RCPsych Publications.

Riding T, Swann C, Swann B (eds) (2005) *The Handbook of Forensic Learning Disabilities*. Radcliffe.

References

Berman G, Dar A (2013) *Prison Population Statistics* (SN/SG/4334). House of Commons Library.

Department of Health (2012) *DH Winterbourne View Review – Concordat: Programme of Action*. Department of Health.

Department of Health (2014) *Positive and Proactive Care: Reducing the Need for Restrictive Interventions*. Department of Health.

Department of Health, Home Office (1992) *Review of Health and Social Services for Mentally Disordered Offenders and Others Requiring Similar Services*. HMSO.

Duggan C (2011) Dangerous and severe personality disorder. *British Journal of Psychiatry*, **198**: 431–3.

Economist (2013) Briefing: falling crime. Where have all the burglars gone? *Economist*, 20 July, pp 21–3.

Gudjonsson G, Clare I, Rutter S, *et al* (1993) *Persons at Risk During Interviews in Police Custody: The Identification of Vulnerabilities*. Royal Commission on Criminal Justice.

Halstead S (1996) Forensic psychiatry for people with learning disability. *Advances in Psychiatric Treatment*, **2**: 76–85.

Halstead S (1997) Risk assessment and management in psychiatric practice: inferring predictors of risk. A view from learning disability. *International Review of Psychiatry*, **9**: 217–24.

Health and Social Care Information Centre (2013) *Inpatients Formally Detained In Hospitals Under The Mental Health Act 1983, And Patients Subject To Supervised Community Treatment* (annual report, England, 2013). Health and Social Care Information Centre.

Herrnstein RJ, Murray C (1994) *The Bell Curve*. Free Press.

Johnston S (2005) Epidemiology of offending in learning disability. In *The Handbook of Forensic Learning Disabilities* (eds T Riding, C Swann, B Swann): pp 15–29. Radcliffe.

Leslie I (2011) *Born Liars: Why We Can't Live Without Deceit*. Quercus.

Ministry of Justice (2013) *Story of the Prison Population: 1993–2012 England and Wales*. Ministry of Justice.

National Institute for Mental Health for England (2003) *Personality Disorder: No Longer a Diagnosis of Exclusion* (Policy Implementation Guidance for the Development of Services for People with Personality Disorder, Gateway Reference 1055). National Institute for Mental Health for England.

Royal College of Psychiatrists (2014) *Forensic Care Pathways for Adults with Intellectual Disability Involved with the Criminal Justice System* (Faculty Report FR/ID/04). Royal College of Psychiatrists.

Talbot J (2008) *No One Knows*. Prison Reform Trust.

World Health Organization (1992) *International Statistical Classification of Diseases and Related Health Problems* (10th revision) (ICD-10). WHO.

Index

Compiled by Linda English

305